MEDICAL TERMINOLOGY FOR HEALTH PROFESSIONS 4.0
© Copyright 2022 by SCOTT J. BARNARD

This document is geared towards providing exact and reliable information with regards to the topic and issue covered. The publication is sold with the idea that the publisher is not required to render accounting, officially permitted, or otherwise, qualified services. If advice is necessary, legal or professional, a practiced individual in the profession should be ordered.

From a Declaration of Principles which was accepted and approved equally by a Committee of the American Bar Association and a Committee of Publishers and Associations.

In no way is it legal to reproduce, duplicate, or transmit any part of this document in either electronic means or in printed format. Recording of this publication is strictly prohibited and any storage of this document is not allowed unless with written permission from the publisher.

All rights reserved.

The information provided herein is stated to be truthful and consistent, in that any liability, in terms of inattention or otherwise, by any usage or abuse of any policies, processes, or directions contained within is the solitary and utter responsibility of the recipient reader. Under no circumstances will any legal responsibility or blame be held against the publisher for any reparation, damages, or monetary loss due to the information herein, either directly or indirectly.

Respective authors own all copyrights not held by the publisher.

The information herein is offered for informational purposes solely, and is universal as so.

The presentation of the information is without contract or any type of guarantee assurance.

The trademarks that are used are without any consent, and the publication of the trademark is without permission or backing by the trademark owner.

All trademarks and brands within this book are for clarifying purposes only and are the owned by the owners themselves, not affiliated with this document.

Copyright © 2022 by Scott J. Barnard
All rights reserved. No part of this book may be reproduced, scanned, or distributed in any printed or electronic form without permission.

First Edition: March 2022

Cover: Illustration made by Diego Gilmar Valenzuela Astudillo

Printed in the United States of America

SCOTT J. BARNARD

MEDICAL TERMINOLOGY FOR HEALTH PROFESSIONS 2.0

Ultimate complete guide
to pass various tests such as the
**NCLEX, MCAT, PCAT, PAX, CEN (Nursing),
EMT (Paramedics),
PANCE (Physician Assistants)**
and many other tests taken by students
in the medical field.

Scott J. Barnard

TABLE OF CONTENTS

ABOUT MY WORK .... Page 1

CHAPTER 1 -
    Introduction to Medical Terminology .... « 3

CHAPTER 2 -
    The Human Body in Health and Disease .... « 21

CHAPTER 3 -
    The Skeletal System .... « 39

CHAPTER 4 -
    The Muscular System .... « 61

CHAPTER 5 -
    The Cardiovascular System .... « 81

CHAPTER 6 -
    The Lymphaticand Immune Systems .... Page 105

CHAPTER 7 -
    The Respiratory System .... « 129

CHAPTER 8 -
    The Digestive System .... « 149

CHAPTER 9 -
    The Urinary System .... « 175

CHAPTER 10 -
    The Nervous System .... « 193

CHAPTER 11 -
    Special Senses: The Eyes and Ears .... « 219

CHAPTER 12 -
    Skin: The Integumentary System .... « 243

CHAPTER 13 -
    The Endocrine System .... « 263

CHAPTER 14 -
    The Reproductive Systems .... « 281

CHAPTER 15 -
    Diagnostic Procedures and Pharmacology .... « 307

CONCLUSION .... « 329

AUTHOR BIO -
    Scott J. Barnard .... « 333

Medical Terminology for Health Professions 4.0

*Dedicated to all my friends and to all the people
who gave me their help.
Thanks a lot
Thanks to all of you for your confidence
in my qualities and what I do.*
Scott J. Barnard

ABOUT MY WORK

Welcome to the world of medical terminology! Learning this special language is an important step in preparing for your career as a health care professional. Here's the good news: Learning medical terms is much easier than learning a foreign language because you are already familiar with a few of the words—such as appendicitis and tonsillectomy. Understanding new words becomes easier with the discovery that many of these terms are made up of interchangeable word parts that are used in different combinations. Once you understand this, you'll be well on your way to translating even the most difficult medical terms, including words you have never seen before. You'll be amazed to see how quickly your vocabulary will grow!

In the current days of economic uncertainty, most of the people are looking for a change in their career path. Above all, there are also fields where employers are worried about obtaining appropriate workforce with the right skill. On the other hand, many workers are left with difficult choices because of forced career changes, layoffs, cost-cutting and off-shoring principles followed by organizations. Some years ago, people were fixed with one employer for their entire careers, but this trend has vanished in the current corporate culture. Therefore, people are always on the lookout for new career path that offers growth potential, stability and enrichment.

In the current circumstances, the workforce is left with no other options other than enriching their marketability by broadening their skill set. Continuing education to enhance the skills has become at the order of the day, so that getting the right type of courses will enhance their employability options in their current working field or get them new opportunities in a new arena as well. Now, the question that might arise in the minds of the readers would be pertaining to the field, where courses can be taken.

It is predicted that health care industry will grow in the near future and therefore taking up courses like medical terminology class will be of great use. From the year 2004, it has been found that the health care industry is one among the top 10 fastest-growing industries. Not only in careers pertaining to direct patient care, but also in supporting professionals like medical transcriptionists, counselors, health information technicians, etc… will be in great demand. So, if you are interested in entering this booming industry, it is better to learn medical terminology. There are great institutions offering this course and not only regular classes, but also online courses are offered by these professional educators in such a way that working professionals can also benefit from it.

In these days of economic uncertainty, career change is a hot button issue. As baby boomers retire and leave the work force, employers are concerned about the shortage of skilled workers. In addition, corporate cost cutting, off-shoring, layoffs, and forced career changes leave many workers with difficult choices. Gone are the days of one job and one employer for life. Following a career path today can mean maneuvering many twists and turns, setbacks, side roads, and blind alleys. Where is the roadmap to a new career that provides enrichment, stability and growth potential?

One of the best ways to ease some of the uncertainty and increase your marketability quotient is to broaden your skill set. Since continuing education is often required to maintain licenses and certifications, make those education hours to be double duty. The right training can mean more opportunities in your current field and serve as a stepping stone to a new career. But which industries offer the best chance for job stability and advancement?

The fundamental requirement to entering into a health-related career is to get a hang on medical terms and this can be achieved by medical terminology classes. In addition to careers directly involved in patient care, demand for support professionals such as medical records and health information technicians, therapists, counselors and medical transcriptionists will increase.

A basic requirement for entry into almost any healthcare-related career is a command of medical terminology. The ability to recognize, understand, spell and pronounce basic medical terms, identify medical abbreviations, and decipher unfamiliar words using roots, suffixes and prefixes is a necessary tool to perform well in any medical setting. Medical terminology courses are widely available in online, home study and instructor-led formats. Because medical technology advances rapidly, medical terminology courses evolve to keep pace. To stay on top of new terminology, consider taking the course again even if you've taken it in the past. To perform well in any medical setting, it is essential that the individual is in a position to identify medical abbreviations, decipher unknown words with the help of root words, prefixes and suffixes and all this can be done only when a person learn medical terminology. Even people, who are already working in the field of medicine, can take up these courses to refresh their knowledge and to enhance their employability chances.

Many other professionals can benefit from an understanding of medical terminology. Lawyers, paralegals, legal secretaries and other legal professionals handling cases involving medical-related issues are better able to litigate these cases when they understand the terminology involved. Health insurance professionals, as well as those working in medical billing and coding positions also benefit from a working knowledge of medical terminology.

Many agencies require certification in medical terminology for pharmacy technicians. Professionals and technicians of biology, dentistry, hospital administration and many others must properly utilize medical terminology to communicate with patients, staff, customers and colleagues. Therapists, technicians, counselors and home health care providers can improve communication, increase the quality of care to patients, and reduce oversights and liability issues with a clear understanding of medical terminology.

A course in medical terminology is a widely accessible mean to broaden your skill set, boost your marketability and increase opportunities for advancement in your current career while helping you map a route to an exciting job in the healthcare industry. Doubling the value of your time and education leads to better employment that will enrich your life.

CHAPTER 1

INTRODUCTION TO MEDICAL TERMINOLOGY

Medical terminology is a special vocabulary used by health care professionals for effective and accurate communication. Because it is based mainly on Greek and Latin words, medical terminology is consistent and uniform throughout the world. It is also efficient; although some of the terms are long, they often reduce an entire phrase to a single word. The one word gastroduodenostomy, for example, stands for "a communication between the stomach and the first part of the small intestine".

The medical vocabulary is vast, and learning it may seem like learning the entire vocabulary of a foreign language. Moreover, like the jargon that arises in all changing fields, it is always expanding. Think of the terms that have been added to our vocabulary with the development of computers, such as software, megabyte, search engine, e-mail, chat room. The task seems overwhelming, but there are methods that can aid in learning and remembering words and can even help in making informed guesses regarding the meanings of unfamiliar words. Most medical terms can be divided into component parts—roots, prefixes, and suffixes—that maintain the same meaning whenever they appear. By learning these meanings, you can analyze and remember many words.

Word Parts

- -algia
- dysh
- -ectomy
- hyperh
- hypoh
- -itis
- -osis
- -ostomy
- -otomy
- -plasty

- -rrhage
- -rrhaphy
- -rrhea
- -rrhexis
- –sclerosis

Medical Terms

- abdominocentesis (ab-dom-ih-noh-sen-TEE-sis)
- acronym (ACK-roh-nim)
- acute
- angiography (an-jee-OG-rah-fee)
- appendectomy (ap-en-DECK-toh-mee)
- arteriosclerosis (ar-tee-ree-oh-skleh-ROH-sis)
- arthralgia (ar-THRAL-jee-ah)
- colostomy (koh-LAHS-toh-mee)
- cyanosis (sigh-ah-NOH-sis)
- dermatologist (der-mah-TOL-oh-jist)
- diagnosis (dye-ag-NOH-sis)
- diarrhea (dye-ah-REE-ah)
- edema (eh-DEE-mah)
- endarterial (end-ar-TEE-ree-al)
- eponym (EP-oh-nim)
- erythrocyte (eh-RITH-roh-sight)
- fissure (FISH-ur)
- fistula (FIS-tyou-lah)
- gastralgia (gas-TRAL-jee-ah)
- gastritis (gas-TRY-tis)
- gastroenteritis (gas-troh-en-ter-EYE-tis)
- gastrosis (gas-TROH-sis)
- hemorrhage (HEM-or-idj)
- hepatomegaly (hep-ah-toh-MEG-ah-lee)
- hypertension (high-per-TEN-shun)
- hypotension (high-poh-TEN-shun)
- infection (in-FECK-shun)
- inflammation (in-flah-MAY-shun)
- interstitial (in-ter-STISH-al)
- intramuscular (in-trah-MUS-kyou-lar)
- laceration (lass-er-AY-shun)
- lesion (LEE-zhun)
- mycosis (my-KOH-sis)
- myelopathy (my-eh-LOP-ah-thee)
- myopathy (my-OP-ah-thee)
- myorrhexis (my-oh-RECK-sis)
- natal (NAY-tal)

- neonatology (nee-oh-nay-TOL-oh-jee)
- neuritis (new-RYE-tis)
- otorhinolaryngology (oh-toh-rye-noh-lar-in-GOLoh-jee)
- palpation (pal-PAY-shun)
- palpitation (pal-pih-TAY-shun)
- pathology (pah-THOL-oh-jee)
- phalanges (fah-LAN-jeez)
- poliomyelitis (poh-lee-oh-my-eh-LYE-tis)
- prognosis (prog-NOH-sis)
- prostate (PROS-tayt)
- pyoderma (pye-oh-DER-mah)
- pyrosis (pye-ROH-sis)
- remission
- sign
- supination (soo-pih-NAY-shun)
- suppuration (sup-you-RAY-shun)
- supracostal (sue-prah-KOS-tal)
- symptom (SIMP-tum)
- syndrome (SIN-drohm)
- tonsillitis (ton-sih-LYE-tis)
- trauma (TRAW-mah)
- triage (tree-AHZH)
- viral (VYE-ral)

Objectives

On completion of this chapter, you should be able to:
1. Identify the roles of the four types of word parts used in forming medical terms.
2. Using your knowledge of word parts, analyze unfamiliar medical terms.
3. Describe the steps in locating a term in a medical dictionary.
4. Define the commonly used prefixes, word roots, combining forms, and suffixes introduced in this chapter.
5. Pronounce medical terms correctly using the "sounds-like" system.
6. Recognize the importance of always spelling medical terms correctly.
7. State why caution is important when using abbreviations.
8. Recognize, define, spell, and pronounce the medical terms in this chapter.

Primary Medical Terms

In this book, you will be introduced to many medical terms; however, mastering them will be easier than you anticipate because this book has this new feature to make learning easier.

Word Parts Are The Key

Learning medical terminology is much easier once you understand how word parts work together to form medical terms. This book includes many aids to help you continue reinforcing your word building skills. The types of word parts and the rules for their use are explained in this chapter. Learn these rules and follow them. When a term is made up of recognizable word parts, these word parts and their meanings are included with the definition of that term.

The Four Types of Word Parts

Four types of word parts may be used to create medical terms.
A word root contains the basic meaning of the term. This word part usually, but not always, indicates the involved body part. For example, the word root meaning stomach is gastr.
A combining form is a word root with a vowel at the end so that a suffix beginning with a consonant can be added. When a combining form appears alone, it is shown with a slash (/) between the word root and the combining vowel. For example, the combining form meaning stomach is gastr/o.

Word Roots

Word roots act as the foundation of most medical terms. They usually, but not always, describe the part of the body that is involved.

Combining Form Vowels

A combining form vowel is added to the end of a word root under certain conditions to make the resulting medical term easier to pronounce.
The letter "o" is the most commonly used combining vowel. When a word root is shown alone as a combining form, it includes a slash (/) and the combining vowel.

Suffixes

A suffix is a word part that is added to the end of a word to complete that term. In medical terminology, suffixes usually, but not always, indicate a procedure, condition, disorder, or disease. For example, tonsil/o means tonsils. The suffix that is added completes the term and tells what is happening to the tonsils.
Tonsillitis (ton-sih-LYE-tis) is an inflammation of the tonsils (tonsil means tonsils, and -itis means inflammation).
A tonsillectomy (ton-sih-LECK-toh-mee) is the surgical removal of the tonsils (tonsil means tonsils, and -ectomy means surgical removal).

Suffixes as Noun Endings

A noun is a word that is the name of a person, place, or thing. In medical terminology, some suffixes change the word root into a noun. For example, the cranium (KRAY-nee-um) is the portion of the skull that encloses the brain (crani means skull, and -um is a noun ending). Other suffixes complete the term by changing the word root into a noun.

Suffixes Meaning "Pertaining To"

An adjective is a word that defines or describes a thing. In medical terminology, many suffixes meaning "pertaining to" change the word root into an adjective. For example, the term cardiac is an adjective that means pertaining to the heart (cardi means heart, and -ac means pertaining to).

Suffixes Meaning Abnormal Condition

In medical terminology, many suffixes, such as -osis, mean "abnormal condition or disease." For example, gastrosis (gas-TROH-sis) means any disease of the stomach (gastr means stomach, and -osis means abnormal condition or disease).

Word Roots/Combining Forms Indicating Color

- cyan/o means blue Cyanosis (sigh-ah-NOH-sis) is blue discoloration of the skin caused by a lack of adequate oxygen in the blood (cyan means blue, and -osis means abnormal condition or disease).
- erythr/o means red An erythrocyte (eh-RITH-roh-sight) is a mature red blood cell (erythr/o means red, and -cyte means cell).
- leuk/o means white A leukocyte (LOO-koh-sight) is a white blood cell (leuk/o means white, and -cyte means cell).
- melan/o means black Melanosis (mel-ah-NOH-sis) is any condition of unusual deposits of black pigment in body tissues or organs (melan means black, and -osis means abnormal condition or disease).
- poli/o means gray Poliomyelitis (poh-lee-oh-my-eh-LYE-tis) is a viral infection of the gray matter of the spinal cord (poli/o means gray, myel means spinal cord, and -itis means inflammation).

Rules For Using Combining Form Vowels

1. A combining vowel is used when the suffix begins with a consonant.
For example, when neur/o (nerve) is joined with the suffix -plasty (surgical repair), the combining vowel "o" is used because -plasty begins with a consonant.
Neuroplasty (NEW-roh-plas-tee) is the surgical repair of a nerve (neur/o means nerve, and -plasty means
surgical repair).

2. A combining vowel is not used when the suffix begins with a vowel (a, e, i, o, u).
For example, when neur/o (nerve) is joined with the suffix -itis (inflammation), no combining vowel is used because -itis begins with a vowel.
Neuritis (new-RYE-tis) is inflammation of a nerve or nerves (neur means nerve, and -itis means
inflammation).

3. A combining vowel is used when two or more word roots are joined.
For example, gastroenteritis combines two word roots with a suffix. When gastr/o (stomach) is joined with enter/o (small intestine), the combining vowel is

used with gastr/o. A combining vowel is not used with enter/o because it is joining the suffix -itis, which begins with a vowel.
Gastroenteritis (gas-troh-en-ter-EYE-tis) is an inflammation of the stomach and small intestine (gastr/o
means stomach, enter means small intestine, and -itis means inflammation).

Suffixes Related to Pathology

Pathology (pah-THOL-oh-jee) is the study of all aspects of diseases (path means disease, and -ology means study of). Suffixes related to pathology describe specific disease conditions.

- -algia means pain and suffering. Gastralgia (gas-TRALjee- ah), also known as stomach ache, means pain in the stomach (gastr means stomach, and -algia means pain).
- -dynia also means pain. Gastrodynia (gas-troh-DINee- ah) also means pain in the stomach (gastr/o means stomach, and -dynia means pain). Although -dynia has the same meaning as -algia, it is not used as commonly.
- -itis means inflammation. Gastritis (gas-TRY-tis) is an inflammation of the stomach (gastr means stomach, and -itis means inflammation).
- -malacia means abnormal softening. Arteriomalacia (ar-tee-ree-oh-mah-LAY-shee-ah) is the abnormal softening of the walls of an artery or arteries (arteri/o means artery, and -malacia means abnormal softening). Notice that -malacia is the opposite of -sclerosis.
- -megaly means enlargement. Hepatomegaly (hep-ahtoh- MEG-ah-lee) is abnormal enlargement of the liver (hepat/o means liver, and -megaly means enlargement).
- -necrosis means tissue death. Arterionecrosis (ar-teeree- oh-neh-KROH-sis) is the tissue death of an artery or arteries (arteri/o means artery, and -necrosis means tissue death).
- -sclerosis means abnormal hardening. Arteriosclerosis (ar-tee-ree-oh-skleh-ROH-sis) is the abnormal hardening of the walls of an artery or arteries (arteri/o means artery, and -sclerosis means abnormal hardening). Notice that -sclerosis is the opposite of -malacia.
- -stenosis means abnormal narrowing. Arteriostenosis (ar-tee–ree-oh-steh-NOH-sis) is the abnormal narrowing of an artery or arteries (arteri/o means artery, and -stenosis means abnormal narrowing.)

Suffixes Related to Procedures

Some suffixes identify the procedure that is performed on the body part identified by the word root.

- -centesis is a surgical puncture to remove fluid for diagnostic purposes or to remove excess fluid.

Abdominocentesis (ab-dom-ih-noh-sen-TEE-sis) is the surgical puncture of the abdominal cavity to remove fluid (abdomin/o means abdomen, and -centesis means a surgical puncture to remove fluid).

- -graphy means the process of producing a picture or record.

Angiography (an-jee-OG-rah-fee) is the process of producing a radiographic (x-ray) study of the blood vessels after the injection of a contrast medium to make these blood vessels visible (angi/o means blood vessel, and -graphy means the process of recording).
- -gram means a picture or record.

An angiogram (AN-jee-oh-gram) is the film produced by angiography (angi/o means blood vessel, and -gram means a picture or record).
- -plasty means surgical repair.

Myoplasty (MY-oh-plastee)
is the surgical repair of a muscle (myo means muscle, and -plasty means surgical repair).
- -scopy means visual examination.

Arthroscopy (ar-THROS-koh-pee) is the visual examination of the internal structure of a joint (arthr/o means joint, and -scopy means visual examination).

The "Double R" Suffixes

Suffixes beginning with two "Rs," which are often referred to as the "double RRs," can be particularly confusing. They are grouped together here to help you understand the word parts and to remember the differences.

- -rrhage and -rrhagia mean bleeding; however, they are most often used to describe sudden, severe bleeding. A hemorrhage (HEM-or-idj) is the loss of a large amount of blood in a short time (hem/o means blood, and -rrhage means bursting forth of blood).
- -rrhaphy means surgical suturing to close a wound and includes the use of sutures, staples, or surgical glue. Myorrhaphy (my-OR-ah-fee) is the surgical suturing of a muscle wound (my/o means muscle, and -rrhaphy means surgical suturing).
- -rrhea means flow or discharge and refers to the flow of most body fluids. Diarrhea (dye-ah-REE-ah) is the frequent flow of loose or watery stools (dia- means through, and -rrhea means flow or discharge).
- -rrhexis means rupture. Myorrhexis (my-oh-RECKsis) is the rupture of a muscle (my/o means muscle, and -rrhexis means rupture).

Prefixes

A prefix is added to the beginning of a word to influence the meaning of that term. Prefixes usually, but not always, indicate location, time, or number. The term natal (NAY-tal) means pertaining to birth (nat means birth, and -al means pertaining to). The following examples
show how prefixes change the meaning of this term.

- Prenatal (pre-NAY-tal) means the time and events before birth (pre- means before, nat means birth, and -al means pertaining to).
- Perinatal (pehr-ih-NAY-tal) refers to the time and events surrounding birth (peri- means surrounding, nat means birth, and -al means pertainingto). This is the time just before, during, and just after birth.

- Postnatal (pohst-NAY-tal) refers to the time and events after birth (post- means after, nat means birth, and -al means pertaining to). This is the time just before, during, and just after birth.
- Postnatal (pohst-NAY-tal) refers to the time and events after birth (post- means after, nat means birth, and -al means pertaining to).

Determining Meanings On The Basis Of Word Parts

Knowing the meaning of the word parts often makes it possible to figure out the definition of an unfamiliar medical term.

Taking Terms Apart

To determine a word's meaning by looking at the component pieces, you must first separate it into word parts.
- Always start at the end of the word, with the suffix, and work toward the beginning.
- As you separate the word parts, identify the meaning of each. Identifying the meaning of each part should give you a definition of the term.
- Because some word parts have more than one meaning, it also is necessary to determine the context in which the term is being used. As used here, context means to determine which body system this term is referring to.
- If you have any doubt, use your medical dictionary to double-check your definition.
- Be aware that not all medical terms are made up of word parts.

An Example

Look at the term otorhinolaryngology (oh-toh-rye-nohlar- in-GOL-oh-jee). It is made up of two combining forms, a word root, and a suffix. This is how it looks when the word parts have been separated by working from the end to the beginning.
- The suffix -ology means the study of.
- The word root laryng means larynx and throat. The combining vowel is not used here because the word root is joining a suffix that begins with a vowel.
- The combining form rhin/o means nose. The combining vowel is used here because the word root rhin is joining another word root.

Contrasting Prefixes

- ab- means away from. Abnormal means not normal or away from normal. ad- means toward or in the direction of. Addiction means drawn toward or a strong dependence on a drug or substance.
- dys- means bad, difficult, or painful. Dysfunctional means an organ or body part that is not working properly.

Medical Terminology for Health Professions 4.0

- eu- means good, normal, well, or easy. Euthyroid (you-THIGH-roid) means a normally functioning thyroid gland.
- hyper- means excessive or increased. Hypertension (high-per-TEN-shun) is higher than normal blood pressure.
- hypo- means deficient or decreased. Hypotension (high-poh-TEN-shun) is lower than normal blood pressure. inter- means between or among.
- Interstitial (in-ter-STISH-al) means between, but not within, the parts of a tissue. intra- means within or inside.
- Intramuscular (in-trah-MUS-kyou-lar) means within the muscle.
- sub- means under, less, or below. Subcostal (sub-KOS-tal) means below a rib or ribs.
- super-, supra- mean above or excessive. Supracostal (sue-prah-KOS-tal) means above or outside the ribs.

The combining form ot/o means ear. The combining vowel is used here because the word root ot is joining another word root.

Together they form otorhinolaryngology, which is the study of the ears, nose, and throat (ot/o means ear, rhin/o means nose, laryng means throat, and -ology means study of). Note: Laryng/o also means larynx. Because this is such a long name, this specialty is frequently referred to as ENT (ears, nose, and throat).

A shortened version of this term is otolaryngology (oh-toh-lar-in-GOL-oh-jee), which is the study of the ears and larynx or throat (ot/o means ears, larynx means larynx, and -ology means study of).

Guessing at Meanings

When you are able to guess at the meaning of a term on the basis of word parts that it is made up of, you must always double-check for accuracy because some terms have more than one meaning. For example, look at the term lithotomy (lih-THOT-oh-mee):

- On the basis of word parts, a lithotomy is a surgical incision for the removal of a stone (lith means stone, and -otomy means a surgical incision).
- However, lithotomy is also the name of an examination position in which the patient is lying on the back with the feet and legs raised and supported in stirrups. The term is used to describe this position because in the early days, this was the preferred position for lithotomy surgery.
- This type of possible confusion is one of the many reasons why a medical dictionary is an important medical terminology tool.

Medical Dictionary Use

Learning to use a medical dictionary and other resources to find the definition of a term is an important part of mastering the correct use of medical terms. The following tips for dictionary use apply whether you are working with a traditional book-form dictionary or with electronic dictionary software on your computer.

If You Know How to Spell the Word

When starting to work with an unfamiliar print dictionary, spend a few minutes reviewing its user guide, table of contents, and appendices. The time you spend reviewing now will be saved later when you are looking up unfamiliar terms.

- On the basis of the first letter of the word, start in the appropriate section of the dictionary. Look at the top of the page for clues. The top left word is the first term on the page. The top right word is the last term on that page.
- Next, look alphabetically for words that start with the first and second letters of the word you are researching. Continue looking through each letter until you find the term you are looking for.
- When you think you have found it, check the spelling very carefully, letter by letter, working from left to right. Terms with similar spellings have very different meanings.
- When you find the term, carefully check all of the definitions.

If You Do Not Know How to Spell the Word

Listen carefully to the term and write it down. If you cannot find the word on the basis of your spelling, start looking for alternative spellings based on the beginning sound.

Note: All of these examples are in this text. However, you could practice looking them up in the dictionary.

Guidelines To Looking Up The Spelling Of Unfamiliar Terms

If it sounds like	It may begin with	Example
F	F	flatus (FLAY-tus)
P	H	phlegm (FLEM)
J	G	gingivitis (jin-jih-VYE-tis)
	J	jaundice (JAWN-dis)
K	C	crepitus (KREP-ih-tus)
	CH	cholera (KOL-er-ah)
	K	kyphosis (kye-FOH-sis)
	QU	quadriplegia (kwad-rih-PLEEjee-ah)
S	C	cytology (sigh-TOL-oh-jee)
	PS	psychologist (sigh-KOL-oh-jist)
	S	serum (SEER-um)
Z	X	xeroderma (zee-roh-DER-mah
	Z	zygote (ZYE-goht)

Pronunciation

A medical term is easier to understand, and remember, when you know how to pronounce it properly. To help you master the pronunciation of new terms, a commonly accepted pronunciation of that word appears (in parentheses) next to the term.

The "sounds-like" pronunciation system is used in this

textbook. Here the word is respelled using normal English letters to create sounds that are familiar. To pronounce a new word, just say it as it is spelled in the parentheses.

- The part of the word that receives the primary (most) emphasis when you say it is shown in uppercase boldface letters. For example, edema (eh-DEE-mah) describes swelling caused by excess fluid in the body tissues.
- A part of the word that receives secondary (less) emphasis when you say it is shown in boldface lowercase letters. For example, appendicitis (ah-

pendih- SIGH-tis) means an inflammation of the appendix (appendic means appendix, and -itis means inflammation).

A Word of Caution

Frequently, there is more than one correct way to pronounce a medical term.
- The pronunciation of many medical terms is based on their Greek, Latin, or other foreign origin. However, there is a trend toward pronouncing terms as they would sound in English.
- The result is more than one "correct" pronunciation for a term. The text shows the most commonly accepted pronunciation.
- If your instructor prefers an alternative pronunciation, follow the instructions you are given.

Spelling Is Always Important

Accuracy in spelling medical terms is extremely important!
- Changing just one or two letters can completely change the meaning of a word—and this difference literally could be a matter of life or death for the patient.
- The section "Look-Alike Sound-Alike Terms and Word Parts" later in this chapter will help you become aware of some terms and word parts that are frequently confused.
- The spelling shown in this text is commonly accepted in the United States (US). You may encounter alternative spellings used in England, Australia, and Canada.

Abbreviations are frequently used as a shorthand way to record long and complex medical terms; Appendix B contains an alphabetized list of many of the more commonly used medical abbreviations.
- Abbreviations can also lead to confusion and errors! Therefore, it is important that you be very careful when using or interpreting an abbreviation.
- For example, the abbreviation BE means both "below elbow" (as in amputation) and "barium enema." Just imagine what a difference a mix-up here would make for the patient!
- Most clinical agencies have policies for accepted abbreviations. It is important to follow this list for the facility where you are working.
- If there is any question in your mind about which abbreviation to use, always follow this rule: When in doubt, spell it out.

Look-Alike Sound-Alike Terms And Word Parts

This section highlights some frequently used terms and word parts that are confusing because they look and sound alike. However, the meanings are very different, and it is important that you pay close attention to these terms and word parts as you encounter them in the text.

arteri/o, ather/o, and arthr/o

- arteri/o means artery. Endarterial (end-ar-TEE-ree-al) means pertaining to the interior or lining of an artery (end- means within, arteri means artery, and -al means pertaining to).
- ather/o means plaque or fatty substance. An atheroma (ath-er-OH-mah) is a fatty deposit within the wall of an artery (ather means fatty substance, and -oma means tumor).
- arthr/o means joint. Arthralgia (ar-THRAL-jee-ah) means pain in a joint or joints (arthr means joint, and -algia means pain).

-ectomy, -ostomy and -otomy

- -ectomy means surgical removal. An appendectomy (ap-en-DECK-toh-mee) is the surgical removal of the appendix (append means appendix, and -ectomy means surgical removal).
- -ostomy means the surgical creation of an artificial opening to the body surface. A colostomy (koh- LAHS-toh-mee) is the surgical creation of an artificial excretory opening between the colon and the body surface (col means colon, and -ostomy means the creation of an artificial opening).
- -otomy means cutting or a surgical incision. A colotomy (koh-LOT-oh-mee) is a surgical incision into the colon (col means colon, and -otomy means a surgical incision).

Basic Medical Terms To Describe Disease Conditions

A sign is objective evidence of disease such as a fever.
Objective means the sign can be evaluated or measured by the patient or others.
A symptom (SIMP-tum) is subjective evidence of a disease, such as pain or a headache. Subjective means that it can be evaluated or measured only by the patient.
A syndrome (SIN-drohm) is a set of the signs and symptoms that occur together as part of a specific disease process.
A diagnosis (dye-ag-NOH-sis) is the identification of a disease (plural, diagnoses).To diagnose is the process of reaching a diagnosis.
A differential diagnosis, which is also known as to rule out (R/O) is an attempt to determine which one of several diseases can be producing the signs and symptoms that are present.
A prognosis (prog-NOH-sis) is a prediction of the probable course
and outcome of a disorder (plural, prognoses).
An acute condition has a rapid onset, a severe course, and a relatively short duration.
A chronic condition is of long duration. Although such diseases can be controlled, they are rarely cured.
A remission is the temporary, partial, or complete disappearance
of the symptoms of a disease without having achieved a cure.
A disease is a condition in which one or more body parts are not functioning normally. Some diseases are named for their signs and symptoms. For example,

chronic fatigue syndrome is a persistent overwhelming fatigue of unknown origin.

An eponym (EP-oh-nim) is a disease, structure, operation, or procedure named for the person who discovered or described it first. For example, Alzheimer's disease is named for German neurologist Alois Alzheimer.

An acronym (ACK-roh-nim) is a word formed from the initial letter of the major parts of a compound term. For example, the acronym laser stands for light amplification by stimulated emission of radiation.

Guidelines To Unusual Plural Forms

- If the singular term ends in the suffix -a, the plural is usually formed by changing the ending to -ae.
- If the singular term ends in the suffix -ex or -ix, the plural is usually formed by changing these endings to -ices.
- If the singular term ends in the suffix -is, the plural is usually formed by changing the ending to -es.
- If the singular term ends in the suffix -itis, the plural is usually formed by changing the -is ending to -ides.
- If the singular term ends in the suffix -nx, the plural is usually formed by the -x ending to -ges.
- If the singular term ends in the suffix -on, the plural is usually formed by changing the ending to -a.
- If the singular term ends in the suffix -um, the plural usually is formed by changing the ending to -a.
- If the singular term ends in the suffix -us, the plural is usually formed by changing the ending to -i.

Fissure and Fistula

- A fissure (FISH-ur) is a groove or crack-like sore of the skin. This term also describes normal folds in the contours of the brain.
- A fistula (FIS-tyou-lah) is an abnormal passage, usually between two internal organs, or leading from an organ to the surface of the body. A fistula may be due to surgery, injury, or the draining of an abscess.

Ileum and Ilium

- The ileum (ILL-ee-um) is the last and longest portion of the small intestine. Memory aid: ileum is spelled with an e as in intestine.
- The ilium (ILL-ee-um) is part of the hip bone. Memory aid: ilium is spelled with an i as in hip.

Infection and Inflammation

- An infection (in-FECK-shun) is the invasion of the body by a pathogenic (disease producing) organism. The infection can remain localized (near the point of entry) or can be systemic (affecting the entire body). Signs and symptoms of infection include malaise, chills and fever, redness,

heat and swelling, or exudate from a wound. Malaise is a feeling of general discomfort or uneasiness that is often the first indication of an infection or other disease. An exudate is fluid, such as pus, that leaks out of an infected wound.
- Inflammation (in-flah-MAY-shun) is a localized response to an injury or destruction of tissues. The cardinal signs (indications) of inflammation are (1) erythema (redness), (2) hyperthermia (heat), (3) edema (swelling), and (4) pain. These are caused by extra blood flowing into the area as part of the healing process.
- Although the suffix -itis means inflammation, it also is commonly used to indicate infection.

Laceration and Lesion
- A laceration (lass-er-AY-shun) is a torn or jagged wound or an accidental cut wound.
- A lesion (LEE-zhun) is a pathologic change of the tissues due to disease or injury.

Mucous and Mucus
- The adjective mucous (MYOU-kus) describes the specialized mucous membranes that line the body cavities.
- The noun mucus (MYOU-kus) is the name of the fluid secreted by the mucous membranes.

myc/o, myel/o, and my/o
- myc/o means fungus. Mycosis (my-KOH-sis) describes any abnormal condition or disease caused by a fungus (myc means fungus, and -osis means abnormal condition or disease).
- myel/o means bone marrow or spinal cord. The term myelopathy (my-eh-LOP-ah-thee) describes any pathologic change or disease in the spinal cord (myel/o means spinal cord or bone marrow, and -pathy means disease).
- my/o means muscle. The term myopathy (my-OP-ahthee) describes any pathologic change or disease of muscle tissue (my/o means muscle, and -pathy means disease).

-ologist and -ology
- -ologist means specialist. A dermatologist (der-mah-TOL-oh-jist) is a physician who specializes in diagnosing and treating disorders of the skin (dermat means skin, and -ologist means specialist).
- -ology means the study of. Neonatology (nee-oh-nay-TOL-oh-jee) is the study of disorders of the newborn (neo- means new, nat means birth, and -ology means study of).

Palpation and Palpitation
- Palpation (pal-PAY-shun) is an examination technique in which the examiner's hands are used to feel the texture, size, consistency, and location of certain body parts.
- Palpitation (pal-pih-TAY-shun) is a pounding or racing heart.

Prostate and Prostrate
- The prostate (PROS-tayt) is a male gland that lies under the urinary bladder and surrounds the urethra.
- Prostrate (PROS-trayt) means to collapse and be lying flat or to be overcome with exhaustion.

pyel/o, py/o, and pyr/o
- pyel/o means renal pelvis, which is part of the kidney. Pyelitis (pye-eh-LYE-tis) is an inflammation of the renal pelvis (pyel means renal pelvis, and -itis means inflammation).
- py/o means pus. Pyoderma (pye-oh-DER-mah) is any acute, inflammatory, pus-forming bacterial skin infection such as impetigo (py/o means pus, and -derma means skin).
- pyr/o means fever or fire. Pyrosis (pye-ROH-sis), also known as heartburn, is discomfort due to the regurgitation of stomach acid upward into the esophagus (pyr means fever or fire, and -osis means abnormal condition or disease).

Supination and Suppuration
- Supination (soo-pih-NAY-shun) is the act of rotating the arm so that the palm of the hand is forward or upward.
- Suppuration (sup-you-RAY-shun) is the formation or discharge of pus.

Triage and Trauma
- Triage (tree-AHZH) is the medical screening of patients to determine their relative priority of need and the proper place of treatment. For example, emergency personnel arriving on an accident scene must identify which of the injured require care first and determine where they can be treated most effectively.
- Trauma (TRAW-mah) means wound or injury. These are the types of injuries that might occur in an accident, shooting, natural disaster, or fire.

Viral and Virile
- Viral (VYE-ral) means pertaining to a virus (vir means virus or poison, and -al means pertaining to).
- Virile (VIR-ill) means having the nature, properties, or qualities of an adult male.

Abbreviations Related To The Introduction To Medical Terminology

- appendectomy or appendicitis = AP
- chronic fatigue syndrome = CFS
- diagnosis = DG, Dg, Diag, diag, DX, Dx DG,
- differential diagnosis= D/D, DD, DDx, diaf. Diag D/D
- hemorrhage = He
- inflammation = Inflam, Inflamm Inflam,
- intramuscular = IM
- pathology = PA, Pa, path Pa,
- postnatal = PN
- prognosis = prog, progn, Prx, Px prog

Critical Thinking Exercise

The following story and questions are designed to stimulate critical thinking through class discussion or as a brief essay response. There are right or wrong answers to these questions.

Baylie Hutchins sits at her kitchen table with her medical terminology book opened to the first chapter, highlighter in hand. Her 2-year-old son, Mathias, plays with a box of Animal Crackersin his highchair, some even finding his mouth. "Arteri/o, ather/o, and arthr/o," she mutters, lips moving to shape unfamiliar sounds. "They're too much alike and they mean totally different things."

Mathias sneezes loudly, and spots of Animal Cracker rain on the page, punctuating her frustration.

"Great job, Thias," she says wiping the text with her finger. "I planned on using the highlighter to mark with, not your lunch." Mathias giggles and peeks through the tunnel made by one small hand.

"Mucous and mucus," she reads aloud, each sounding the same. Then she remembers her teacher's tip for remembering the difference, "The long word's the membrane and the short one's the secretion."

Mathias picks up an Animal Crackerand excitedly shouts "Tiger, Mommy! Tiger!"

"That's right,

Thias. Good job!"

Turning back to the page she stares at the red words -rrhagia, -rrhaphy, -rrhea, and -rrhexis.

Stumbling over the pronunciation, Baylie closes her eyes and tries to silence the voices in her head. "You can't do anything right," her ex-husband says. "Couldn't finish if your life depended on it," her mother's voice snaps.

Baylie keeps at it. "Rhin/o means nose," highlighting those three words, "and a rhinoceros has a big horn on his nose."

"Rhino!" Matthias shouts, holding up an AnimalCracker. Baylie laughs. We both have new things to learn, she realizes. And we can do it!

Suggested Discussion Topics

1. Baylie needs to learn medical terminology because she wants a career in the medical field. What study habits would help Baylie accomplish this task?
2. A support group could help empower Baylie to accomplish her goals. What people would you
3. suggest for this group and why?
4. How can this textbook and other resource materials help her, and you, learn medical terminology?
5. Discuss strategies that the instructor could use, and has already used, to help Baylie improve her terminology skills.

CHAPTER 2

THE HUMAN BODY IN HEALTH AND DISEASE

This list contains essential word parts and medical terms for this chapter.

Word Parts
- aden/o
- adip/o
- anter/o
- caud/o
- cephal/o
- cyt/o
- endoh
- exoh
- hist/o
- -ologist
- -ology
- path/o
- -plasia
- poster/o
- –stasis

Medical Terms
- abdominal cavity (ab-DOM-ih-nal)
- adenectomy (ad-eh-NECK-toh-mee)
- adenocarcinoma (ad-eh-noh-kar-sih-NOH-mah)
- adenoma (ad-eh-NOH-mah)
- adenomalacia (ad-eh-noh-mah-LAY-shee-ah)
- adenosclerosis (ad-eh-noh-skleh-ROH-sis)
- anaplasia (an-ah-PLAY-zee-ah)
- anatomy (ah-NAT-oh-mee)
- anomaly (ah-NOM-ah-lee)
- anterior (an-TEER-ee-or)

- aplasia (ah-PLAY-zee-ah)
- bloodborne transmission
- caudal (KAW-dal)
- cephalic (seh-FAL-ick)
- chromosomes (KROH-moh-sohmes)
- communicable disease (kuh-MEWnih-kuh-bul)
- congenital disorder (kon-JEN-ih-tahl)
- cytoplasm (SIGH-toh-plazm)
- distal (DIS-tal)
- dorsal (DOR-sal)
- dysplasia (dis-PLAY-see-ah)
- endemic (en-DEM-ick)
- endocrine glands (EN-doh-krin)
- epidemic (ep-ih-DEM-ick)
- epigastric region (ep-ih-GAS-trick)
- etiology (ee-tee-OL-oh-jee)
- exocrine glands (ECK-soh-krin)
- functional disorder
- genetic disorder
- geriatrician (jer-ee-ah-TRISH-un)
- hemophilia (hee-moh-FILL-ee-ah)
- histology (hiss-TOL-oh-jee)
- homeostasis (hoh-mee-oh-STAY-sis)
- hyperplasia (high-per-PLAY-zee-ah)
- hypertrophy (high-PER-troh-fee)
- hypogastric region (high-poh-GAS-trick)
- hypoplasia (high-poh-PLAY-zee-ah)
- iatrogenic illness (eye-at-roh-JEN-ick)
- idiopathic disorder (id-ee-oh-PATH-ick)
- infectious disease (in-FECK-shus)
- inguinal (ING-gwih-nal)
- medial (MEE-dee-al)
- mesentery (MESS-en-terr-ee)
- midsagittal plane (mid-SADJ-ih-tal)
- nosocomial infection (nos-oh-KOH-mee-al in-FECK-shun)
- pandemic (pan-DEM-ick)
- pelvic cavity (PEL-vick)
- peritoneum (pehr-ih-toh-NEE-um)
- peritonitis (pehr-ih-toh-NIGH-tis)
- phenylketonuria (fen-il-kee-toh-NEW-ree-ah)
- physiology (fiz-ee-OL-oh-jee)
- posterior (pos-TEER-ee-or)
- proximal (PROCK-sih-mal)
- retroperitoneal (ret-roh-pehr-ih-toh-NEE-al)

- stem cells
- thoracic cavity (thoh-RAS-ick)
- transverse plane (trans-VERSE)
- umbilicus (um-BILL-ih-kus)
- vector-borne transmission
- ventral (VEN-tral)

Objectives

On completion of this chapter, you should be able to:
1. Define anatomy and physiology and the uses of anatomic reference systems to identify the anatomic position plus body planes, directions, and cavities.
2. Recognize, define, spell, and pronounce the terms related to cells, and genetics.
3. Recognize, define, spell, and pronounce the terms related to the structure, function, pathology, and procedures of tissues, and glands.
4. Identify the major organs and functions of the body systems.
5. Recognize, define, spell, and pronounce the terms used to describe pathology, the modes of transmission, and the types of diseases.

Anatomic Reference Systems

Anatomic reference systems are used to describe the locations of the structural units of the body. The simplest anatomic reference is the one we learn in childhood: our right hand is on the right, and our left hand on the left. In medical terminology, there are several additional ways to describe the location of different body parts. These anatomical reference systems include:
- Body planes
- Body directions
- Body cavities
- Structural units

When body parts function together to perform a related function they are grouped together and are known as a body system.

Anatomy and Physiology Defined

Anatomy (ah-NAT-oh-mee) is the study of the structures of the body.
Physiology (fiz-ee-OL-oh-jee) is the study of the functions of the structures of the body (physi means nature or physical, and -ology means study of).

The Anatomic Position

The anatomic position describes the body assuming that the individual is standing in the standard position that includes:
- Standing up straight so that the body is erect and facing forward.
- Holding the arms at the sides with the hands turned with the palms turned toward the front.

The Body Planes
Body planes are imaginary vertical and horizontal lines used to divide the body into sections for descriptive purposes. These planes are aligned to a body standing in the anatomic position.

The Vertical Planes
A vertical plane is an up-and-down plane that is a right angle to the horizon.
- The midsagittal plane (mid-SADJ-ih-tal), also known as the midline, is the sagittal plane A sagittal plane (SADJ-ih-tal) is a vertical plane that divides the body into unequal left and right portions.
- A frontal plane is a vertical plane that divides the body into anterior (front) and posterior (back) portions. Also known as the coronal plane, it is located at right angles to the sagittal plane.

The Horizontal Plane
A horizontal plane is a flat crosswise plane, such as the horizon.
- A transverse plane (trans-VERSE) is a horizontal plane that divides the body into superior (upper) and inferior (lower) portions. A transverse plane can be at the waist or at any other level across the body.

Body Direction Terms
The relative location of sections of the body, or of an organ, can be described through the use of pairs of contrasting body direction terms.
- Ventral (VEN-tral) refers to the front, or belly side, of the organ or body (ventr means belly side of the body, and -al means pertaining to). Ventral is the opposite of dorsal.
- Dorsal (DOR-sal) refers to the back of the organ or body (dors means back of the body, and -al means pertaining to). Dorsal is the opposite of ventral.
- Anterior (an-TEER-ee-or) means situated in the front. It also means on the front or forward part of an organ (anter means front or before, and -ior means pertaining to). For example, the stomach is located anterior to (in front of) the pancreas. Anterior is also used in reference to the ventral surface of the body. Anterior is the opposite of posterior.
- Posterior (pos-TEER-ee-or) means situated in the back. It also means on the back part of an organ (poster means back or toward the back, and -ior means pertaining to). For example, the pancreas is located posterior to (behind) the stomach. The term posterior is also used in reference to the dorsal surface of the body. Posterior is the opposite of anterior.
- Superior means uppermost, above, or toward the head. For example, the lungs are located superior to (above) the diaphragm. Superior is the opposite of inferior.
- Inferior means lowermost, below, or toward the feet. For example, the stomach is located inferior to (below) the diaphragm. Inferior is the opposite of superior.

- Cephalic (seh-FAL-ick) means toward the head (cephal means head, and -ic means pertaining to). Cephalic is the opposite of caudal.
- Caudal (KAW-dal) means toward the lower part of the body (caud means tail or lower part of the body, and -al means pertaining to). Caudal is the opposite of cephalic.
- Proximal (PROCK-sih-mal) means situated nearest the midline or beginning of a body structure. For example, the proximal end of the humerus (bone of the upper arm) forms part of the shoulder. Proximal is the opposite of distal.
- Distal (DIS-tal) means situated farthest from the midline or beginning of a body structure. For example,
- n Medial (MEE-dee-al) means the direction toward, or nearer, the midline. For example, the medial ligament of the knee is near the inner surface of the leg. Medial is the opposite of lateral.
- Lateral means the direction toward or nearer the side and away from the midline. For example, the lateral ligament of the knee is near the side of the leg. Lateral is the opposite of medial. Bilateral means relating to, or having, two sides.

Major Body Cavities

The two major body cavities, which are the dorsal and the ventral cavities, are spaces within the body that contain and protect internal organs

The Dorsal Cavity

The dorsal cavity, which is located along the back of the body and head, contains organs of the nervous system that coordinate body functions and is divided into two portions:
- The cranial cavity, which is located within the skull, surrounds and protects the brain. Cranial means pertaining to the skull.
- The spinal cavity, which is located within the spinal column, surrounds and protects the spinal cord.

The Ventral Cavity

The ventral cavity, which is located along the front of the body, contains the body organs that maintain homeostasis.
- Homeostasis (hoh-mee-oh-STAY-sis) is the processes through which the body maintains a constant internal environment (home/o means constant, and -stasis means control).
- The thoracic cavity (thoh-RAS-ick), also known as the chest cavity or thorax, surrounds and protects the heart and the lungs. The diaphragm is a muscle that separates the thoracic and abdominal cavities.
- The abdominal cavity (ab-DOM-ih-nal) contains primarily the major organs of digestion. This cavity is frequently referred to simply as the abdomen (AB-doh-men).

- The pelvic cavity (PEL-vick) is the space formed by the hip bones and it contains primarily the organs of the reproductive and excretory systems.
- There is no physical division between the abdominal and pelvic cavities. The term abdominopelvic cavity (ab-dom-ih-noh-PEL-vick) refers to as these two cavities as a single unit (abdomin/o means abdomen, pelv means pelvis, and -ic means pertaining to).
- The term inguinal (ING-gwih-nal), which means relating to the groin, refers to the entire lower area of the abdomen. This includes the groin which is the crease at the junction of the trunk with the upper end of the thigh.

Regions of the Thorax and Abdomen

Regions of the thorax and abdomen are a descriptive system that divides the abdomen and lower portion of the thorax into nine parts.
- The hypochondriac regions (high-poh-KON-dree-ack) are located on the left and right sides of the body and are covered by the lower ribs (hypo- means below, chondr/i means cartilage, and -ac means pertaining to). As used here, the term hypochondriac means below the ribs. This term also describes an individual with an abnormal concern about his or her health.
- The epigastric region (ep-ih-GAS-trick) is located above the stomach (epi- means above, gastr means stomach, and -ic means pertaining to).
- The lumbar regions (LUM-bar) are located on the left and right sides near the inward curve of the spine (lumb means lower back, and -ar means pertaining to). The term lumbar describes the part of the back between the ribs and the pelvis.
- The umbilical region (um-BILL-ih-kal) surrounds the umbilicus (um-BILL-ih-kus) which is commonly known as the belly button or navel. This pit in the center of the abdominal wall marks the point where the umbilical cord was attached before birth.
- The iliac regions (ILL-ee-ack) are located on the left and right sides over the hip bones (ili means hip bone, and -ac mean pertaining to). The iliac region is named for the wide portion of the hip bone.
- The hypogastric region (high-poh-GAS-trick) is located below the stomach (hypo- means below, gastr means stomach, and -ic means pertaining to).

Quadrants of the Abdomen

Describing where an abdominal organ or pain is located is made easier by dividing the abdomen into four imaginary quadrants. The term quadrant means divided into four. The quadrants of the abdomen are the:
- Right upper quadrant (RUq)
- Left upper quadrant (LUq)
- Right lower quadrant (RLq)

- Left lower quadrant (LLq)

The Peritoneum

The peritoneum (pehr-ih-toh-NEE-um) is a multilayered membrane that protects and holds the organs in place within the abdominal cavity. A membrane is a thin layer of tissue that covers a surface, lines a cavity, or divides a space or organ.
- The parietal peritoneum (pah-RYE-eh-tal pehr-ih-toh- NEE-um) is the outer layer of the peritoneum that lines the interior of the abdominal wall. Parietal means cavity wall.
- The visceral peritoneum (VIS-er-al pehr-ih-toh-NEEum) is the inner layer of the peritoneum that surrounds the organs of the abdominal cavity. Visceral means relating to the internal organs.
- The mesentery (MESS-en-terr-ee) is a fused double layer of the parietal peritoneum that attaches parts of the intestine to the interior abdominal wall.
- Retroperitoneal (ret-roh-pehr-ih-toh-NEE-al) means located behind the peritoneum (retro- means behind, periton means peritoneum, and -eal means pertaining to). For example, the location of the kidneys is retroperitoneal with one on each side of the spinal column.
- Peritonitis (pehr-ih-toh-NIGH-tis) is inflammation of the peritoneum (periton means peritoneum, and -itis means inflammation).

Structures Of The Body

The body is made up of increasing larger, and more complex, structural units. From smallest to largest these are: cells, tissues, organs, and the body systems. Working together, these structures form the complete body and enable it to function properly.

Cells

Cells are the basic structural and functional units of the body. Cells are specialized and grouped together to form tissues and organs.
- Cytology (sigh-TOL-oh-jee) is the study of the anatomy, physiology, pathology, and chemistry of the cell (cyt means cell, and -ology means study of).

The Structure of Cells

- The cell membrane (MEM-brain) is the tissue that surrounds and protects the contents of the cell by separating them from its external environment.
- Cytoplasm (SIGH-toh-plazm) is the material within the cell membrane that is not part of the nucleus (cyt/o means cell, and -plasm means formative material of cells).
- The nucleus (NEW-klee-us), which is surrounded by the nuclear membrane, is a structure within the cell that has two important

functions: (1) it controls the activities of the cell, and (2) it helps the cell divide.

Stem Cells

Stem cells differ from other kinds of cells in the body because of two characteristics:

Stem cells are unspecialized cells that are able to renew themselves for long periods of time by cell division. This is in contrast to other types of cells that have a specialized role and die after a determined lifespan.

Under certain conditions stem cells can be transformed into cells with special functions such as the cells of the heart muscle that make the heartbeat possible or the specialized cells of the pancreas that are capable of producing insulin.

Adult Stem Cells

Adult stem cells, also known as somatic stem cells, are undifferentiated cells found among differentiated cells in a tissue or organ. Normally the primary role of these cells is to maintain and repair the tissue in which they are found. The term undifferentiated means not having a specialized function or structure. In contrast the term differentiated means having a specialized function or structure.

Stem cells potentially have many therapeutic uses, including being transplanted from one individual to

another. Cells for this purpose are harvested from the hemopoietic (blood forming) tissue of the donor's bone marrow. However unless there is an excellent match between the donor and recipient, there is the possibility of rejection known as graft versus host disease.

Embryonic Stem Cells

Embryonic stem cells are undifferentiated cells that are unlike any specific adult cell; however, they have the important ability to form any adult cell.

These cells can proliferate (grow rapidly) indefinitely in a laboratory, and could therefore potentially provide a source for adult muscle, liver, bone, or blood cells. Because these cells are more primitive than adult stem cells, an embryonic stem cell transplant does not require as perfect a match between the patient and donor as the transplantation of adult stem cells.

Embryonic stem cells come from the cord blood found in the umbilical cord and placenta of a newborn infant. Embryonic stem cells from cord blood can be harvested at the time of birth without danger to mother or child. These cells are kept frozen until needed for treatment purposes.

Embryonic stem cells can also be obtained from surplus embryos produced by in vitro (test tube) fertilization. With the informed consent of the donor couple, stem cells obtained in this manner are being used for important medical and scientific research.

Genetics

A gene is a fundamental physical and functional unit of heredity. Genes control hereditary disorders and all physical traits such as hair, skin, and eye color. Genetics is the study of how genes are transferred
from parents to their children and the role of genes in health and disease (gene means producing, and tics means pertaining to).
- A specialist in this field is known as a geneticist (jeh-NET-ih-sist).

Dominant and Recessive Genes

Each newly formed individual receives two genes of each genetic trait: one from the father and one from the mother.

When a dominant gene is inherited from either parent, the offspring will inherit that genetic condition or characteristic. For example, freckles are a physical trait that is transmitted by a dominant gene. So too is the hereditary disorder Huntington's disease which is discussed later in this chapter.

When the same recessive gene is inherited from both parents, the offspring will have that condition. For example, sickle cell anemia is a group of inherited red blood cell disorders that are transmitted by a recessive gene. When this gene is transmitted by both parents, the child will have sickle cell anemia.

When a recessive gene is inherited from only one parent, and a normal gene is inherited for the other
parent, the offspring will not have the condition. Although this child will not develop sickle cell anemia, he or she does have sickle cell anemia trait. Children with this trait can transmit the sickle cell gene to their offspring.

The Human Genome

A genome (JEE-nohm) is the complete set of genetic information of an individual. The Human Genome Project was formed to study this genetic code in all people, and found that it is over 99% identical among humans throughout the world. The first complete mapping of the human genome was just published in 2003. Having access to this data is a very important step in studying the use of genetics in health and science.

Chromosomes

Chromosomes (KROH-moh-sohmes) are the genetic structures located within the nucleus of each cell. These chromosomes are made up of the DNA molecules containing the body's genes. Packaging genetic
information into chromosomes helps a cell keep a large amount of genetic information neat, organized, and compact. Each chromosome contains about 100,000 genes.

A somatic cell is any cell in the body except the gametes (sex cells). Somatic means pertaining to the body in general. Somatic cells contain 46 chromosomes arranged into 23 pairs. There are 22 identical
pairs of chromosomes, plus another pair. In a typical female, this pair consists of XX chromosomes. In a

typical male, this pair consists of an XY chromosome pair. It is this chromosome pair that determines the sex of the individual.

A sex cell (sperm or egg), also known as a gamete, is the only type of cell that does not contain 46 chromosomes. Instead each ovum (egg) or sperm has 23 single chromosomes. In a female, one of these will be an X chromosome. In a male one of these will be either an X or a Y chromosome. When a sperm and ovum join, the newly formed offspring receives 23 chromosomes from each parent, for a total of 46.

It is the X or Y chromosome from the father that determines the gender of the child.

A defect in chromosomes can lead to birth defects. For example, individuals with Down syndrome have 47 chromosomes instead of the usual 46. Down syndrome is discussed later in this chapter.

DNA

DNA is the abbreviation for deoxyribonucleic acid. The basic structure of the DNA molecule, which is located on the pairs of chromosomes in the nucleus of each cell, is the same for all living organisms. Human DNA contains thousands of genes that provide the information essential for heredity, determining our physical appearance, disease risks, and other traits.

DNA is packaged in a chromosome as two spiraling strands that twist together to form a double helix. A

helix is a shape twisted like a spiral staircase. A double helix consists of two of these strands twisted together. DNA is found in the nucleus of all types of cells except erythrocytes (red blood cells). The difference here is due to the fact that erythrocytes do not have a nucleus.

The DNA for each individual is different and no two DNA patterns are exactly the same. The only exception to this rule is identical twins, which are formed from one fertilized egg that divides. Although their DNA is identical, these twins do develop fingerprints and other characteristics that make each of them unique.

A very small sample of DNA, such as from human hair or tissue can be used to identify individuals in criminal investigations, paternity suits, or genealogy research.

Genetic Mutation

A genetic mutation is a change of the sequence of a DNA molecule. Potential causes of genetic mutation include exposure to radiation or environmental pollution.

A somatic cell mutation is a change within the cells of the body. These changes affect the individual but cannot be transmitted to the next generation.

A gametic cell mutation is a change within the genes in a gamete (sex cell) that can be transmitted by a parent to his or her children.

Genetic engineering is the manipulating or splicing of genes for scientific or medical purposes. The production of human insulin from modified bacteria is an example of one result of genetic engineering.

Genetic Disorders

A genetic disorder, also known as a hereditary disorder, is a pathological condition caused by an absent or defective gene. Some genetic disorders are obvious at birth. Other may manifest (become evident) at any time in life. The following are examples of genetic disorders.

- Cystic fibrosis (CF) is a genetic disorder that is present at birth and affects both the respiratory and digestive systems.
- Down syndrome (DS) is a genetic variation that is associated with characteristic facial appearance, learning disabilities, and physical abnormalities such as heart valve disease.
- Hemophilia (hee-moh-FILL-ee-ah) is a group of hereditary bleeding disorders in which a blood-clotting factor is missing. This blood coagulation disorder is characterized by spontaneous hemorrhages or severe bleeding following an injury.
- Huntington's disease (HD) is a genetic disorder that is passed fromparent to child. Each child of a parent with the gene for Huntington's disease has a 50–50 chance of inheriting this defective gene. This condition causes nerve degeneration with symptoms that most often appear in midlife. (Degeneration means worsening condition.) This damage eventually results in uncontrolled movements and the loss of some mental abilities.
- Muscular dystrophy (DIS-troh-fee) is the term used to describe a group of genetic diseases that are characterized by progressive weakness and degeneration of the skeletal muscles that control movement.
- Phenylketonuria (fen-il-kee-toh-NEW-ree-ah), which is commonly known as PKU, is a genetic disorder in which the essential digestive enzyme phenylalanine hydroxylase is missing. PKU can be detected by a blood test performed on infants at birth. With careful dietary supervision, children born with PKU can lead normal lives. Without early detection and treatment, PKU causes severe mental retardation.
- Tay-Sachs disease (TAY SAKS) is a fatal genetic disorder in which harmful quantities of a fatty substance build up in tissues and nerve cells in the brain. Both parents must carry the mutated gene in order to have an affected child. The most common form of the disease affects babies who appear healthy at birth and seem to develop normally for the first few months. Development then slows and a relentless deterioration of mental and physical abilities results in progressive blindness, paralysis, and early death.

Tissues

A tissue is a group or layer of similarly specialized cells that join together to perform certain specific functions. The four main types of tissue are epithelial, connective, muscle, and nerve.

- Histology (hiss-TOL-oh-jee) is the study of the structure, composition, and function of tissues (hist means tissue, and -ology means a study of).

- A histologist (hiss-TOL-oh-jist) is a specialist in the study of the organization of tissues at all levels (hist means tissue, and -ologist means specialist).

Epithelial Tissues
- Epithelial tissues (ep-ih-THEE-lee-al) form a protective covering for all of the internal and external surfaces of the body. These tissues also form glands.
- Epithelium (ep-ih-THEE-lee-um) is the specialized epithelial tissue that forms the epidermis of the skin and the surface layer of mucous membranes. The epidermis, which is the outer layer of the skin, is discussed.
- Endothelium (en-doh-THEE-lee-um) is the specialized epithelial tissue that lines the blood and lymph vessels, body cavities, glands, and organs.

Connective Tissues
Connective tissues support and connect organs and other body tissues. The four kinds of connective tissue are:
- Dense connective tissues, such as bone and cartilage, formthe joints and framework of the body.
- Adipose tissue, also known as fat, provides protective padding, insulation, and support (adip means fat, and -ose means pertaining to).
- Loose connective tissue surrounds various organs and supports both nerve cells and blood vessels.
- Liquid connective tissues, which are blood and lymph, transport nutrients and waste products throughout the body.

Muscle Tissue
Muscle tissue contains cells with the specialized ability to contract and relax

Nerve Tissue
Nerve tissue contains cells with the specialized ability to react to stimuli and to conduct electrical impulses.

Pathology of Tissue Formation
Disorders of the tissues, which are frequently due to unknown causes, can occur before birth as the tissues are forming or appear later in life.

Incomplete Tissue Formation
- Aplasia (ah-PLAY-zee-ah) is the defective development, or the congenital absence, of an organ or tissue (a- means without, and -plasia means formation). Compare aplasia with hypoplasia.
- Hypoplasia (high-poh-PLAY-zee-ah) is the incomplete development of an organ or tissue usually due to a deficiency in the number of cells (hypo-

means deficient, and -plasia means formation). Compare hypoplasia with aplasia.

Abnormal Tissue Formation

- Anaplasia (an-ah-PLAY-zee-ah) is a change in the structure of cells and in their orientation to each other (ana- means excessive, and -plasia means formation). This abnormal cell development is characteristic of tumor formation in cancers. Contrast anaplasia with hypertrophy.
- Dysplasia (dis-PLAY-see-ah) is abnormal development or growth of cells, tissues, or organs (dys- means bad, and -plasia means formation).
- Hyperplasia (high-per-PLAY-zee-ah) is the enlargement of an organ or tissue because of an abnormal increase in the number of cells in the tissues (hypermeans excessive, and -plasia means formation). Contrast hyperplasia with hypertrophy.
- Hypertrophy (high-PER-troh-fee) is a general increase in the bulk of a body part or organ that is due to an increase in the size, but not in the number, of cells in the tissues (hyper- means excessive, and -trophy means development). This enlargement is not due to tumor formation. Contrast hypertrophy with anaplasia and hyperplasia.

GLANDS

A gland is a group of specialized epithelial cells that are capable of producing secretions. A secretion is the substance produced by a gland. The two major types of glands are exocrine and endocrine glands.

- Exocrine glands (ECK-soh-krin), such as sweat glands, secrete chemical substances into ducts that lead either to other organs or out of the body (exo- means out of, and -crine means to secrete).
- Endocrine glands (EN-doh-krin), which produce hormones, do not have ducts (endo- means within, and -crine means to secrete). These hormones are secreted directly into the bloodstream, which are then transported to organs and structures throughout the body.

Pathology and Procedures of the Glands

- Adenitis (ad-eh-NIGH-tis) is the inflammation of a gland (aden means gland, and -itis means inflammation).
- An adenocarcinoma (ad-eh-noh-kar-sih-NOH-mah) is a malignant tumor that originates in glandular tissue (aden/o means gland, carcin means cancerous, and -oma means tumor). Malignant means harmful, capable of spreading, and potentially life threatening.
- An adenoma (ad-eh-NOH-mah) is a benign tumor that arises in, or resembles, glandular tissue (aden means gland, and -oma means tumor). Benign means not life threatening.
- Adenomalacia (ad-eh-noh-mah-LAY-shee-ah) is the abnormal softening of a gland (aden/o means gland, and -malacia means abnormal softening). Adenomalacia is the opposite of adenosclerosis.

- Adenosis (ad-eh-NOH-sis) is any disease condition of a gland (aden means gland, and -osis means an abnormal condition or disease).
- Adenosclerosis (ad-eh-noh-skleh-ROH-sis) is the abnormal hardening of a gland (aden/o means gland, and -sclerosis means abnormal hardening). Adenosclerosis is the opposite of adenomalacia.
- An adenectomy (ad-eh-NECK-toh-mee) is the surgical removal of a gland (aden means gland, and -ectomy means surgical removal).

Body Systems And Related Organs

A body organ is a somewhat independent part of the body that performs a specific function. For purposes of description, the related tissues and organs are described as being organized into body systems with specialized functions.

Pathology

Pathology (pah-THOL-oh-jee) is the study of the nature and cause of disease that involves changes in structure and function. Pathology also means a condition produced by disease. The word root (combining form) path/o and the suffix -pathy mean disease; however, they also mean suffering, feeling, and emotion.
- A pathologist (pah-THOL-oh-jist) specializes in the laboratory analysis of tissue samples to confirm or establish a diagnosis (path means disease, and -ologist means specialist). These tissue specimens can be removed in biopsies, during operations, or in postmortem examinations. Postmortem means after death and a postmortem examination is also known as an autopsy (AW-top-see).
- Etiology (ee-tee-OL-oh-jee) is the study of the causes of diseases (eti- means cause, and -ology means study of).

Disease Transmission

A pathogen is a disease-producing microorganism such as a virus. Transmission is the spread of a disease. Contamination means that a pathogen is possibly present. Contamination occurs through a lack of proper hygiene standards or by failure to take appropriate infection control precautions.
- A communicable disease (kuh-MEW-nih-kuh-bul), also known as a contagious disease, is any condition that is transmitted from one person to another either by direct or by indirect contact with contaminated objects. Communicable means capable of being transmitted.
- Indirect contact transmission refers to situations in which a susceptible person is infected by contact with a contaminated surface.
- Bloodborne transmission is the spread of a disease through contact with blood or other body fluids that are contaminated with blood. Examples of bloodborne transmission are human immunodeficiency virus (HIV), hepatitis B, and most sexually transmitted diseases (STDs).
- Airborne transmission occurs through contact withcontaminated respiratory droplets spread by a cough or sneeze. Examples include tuberculosis, flu, colds, and measles.

- Food-borne and waterborne transmission, also known as fecal–oral transmission, is caused by eating or drinking contaminated food or water that has not been properly treated to remove contamination or kill pathogens that are present.
- Vector-borne transmission is the spread of certain disease due to the bite of a vector. As used here, the term vector describes insects or animals such as flies, mites, fleas, ticks, rats, and dogs that are capable of transmitting a disease. Mosquitoes are the most common vectors, and the diseases they transmit include malaria and West Nile virus.

Outbreaks of Diseases

- An epidemiologist (ep-ih-dee-mee-OL-oh-jist) is a specialist in the study of outbreaks of disease within a population group (epi- means above, dem means population, and -ologist means specialist).
- Endemic (en-DEM-ick) refers to the ongoing presence of a disease within a population, group, or area (enmeans within, dem means population, and -ic means pertaining to). For example, the common cold is endemic because it is always present within the general population.
- An epidemic (ep-ih-DEM-ick) is a sudden and widespread outbreak of a disease within a specific population group or area (epi- means above, dem means population, and -ic means pertaining to). For example, a sudden widespread outbreak of measles is an epidemic.
- Pandemic (pan-DEM-ick) refers to an outbreak of a disease occurring over a large geographic area, possibly worldwide (pan- means entire, dem means population, and -ic means pertaining to). For example, the worldwide spread of AIDS is pandemic.

Types of Diseases

- A functional disorder produces symptoms for which no physiological or anatomical cause can be identified. For example, a panic attack is a functional disorder.
- An iatrogenic illness (eye-at-roh-JEN-ick) is an unfavorable response due to prescribed medical treatment. For example, severe burns resulting from radiation therapy are iatrogenic.
- An idiopathic disorder (id-ee-oh-PATH-ick) is an illness without known cause (idi/o means peculiar to the individual, path means disease, and -ic means pertaining to). Idiopathic means without known cause.
- An infectious disease (in-FECK-shus) is an illness caused by living pathogenic organisms such as bacteria and viruses.
- A nosocomial infection (nos-oh-KOH-mee-al in- FECK-shun) is a disease acquired in a hospital or clinical setting. Nosocomial means hospital-acquired. For example, MRSA infections are often spread in Hospitals.
- An organic disorder (or-GAN-ick) produces symptoms caused by detectable physical changes in the body. For example, chickenpox, which has a characteristic rash, is an organic disorder caused by a virus.

Congenital Disorders

A congenital disorder (kon-JEN-ih-tahl) is an abnormal condition that exists at the time of birth. Congenital means existing at birth. These conditions can be caused by a developmental disorder before birth, prenatal influences, premature birth, or injuries during the birth process.

Developmental Disorders

A developmental disorder, also known as a birth defect, can result in an anomaly or malformation such as the absence of a limb or the presence of an extra toe. An anomaly (ah-NOM-ah-lee) is a deviation from what is regarded as normal.
- The term atresia (at-TREE-zee-ah) describes the congenital absence of a normal opening or the failure of a structure to be tubular. For example, an anal atresia is the congenital absence of the opening at the bottom end of the anus.

Prenatal Influences
Prenatal influences are the mother's health, behavior, and the prenatal medical care she does, or does not, receive before delivery.
- An example of a problem with the mother's health is an rubella infection. Birth defects often develop if a pregnant woman contracts this viral infection early in her pregnancy.
- An example of a problem caused by the mother's behavior is fetal alcohol syndrome (FAS) which is caused by the mother's consumption of alcohol during the pregnancy. This resulting condition of the baby is characterized by physical and behavioral traits, including growth abnormalities, mental retardation, brain damage, and socialization difficulties.
- An example of a problem caused by the lack of adequate prenatal medical care is premature delivery or a low birth-weight baby.

Premature Birth and Birth Injuries

- Premature birth, which is a birth that occurs earlier than 37 weeks of development, can cause serious health problems because the baby's body systems have not had time to form completely. Breathing difficulties and heart problems are common in premature babies.
- Birth injuries are congenital disorders that were not present before the events surrounding the time of birth. For example, cerebral palsy, which is the result of brain damage, can be caused by premature birth or inadequate oxygen to the brain during the birth process.

Aging

Aging is the normal progression of the life cycle that will eventually end in death. During the latter portion of life, individuals become increasingly at higher risk of developing health problems that are chronic or eventually fatal. As the average life span is becoming longer, a larger portion of the population is affected by such disorders related to aging.

- The study of the medical problem and care of the aged is known as geriatrics (jer-ee-AT-ricks) or as gerontology. Both of these terms have the same meaning; however, geriatrics is the preferred term.
- A physician who specializes in the care of older people is known as a geriatrician (jer-ee-ah-TRISH-un) or as a gerontologist. Both of these terms have the same meaning; however, geriatrician is the preferred term.

Abbreviations Related To The Human Body In Health And Disease

- anterior = A
- abdomen = Abd, Abdo
- anatomy = anat
- communicable disease = CD
- chromosome or chromosomes = CH, chr
- cytology, cytoplasm = cyt
- dorsal = D
- epidemic = epid
- hemophilia = HEM, hemo
- histology = HIS, Histo, histol
- physiology, posterior = P
- umbilical = umb
- ventral = V, vent, ventr

Critical Thinking Exercise

The following story and questions are designed to stimulate critical thinking through class discussion or as a brief essay response. There are no right or wrong answers to these questions.

The sign read in the fifth floor restroom read, "Dirty hands spread disease. Always use soap." Dave rinsed his hands with water, gave his hair a quick "finger-comb," and then rushed into the hallway, already late for biology class.

There was an overwhelming smell as he entered the classroom, and he could immediately tell why: on each counter was sitting the day's project, a fetal pig. "Do these things have to stink?" he asked his teacher. "Well, Dave, if they didn't 'stink' of the formaldehyde, they would be rotting and could be spreading diseases. Now let's get started," the teacher said. At the end of class period, they were told, "Be sure to wash your hands thoroughly before leaving this classroom."

This reminded Dave of the lectures they had earlier in the semester about diseases caused by pathogens and how these diseases are spread. As he looked around the classroom, Dave was aware of the other students. Most were gathering up their books to go directly to lunch without washing their hands, Gail and Susan were sharing a bottle of water, Beth was rubbing her eyes, and Jim was coughing without covering his mouth! Suddenly, Dave had a mental image of pathogens everywhere: lying on hands and counter tops, floating in the air—and all of these pathogens were looking for someone to infect! Dave shook his head to get rid of this mental image. Then he went to the sink and carefully washed his hands again—this time with soap.

Suggested Discussion Topics

1. Identify and discuss the examples of the potential disease transmission methods that are included in Dave's story and describe what should have been done to eliminate these risks.
2. Describe how bloodborne, airborne, and food-borne diseases are transmitted and give an example of each type of transmission.
3. Discuss what might happen in a school if a cafeteria worker has a food-borne disease, and after a trip to the lavatory, did not wash his or her hands. Instead, the worker went right back to work without putting on gloves, preparing salads and putting fresh fruit out for lunch.
4. When treating a bloody wound the caregiver is required to wear protective gloves. Discuss the possible reasons for this. Is this step taken to protect the patient against diseases on the caregiver's hands? Is this step required to protect the caregiver from a bloodborne disease that the patient might have?

Medical Terminology for Health Professions 4.0

CHAPTER 3

THE SKELETAL SYSTEM

This list contains essential word parts and medical terms for this chapter.

Word Parts
- ankyl/o
- arthr/o
- chondr/o
- cost/o
- crani/o
- -desis
- kyph/o
- lord/o
- -lysis
- myel/o
- oss/e, oss/i, ost/o, oste/o
- scoli/o
- spondyl/o
- synovi/o, synov/o
- -um

Medical Terms
- acetabulum (ass-eh-TAB-you-lum)
- allogenic (al-oh-JEN-ick)
- ankylosing spondylitis (ang-kih-LOH-sing spon-dih-LYE-tis)
- arthrodesis (ar-throh-DEE-sis)
- arthrolysis (ar-THROL-ih-sis)
- arthroscopy (ar-THROS-koh-pee)
- autologous (aw-TOL-uh-guss)
- chondroma (kon-DROH-mah)
- chondromalacia (kon-droh-mah-LAY-shee-ah)
- comminuted fracture (KOM-ih-newt-ed)
- compression fracture
- costochondritis (kos-toh-kon-DRIGH-tis)

- craniostenosis (kray-nee-oh-steh-NOH-sis)
- crepitation (krep-ih-TAY-shun)
- dual x-ray absorptiometry (ab-sorp-shee-OM-ehtree)
- fibrous dysplasia (dis-PLAY-see-ah)
- hallux valgus (HAL-ucks VAL-guss)
- hemarthrosis (hem-ar-THROH-sis)
- hemopoietic (hee-moh poy-ET-ick)
- internal fixation
- juvenile rheumatoid arthritis (ROO-mah-toyd ar-THRIGH-tis)
- kyphosis (kye-FOH-sis)
- laminectomy (lam-ih-NECK-toh-mee)
- lordosis (lor-DOH-sis)
- lumbago (lum-BAY-goh)
- malleolus (mal-LEE-oh-lus)
- manubrium (mah-NEW-bree-um)
- metacarpals (met-ah-KAR-palz)
- metatarsals (met-ah-TAHR-salz)
- myeloma (my-eh-LOH-mah)
- open fracture
- orthopedic surgeon (or-thoh-PEE-dick)
- orthotic (or-THOT-ick)
- osteitis (oss-tee-EYE-tis)
- osteoarthritis (oss-tee-oh-ar-THRIGH-tis)
- osteochondroma (oss-tee-oh-kon -DROH-mah)
- osteoclasis (oss-tee-OCK-lah-sis)
- osteomalacia (oss-tee-oh-mah-LAY-shee-ah)
- osteomyelitis (oss-tee-oh-my-eh-LYE-tis)
- osteonecrosis (oss-tee-oh-neh-KROH-sis)
- osteopenia (oss-tee-oh-PEE-nee-ah)
- osteoporosis (oss-tee-oh-poh-ROH-sis)
- osteoporotic hip fracture (oss-tee-oh-pah- ROT-ick)
- osteorrhaphy (oss-tee-OR-ah-fee)
- Paget's disease (PAJ-its)
- pathologic fracture
- percutaneous vertebroplasty (per-kyou-TAY-neeus VER-tee-broh-plas-tee)
- periostitis (pehr-ee-oss-TYE-tis)
- podiatrist (poh-DYE-ah-trist)
- prosthesis (pros-THEE-sis)
- rheumatoid arthritis (ROO-mah-toyd ar- THRIGH-tis)
- rickets (RICK-ets)
- scoliosis (skoh-lee-OH-sis)
- spina bifida (SPY-nah BIF-ih-dah)
- spiral fracture

- spondylolisthesis (spon-dih-loh-liss-THEE-sis)
- spondylosis (spon-dih-LOH-sis)
- subluxation (sub-luck-SAY-shun)
- synovectomy (sin-oh-VECK-toh-mee)
- vertebrae (VER-teh-bray)

The Structure Of Bones

Bone is the form of connective tissue that is the second hardest tissue in the human body. Only dental enamel is harder than bone.

The Tissues of Bone

Although it is a dense and rigid tissue, bone is also capable of growth, healing, and reshaping itself.
- Periosteum (pehr-ee-OSS-tee-um) is the tough, fibrous tissue that forms the outermost covering of bone (perimeans surrounding, oste means bone, and -um is a noun ending).
- Compact bone is the dense, hard, and very strong bone that forms the protective outer layer of bones.
- Spongy bone is lighter, and not as strong, as compact bone. This type of bone is commonly found in the ends and inner portions of long bones such as the femur. Red bone marrow is located within this spongy bone.
- The medullary cavity (MED-you-lehr-ee) is located in the shaft of a long bone and is surrounded by compactbone. Medullary means pertaining to the inner section.
- The endosteum (en-DOS-tee-um) is the tissue that lines the medullary cavity (end- means within, oste means bone, and -um is a noun ending).

Bone Marrow

- Red bone marrow, which is located within the spongy bone, is hemopoietic tissue that manufactures red blood cells, hemoglobin, white blood cells, and thrombocytes.
- Hemopoietic (hee-moh poy-ET-ick) means pertaining to the formation of blood cells (hem/o means blood, and -poietic means pertaining to formation). This term is also spelled hematopoietic.
- Yellow bone marrow, which functions as a fat storage area, is composed chiefly of fat cells and is located in the medullary cavity.

Cartilage

- Cartilage (KAR-tih-lidj) is the smooth, rubbery, blue-white connective tissue that acts as a shock absorber between bones. Cartilage, which is more elastic than bone, also makes up the flexible parts of the skeleton such as the outer ear and the tip of the nose.
- Articular cartilage (ar-TICK-you-lar KAR-tih-lidj) covers the surfaces of bones where they come together to form joints. This cartilage makes

smooth joint movement possible and protects the bones from rubbing against each other.
- The meniscus (meh-NIS-kus) is the curved fibrous cartilage found in some joints, such as the knee and the temporomandibular joint of the jaw.

Anatomic Landmarks of Bones
- The diaphysis (dye-AF-ih-sis) is the shaft of a long bone.
- The epiphysis (eh-PIF-ih-sis), which is covered with articular cartilage, is the wide end of a long bone. The proximal epiphysis is the end of the bone located nearest to the midline of the body. The distal epiphysis is the end of the bone located farthest away from the midline.
- A foramen (foh-RAY-men) is an opening in a bone through which blood vessels, nerves, and ligaments pass (plural, foramina). For example, the spinal cord passes through the foramen magnum of the occipital bone.
- A process is a normal projection on the surface of a bone that serves as an attachment for muscles and tendons. For example, the mastoid process is the bony projection located on temporal bones just behind the ears.

Joints
Joints, which are also known as articulations, are the place of union between two or more bones. Joints are classified according to either their construction or based on the degree of movement they allow.

Fibrous Joints
Fibrous joints, consisting of inflexible layers of dense connective tissue, hold the bones tightly together. In adults these joints, which are also known as sutures, do not allow any movement. In newborns and very young children some fibrous joints are movable before they have solidified.
- The fontanelles (fon-tah-NELLS), also known as the soft spots, are normally present on the skull of a newborn. These flexible soft spots facilitate the passage of the infant through the birth canal. They also allow for the growth of the skull during the first year. As the child matures, and the sutures close, the fontanelles gradually harden.

Cartilaginous Joints
Cartilaginous joints (kar-tih-LADJ-ih-nus) allow only slight movement and consist of bones connected entirely by cartilage. Examples include:
- Cartilaginous joints, such as where the ribs connect to the sternum (breast bone). These joints allow movement during breathing.
- The pubic symphysis (PEW-bick SIM-fih-sis) is the cartilaginous joint known that allows some movement to facilitate childbirth. This joint is located between the pubic bones in the anterior (front) of the pelvis.

Synovial Joints

Asynovial joint (sih-NOH-vee-al) is createdwhere two bones articulate to permit a varietyofmotions.Asusedhere the term articulate means to come together. These joints are also described based on their type of motion.

- Ball and socket joints, such as the hips and shoulders, allow a wide range of movement in many directions.
- Hinge joints, such as the knees and elbows, are synovial joints that allow movement primarily in one direction or plane. Synovial joints consist of several components that make complex movements possible.
- The synovial capsule is the outermost layer of strong fibrous tissue that resembles a sleeve as it surrounds the joint.
- Synovial membrane lines the capsule and secretes synovial fluid.
- Synovial fluid, which flows within the synovial cavity, acts as a lubricant to make the smooth movement of the joint possible.
- Ligaments (LIG-ah-mentz) are bands of fibrous tissue that form joints by connecting one bone to another bone, or joining a bone to cartilage. Complex hinge joints, such as the knee, are made up of a series of ligaments that permit movement in different directions.
- A bursa (BER-sah) is a fibrous sac that acts as a cushion to ease movement in areas that are subject to friction such as in the shoulder, elbow, and knee joints where a tendon passes over a bone (plural, bursae).

The Skeleton

The typical adult human skeleton consists of approximately 206 bones. Depending upon the age of the individual, the exact number of ranges from 206 to 350 bones. For descriptive purposes, the skeleton is divided into the axial and appendicular skeletal systems.

Axial Skeleton

The axial skeleton protects the major organs of the nervous, respiratory, and circulatory systems. Axial means pertaining to an axis, which is an imaginary line that runs lengthwise through the center of the body. The axial skeleton consists of 80 bones including those of the skull; the ribs, sternum, and thoracic vertebrae of the thoracic cavity; and the other vertebrae of the spinal column.

Appendicular Skeleton

The appendicular skeleton makes body movement possible and also protects the organs of digestion, excretion, and reproduction. The term appendicular means referring to an appendage. An appendage is anything that is attached to a major part of the body. The appendicular skeleton consists of 126 bones that are organized into the upper extremities (shoulders, arms, forearms, wrists, and hands) and the lower extremities (hips, thighs, legs, ankles, and feet).

Bones of the Skull

The skull consists of the eight bones that form the cranium, 14 bones that form the face, and six bones in the middle ear.

Bones of the Cranium

The cranium (KRAY-nee-um), which is made up of the following eight bones, is the portion of the skull that encloses the brain (crani means skull, and -um is a noun ending).
- The frontal bone forms the forehead.
- The two parietal bones (pah-RYE-eh-tal) form most of the roof and upper sides of the cranium.
- The occipital bone (ock-SIP-ih-tal) forms the posterior floor and walls of the cranium.
- The two temporal bones form the sides and base of the cranium.
- The sphenoid bone (SFEE-noid) forms part of the base of the skull and parts of the floor and sides of the orbit. The orbit is the bony socket that surrounds and protects the eyeball.
- The ethmoid bone (ETH-moid) forms part of the posterior portion of the nose, the orbit, and the floor of the cranium.

Auditory Ossicles

The six tiny bones of the middle ear, known as the auditory ossicles (OSS-ih-kulz), n The external auditory meatus (mee-AY-tus), which is located in the temporal bone on each side of the skull, is the opening of the external auditory canal of the outer ear. A meatus is the external opening of a canal.

Bones of the Face

The face is made up of the following 14 bones:
- The two nasal bones that form the upper part of the bridge of the nose.
- The two zygomatic bones (zye-goh-MAT-ick), also known as the cheekbones, articulate with the frontal bone (forehead).
- The two maxillary bones (MACK-sih-ler-ee), also known as the maxillae, form most of the upper jaw (singular, maxilla).
- The two palatine bones (PAL-ah-tine) form part of the hard palate of the mouth and the floor of the nose.
- The two lacrimal bones (LACK-rih-mal) make up part of the orbit at the inner angle of the eye.
- The two inferior conchae (KONG-kee or KONG-kay) are the thin, scroll-like bones that form part of the interior of the nose (singular, concha).
- The vomer bone (VOH-mer) forms the base for the nasal septum. The nasal septum is the cartilage wall that divides the two nasal cavities.
- The mandible (MAN-dih-bul), also known as the jawbone, is the only movable bone of the skull. The mandible is attached to the skull at the

temporomandibular joint (tem-poh-roh-man-DIB-you-lar), which is also known as the TMJ.

Thoracic Cavity

The thoracic cavity (thoh-RAS-ick), also known as the rib cage, is the bony structure that protects the heart and lungs. It consists of the ribs, sternum, and upper portion of the spinal column extending from the neck to the diaphragm, not including the arms.

Ribs

The 12 pairs of ribs, which are also known as costals, attach posteriorly to the thoracic vertebrae (cost means rib, and -al means pertaining to).
- The first seven pairs of ribs, called true ribs, are attached anteriorly to the sternum.
- The next three pairs of ribs, called false ribs, are attached anteriorly to cartilage that joins with the sternum.
- The last two pairs of ribs, called floating ribs, are only attached posteriorly.

Sternum

The sternum (STER-num), also known as the breastbone, forms the middle of the front of the rib cage and is divided into three parts.
- The manubrium (mah-NEW-bree-um) is the bony structure that forms the upper portion of the sternum.
- The body of the sternum is the bony structure that forms the middle portion of the sternum.
- The xiphoid process (ZIF-oid) is the structure made of cartilage that forms the lower portion of the sternum.

Shoulders

The shoulders form the pectoral girdle (PECK-toh-rahl), which supports the arms and hands; this also known as the shoulder girdle. As used here, the term girdle means a structure that encircles the body. As you study the bones of the shoulder.
- The clavicle (KLAV-ih-kul), also known as the collar bone, is a slender bone that connects the manubrium of the sternum to the scapula.
- The scapula (SKAP-you-lah) is also known as the shoulder blade (plural, scapulae).
- The acromion (ah-KROH-mee-on) is an extension of the scapula that forms the high point of the shoulder.

Arms
- The humerus (HEW-mer-us) is the bone of the upper arm (plural, humeri).

- The radius (RAY-dee-us) is the smaller and shorter bone in the forearm. The radius runs up the thumb side of the forearm.
- The ulna (ULL-nah) is the larger and longer bone of the forearm. The proximal end of the ulna articulates with the distal end of the humerus to form the elbow joint.
- The olecranon process (oh-LEK-rah-non), commonly known as the funny bone, is a large projection on the upper end of the ulna. This forms the point of the elbow and exposes a nerve that tingles when struck.

Wrists, Hands, and Fingers
- The eight carpals (KAR-palz) are the bones that form the wrist. These bones form the carpal tunnel, a narrow bony passage through which passes the median nerve and the tendons of the fingers.
- The metacarpals (met-ah-KAR-palz) are the five bones that form the palms of the hand.
- The phalanges (fah-LAN-jeez) are the 14 bones of the fingers (singular, phalanx). The bones of the toes are also known as phalanges.
- Each of the four fingers has three bones. These are the distal (outermost), middle, and proximal (nearest the hand) phalanges.
- The thumb has two bones. These are the distal and proximal phalanges.

The Spinal Column
The spinal column, also known as the vertebral column, supports the head and body, and protects the spinal cord. This structure consists of 26 vertebrae (VER-teh-bray). A vertebra is a single segment of the spinal column. Vertebral means pertaining to the vertebrae.

Structures of a Vertebra
The vertebrae (VER-teh-bray) are the bony structure units of the spinal column.
- The body of the vertebra is the solid anterior portion.
- The lamina (LAM-ih-nah) is the posterior portion of a vertebra (plural, laminae). The transverse and spinous processes extend from this area.
- The vertebral foramen is the opening in the middle of the vertebra. The spinal cord passes through this opening.

Types of Vertebrae
- The cervical vertebrae (SER-vih-kal) are the first set of seven vertebrae that form the neck. They are also known as C1 through C7. Cervical means pertaining to the neck.
- The thoracic vertebrae (thoh-RASS-ick) make up the second set of 12 vertebrae. They form the outward curve of the spine and are known as T1 through T12. Thoracic means pertaining to the thoracic cavity.
- The lumbar vertebrae (LUM-bar) make up the third set of five vertebrae and form the inward curve of the lower spine. They are known as L1 through L5. The lumbar vertebrae are the largest and strongest of the

vertebrae and bear most of the body's weight. Lumbar means relating to the part of the back and sides between the ribs and the pelvis.

Sacrum and Coccyx

The remaining two vertebrae are the sacrum and coccyx.
- The sacrum (SAY-krum) is the slightly curved, triangular-shaped bone near the base of the spine that forms the lower portion of the back. At birth, the sacrum is composed of five separate bones; however they fuse together in the young child to form a single bone.
- The coccyx (KOCK-sicks), also known as the tailbone, forms the end of the spine and is actually made up of four small vertebrae that are fused together.

Intervertebral Disks

The intervertebral disks (in-ter-VER-teh-bral), which are made of cartilage, separate and cushion the vertebrae from each other. These disks act as shock absorbers and allow for movement of the spinal column.

Pelvic Girdle

The pelvic girdle, which protects internal organs and supports the lower extremities, is also known as the pelvis or hips. The pelvis is a cup-shaped ring of bone at the lower end of the trunk that consists of the ilium, ischium, and pubis.
- The ilium (ILL-ee-um) is the broad blade-shaped bone that forms the back and sides of the pubic bone.
- The sacroiliac (say-kroh-ILL-ee-ack) is the slightly movable articulation between the sacrum and posterior portion of the ilium (sacr/o means sacrum, ili means ilium, and -ac means pertaining to).
- The ischium (ISS-kee-um), which forms the lower posterior portion of the pubic bone, bears the weight of the body when sitting.
- The pubis (PEW-bis), which forms the anterior portion of the pubic bone, is located just below the urinary bladder.
- The ileum, ischium, and pubis are separate at birth; however, they fuse to form the left and right pubic bones. These bones are held securely together by the pubic symphysis.
- The acetabulum (ass-eh-TAB-you-lum), also known as the hip socket, is the large circular cavity in each side of the pelvis that articulates with the head of the femur to form the hip joint.

Femur

The femur (FEE-mur) is the upper leg bone. Also known as the thigh bone, it is the largest bone in the body.
- The head of the femur articulates with the acetabulum (hip socket).
- The femoral neck is the narrow area just below the head of the femur. Femoral means pertaining to the femur.

Knees

The knees are the complex joints that make possible movement between the upper and lower leg.
- The patella (pah-TEL-ah), also known as the kneecap, is the bony anterior portion of the knee.
- The term popliteal (pop-LIT-ee-al) means referring to the posterior space behind the knee where the ligaments, vessels, and muscles related to this joint are located.
- The cruciate ligaments (KROO-shee-ayt), make possible the movements of the knee. These are known as the anterior and posterior cruciate ligaments because they are shaped like a cross.

Lower Leg

The lower leg is made up of two bones: the tibia and the Fibula.
- The tibia (TIB-ee-ah), also known as the shinbone, is the larger weight-bearing bone in the anterior of the lower leg.
- The fibula (FIB-you-lah) is the smaller of the two bones of the lower leg.
- The malleolus (mal-LEE-oh-lus) is the rounded bony protuberance on each side of the ankle (plural, malleoli).

The Ankles

The ankles, which form the joint between the lower leg and the foot, are each made up of seven short tarsal (TAHR-sal) bones. These bones are similar to the bones of the wrist, but are larger in size.
- The talus (TAY-luss) is the anklebone that articulates with the tibia and fibula.
- The calcaneus (kal-KAY-nee-uss), also known as the heel bone, is the largest of the tarsal bones.

The Feet and Toes

The feet and toes are made up of the following bones.
- The five metatarsals (met-ah-TAHR-salz) form that part of the foot to which the toes are attached.
- The phalanges are the bones of the toes. The great toe has two phalanges. Each of the other toes has three phalanges. The bones of the fingers are also called phalanges.

Medical Specialties Related To The Skeletal System

- A chiropractor (KYE-roh-prack-tor) holds a Doctor of Chiropractic degree and specializes in the manipulative treatment of disorders originating from misalignment of the spine. Manipulative treatment involves manually adjusting the positions of the bones.
- An orthopedic surgeon (or-thoh-PEE-dick), also known as an orthopedist, is a physician who specializes in diagnosing and treating diseases and disorders involving the bones, joints, and muscles.

- An osteopath (oss-tee-oh-PATH) holds a Doctor of Osteopathy (DO) degree and uses traditional forms of medical treatment in addition to specializing in treating health problems by spinal manipulation (oste/o means bone, and -path means disease). This type of medical practice is known as osteopathy; however, that term is also used to mean any bone disease.
- A podiatrist (poh-DYE-ah-trist) holds a Doctor of Podiatry (DP) or Doctor of Podiatric Medicine (DPM) degree and specializes in diagnosing and treating disorders of the foot (pod mean foot, and -iatrist means specialist).

Pathology Of The Skeletal System

Joints

- Ankylosis (ang-kih-LOH-sis) is the loss, or absence, of mobility in a joint due to disease, injury, or a surgical procedure (ankyl means crooked, bent, or stiff, and -osis means abnormal condition or disease). Mobility means being capable of movement.
- Arthrosclerosis (ar-throh-skleh-ROH-sis) is stiffness of the joints, especially in the elderly (arthr/o means joint, and -sclerosis means abnormal hardening).
- Bursitis (ber-SIGH-tis) is an inflammation of a bursa (burs means bursa, and -itis means inflammation).
- Chondromalacia (kon-droh-mah-LAY-shee-ah) is the abnormal softening of cartilage (chondr/o means cartilage, and -malacia means abnormal softening).
- A chondroma (kon-DROH-mah) is a slow-growing benign tumor derived from cartilage cells (chondr means cartilage, and -oma means tumor).
- Costochondritis (kos-toh-kon-DRIGH-tis) is an inflammation of the cartilage that connects a rib to the sternum (cost/omeans rib, chondr means cartilage, and -itis means inflammation).
- Hallux valgus (HAL-ucks VAL-guss), also known as a bunion, is an abnormal enlargement of the joint at the base of the great toe (hallux means big toe, and valgus means bent).
- Hemarthrosis (hem-ar-THROH-sis) is blood within a joint (hem means blood, arthr means joint, and -osis means abnormal condition or disease). This condition is frequently due to a joint injury. It also can occur spontaneously in patients taking blood-thinning medications or those having a blood clotting disorder such as hemophilia.
- Synovitis (sin-oh-VYE-tiss) is inflammation of the synovial membrane that results in swelling and pain of the affected joint (synov means synovial membrane, and -itis means inflammation). This condition can be caused by arthritis, trauma, infection, or irritation produced by damaged cartilage.

Dislocation
- Dislocation, also known as luxation (luck-SAY-shun), is the total displacement of a bone from its joint.
- Subluxation (sub-luck-SAY-shun) is the partial displacement of a bone from its joint.

Arthritis
Arthritis (ar-THRIGH-tis) is an inflammatory condition of one or more joints (arthr means joint, and -itis means inflammation). There are many different forms and causes of arthritis. Rheumatism is an obsolete term for arthritis to describe any painful disorder of the joints; however, in lay language, this word is still in use.

Osteoarthritis
Osteoarthritis (oss-tee-oh-ar-THRIGH-tis), also known as wear-and-tear arthritis, is most commonly associated with aging (oste/o means bone, arthr means joint, and -itis means inflammation).
- This condition is described as a degenerative joint disease because it is characterized by the wearing away of the articular cartilage within the joints. Degenerative means the breaking down or impairment of a body part.
- Spondylosis (spon-dih-LOH-sis), which is also known as spinal osteoarthritis, is a degenerative disorder that can cause the loss of normal spinal structure and function (spondyl means vertebrae, and -osis means abnormal condition or disease).

Gouty Arthritis
Gouty arthritis (GOW-tee ar-THRIGH-tis), also known as gout, is a type of arthritis characterized by deposits of uric acid in the joints. Uric acid is a byproduct that is normally excreted by the kidneys. Gout develops when excess uric acid, which is present in the blood, forms crystals in the joints of the feet and legs.

Rheumatoid Arthritis
Rheumatoid arthritis (ROO-mah-toyd ar-THRIGH-tis), commonly known by its abbreviation RA, is a chronic autoimmune disorder in which the joints and some organs of other body systems are attacked.
As RA progressively attacks the synovial membranes they inflamed and thickened so that the joints are increasingly swollen, painful, and immobile.

Ankylosing Spondylitis
Ankylosing spondylitis (ang-kih-LOH-sing spon-dih-LYEtis) is a form of rheumatoid arthritis that primarily causes inflammation of the joints between the vertebrae. Ankylosing means the progressive stiffening of a joint or joints, and spondylitis means inflammation of the vertebrae.

Juvenile Rheumatoid Arthritis

Juvenile rheumatoid arthritis is an autoimmune disorder that affects children aged 16 years or less with symptoms that include stiffness, pain, joint swelling, skin rash, fever, slowed growth, and fatigue.

The Spinal Column

- A herniated disk (HER-nee-ayt-ed), also known as a slipped or ruptured disk, is the breaking apart of an intervertebral disk that results in pressure on spinal nerve roots.
- Lumbago (lum-BAY-goh), also known as low back pain, is pain of the lumbar region of the spine (lumb means lumbar, and -ago means diseased condition).
- Spondylolisthesis (spon-dih-loh-liss-THEE-sis) is the forward slipping movement of the body of one of the lower lumbar vertebrae on the vertebra or sacrum below it (spondyl/o means vertebrae, and -listhesis means slipping).
- Spina bifida (SPY-nah BIF-ih-dah) is a congenital defect that occurs during early pregnancy when the spinal canal fails to close completely around the spinal cord to protect it. Spina means pertaining to the spine. Bifida means split. Some cases of spina bifida are due to a lack of the nutrient folic acid during the early stages of pregnancy.

Curvatures of the Spine

- Kyphosis (kye-FOH-sis) is an abnormal increase in the outward curvature of the thoracic spine as viewed from the side (kyph means hump and -osis means abnormal condition or disease). This condition, also known as humpback or dowager's hump, is frequently associated with aging
- Lordosis (lor-DOH-sis) is an abnormal increase in the forward curvature of the lumbar spine (lord means bent backward, and -osis means abnormal condition or disease). This condition is also known as swayback.
- Scoliosis (skoh-lee-OH-sis) is an abnormal lateral (sideways) curvature of the spine (scoli means curved, and -osis means abnormal condition or disease).

Bones

- Craniostenosis (kray-nee-oh-steh-NOH-sis) is a malformation of the skull due to the premature closure of the cranial sutures (crani/o means skull, and -stenosis means abnormal narrowing).
- Fibrous dysplasia (dis-PLAY-see-ah) is a bone disorder of unknown cause that destroys normal bone structure and replaces it with fibrous (scar-like) tissue. This leads to uneven growth, brittleness, and deformity of the affected bones.
- Ostealgia (oss-tee-AL-jee-ah), also known as osteodynia, mean pain in a bone (oste means bone, and -algia means pain).

- Osteitis (oss-tee-EYE-tis), also spelled ostitis, is an inflammation of bone (oste means bone, and -itis means inflammation).
- Osteomalacia (oss-tee-oh-mah-LAY-shee-ah), also known as adult rickets, is abnormal softening of bones in adults (oste/o means bone, and -malacia means abnormal softening). This condition is usually caused by a deficiency of vitamin D, calcium, and/or phosphate. Compare with rickets.
- Osteomyelitis (oss-tee-oh-my-eh-LYE-tis) is an inflammation of the bone marrow and adjacent bone (oste/o means bone, myel means bone marrow, and -itis means inflammation). The bacterial infection that causes osteomyelitis often originates in another part of the body and spreads to the bone via the blood.
- Osteonecrosis (oss-tee-oh-neh-KROH-sis) is the death of bone tissue due to a lack of insufficient blood supply (oste/o means bone, and -necrosis means tissue death).
- Paget's disease (PAJ-its), also known as osteitis deformans, is a bone disease of unknown cause. This condition is characterized by the excessive breakdown of bone tissue, followed by abnormal bone formation. The new bone is structurally enlarged, but weakened and filled with new blood vessels.
- Periostitis (pehr-ee-oss-TYE-tis) is an inflammation of the periosteum (peri- means surrounding, ost means bone, and -itis means inflammation). This condition is often associated with shin splints.
- Rickets (RICK-ets), also known as infantile osteomalacia, is a deficiency disease occurring in children. This condition, which is characterized by defective bone growth, results from a vitamin D deficiency that is sometimes due to insufficient exposure to sunlight.
- Short stature, formerly known as dwarfism, is condition resulting from the failure of the bones of the limbs to grow to an appropriate length. The average adult height is no more than 4'10" and these individuals are appropriately referred to as "little people."
- The term talipes (TAL-ih-peez), also known as clubfoot, describes any congenital deformity of the foot involving the talus (ankle bones).

Bone Tumors

- Primary bone cancer is a relatively rare malignant tumor that originates in a bone. Malignant means becoming progressively worse and life-threatening. As an example, Ewing's sarcoma is a tumor that occurs in the bones of the upper arm, legs, pelvis, or rib. The peak incidence is between ages 10 and 20 years.
- The term secondary bone cancer describes tumors that have metastasized (spread) to bones from other organs such as the breasts and lungs.
- A myeloma (my-eh-LOH-mah) is a type of cancer that occurs in blood-making cells found in the red bone marrow (myel means bone marrow,

and -oma means tumor). This condition can cause pathologic fractures and is often fatal.
- An osteochondroma (oss-tee-oh-kon-DROH-mah) is a benign bony projection covered with cartilage (oste/o means bone, chondr means cartilage, and -oma means tumor). Benign means something that is not lifethreatening and does not recur. This type of tumor is also known as an exostosis (plural, exostoses).

Osteoporosis

Osteoporosis (oss-tee-oh-poh-ROH-sis) is a marked loss of bone density and an increase in bone porosity that is frequently associated with aging (oste/o means bone, por means small opening, and -osis means abnormal condition or disease).
- Osteopenia (oss-tee-oh-PEE-nee-ah) is thinner than average bone density in a young person (oste/o means bone, and -penia means deficiency). This term is used to describe the condition of someone who does not yet have osteoporosis, but is at risk for developing it.

Osteoporosis Related Fractures

Osteoporosis is primarily responsible for three types of fractures:
- A compression fracture, also known as a vertebral crush fracture, occurs when the bone is pressed together (compressed) on itself. These fractures are sometimes caused by the spontaneous collapse of weakened vertebrae or can be due to an injury. This results in pain, loss of height, and development of the spinal curvature known as dowager's hump
- A Colles' fracture, which is named for the Irish surgeon Abraham Colles, is also known as a fractured wrist. This fracture occurs at the lower end of the radius when a person tries to stop a fall by landing on his or her hands. The impact of this fall causes the bone weakened by osteoporosis to break
- An osteoporotic hip fracture (oss-tee-oh-pah-ROTick), also known as a broken hip, is usually caused by weakening of the bones due to osteoporosis and can occur either spontaneously or as the result of a fall. Complications from these fractures can result in the loss of function, mobility, independence, or death. Osteoporotic means pertaining to or caused by the porous condition of bones.

Fractures

A fracture, which is a broken bone, is described in terms of its complexity.
- A closed fracture, also known as a simple fracture or a complete fracture, is one in which the bone is broken, but there is no open wound in the skin.
- An open fracture, also known as a compound fracture, is one in which the bone is broken and there is an open wound in the skin.

- A comminuted fracture (KOM-ih-newt-ed) is one in which the bone is splintered or crushed. Comminuted means crushed into small pieces.
- A greenstick fracture, or incomplete fracture, is one in which the bone is bent and only partially broken. This type of fracture occurs primarily in children.
- An oblique fracture occurs at an angle across the bone.
- A pathologic fracture occurs when a weakened bone breaks under normal strain. This is due to bones being weakened by osteoporosis or to a disease process such as cancer.
- A spiral fracture is a fracture in which the bone has been twisted apart. This type of fracture occurs as the result of a severe twisting motion such as in a sports injury.
- A stress fracture, which is an overuse injury, is a small crack in the bone that often develops from chronic, excessive impact.
- A transverse fracture occurs straight across the bone.

Additional Terms Associated with Fractures
- A fat embolus (EM-boh-lus) can form when a long bone is fractured and fat cells from yellow bone marrow are released into the blood. An embolus is any foreign matter circulating in the blood that can become lodged and block the blood vessel.
- Crepitation (krep-ih-TAY-shun), also known as crepitus, is the grating sound heard when the ends of a broken bone move together. This term also describes the crackling sound heard in lungs affected with pneumonia and the clicking sound heard in the movements of some joints.
- As the bone heals, a callus (KAL-us) forms as a bulging deposit around the area of the break. This tissue eventually becomes bone. A callus is also a thickening of the skin caused by repeated rubbing.

Skeletal System
- A radiograph, also known as an x-ray, is the use of x-radiation to visualize bone fractures and other abnormalities
- Arthroscopy (ar-THROS-koh-pee) is the visual examination of the internal structure of a joint (arthr/o means joint, and -scopy means visual examination) using an arthroscope.
- A bone marrow biopsy is a diagnostic test that may be necessary after abnormal types or numbers of red or white blood cells are found in a complete blood count test.
- Bone marrow aspiration is the use of a syringe to withdraw the liquid bone marrow. This procedure is used to obtain tissue for diagnostic purposes or to collect bone marrow for medical procedures such as stem cell transplantation.

- Magnetic resonance imaging (MRI) is used to image soft tissue structures such as the interior of complex joints. It is not the most effective method of imaging hard tissues such as bone.

Bone Density Testing

Bone density testing is used to determine losses or changes in bone density. These tests are used to diagnose conditions such as osteoporosis, osteomalacia, osteopenia, and Paget's disease.
- Ultrasonic bone density testing is a screening test for osteoposoris or other conditions that cause a loss of bone mass. In this procedure, sound waves are used to take measurements of the calcenaeous (heel) bone. If the results indicate risks, more definitive testing is indicated.
- Dual x-ray absorptiometry (ab-sorp-shee-OM-ehtree) is a low-exposure radiographic measurement of the spine and hips to measure bone density. This test produces more accurate results than ultrasonic bone density testing.

Skeletal System

Bone Marrow Transplants
- A bone marrow transplant (BMT) is used to treat certain types of cancers, such as leukemia and lymphomas, that affect bone marrow. In this treatment, initially both the cancer cells and the patient's bone marrow are destroyed with high-intensity radiation and chemotherapy.
- Next, healthy bone marrow stem cells are transfused into the recipient's blood. These cells migrate to the spongy bone, where they multiply to form cancer-free red bone marrow.

Allogenic Bone Marrow Transplant

An allogenic bone marrow transplant uses healthy bone marrow cells from a compatible donor, often a sibling. However, unless this is a perfect match, there is the danger that the recipient's body will reject the transplant. Allogenic (al-oh-JEN-ick) means originating within another.

Autologous Bone Marrow Transplant

In an autologous bone marrow transplant, the patient receives his own bone marrow cells which have been harvested, cleansed, treated, and then stored before the remaining bone marrow is destroyed. Autologous (aw- TOL-uh-guss) means originating within an individual.

Medical Devices

- An orthotic (or-THOT-ick) is a mechanical appliance, such as a leg brace or splint, that is specially designed to control, correct, or compensate for impaired limb function.
- A prosthesis (pros-THEE-sis) is a substitute for a diseased or missing body part, such as a leg that has been amputated (plural, prostheses).

Joints

- Arthrodesis (ar-throh-DEE-sis), also known as surgical ankylosis, is the surgical fusion (joining together) of two bones to stiffen a joint, such as an ankle, elbow, or shoulder (arthr/o means joint, and -desis means surgical fixation of bone or joint). This procedure is performed to treat severe arthritis or a damaged joint. Compare with arthrolysis.
- Arthrolysis (ar-THROL-ih-sis) is the surgical loosening of an ankylosed joint (arthr/o means joint, and -lysis means loosening or setting free). Note: The suffix -lysis also means breaking down or destruction and may indicate either a pathologic state or a therapeutic procedure. Compare with arthrodesis.
- Arthroscopic surgery (ar-throh-SKOP-ick) is a minimally invasive procedure for the treatment of the interior of a joint. For example, torn cartilage can be removed with the use of an arthroscope and instruments inserted through small incisions.
- A bursectomy (ber-SECK-toh-mee) is the surgical removal of a bursa (burs means the bursa, and -ectomy means surgical removal).
- Chondroplasty (KON-droh-plas-tee) is the surgical repair of damaged cartilage (chondr/o means cartilage, and -plasty means surgical repair).
- A synovectomy (sin-oh-VECK-toh-mee) is the surgical removal of a synovial membrane from a joint (synov means synovial membrane, and -ectomy means surgical removal). One use of this procedure, which can be performed endoscopically, is to repair joint damage caused by rheumatoid arthritis.

Joint Replacement

Based on its word parts, the term arthroplasty (AR-throhplas- tee) means the surgical repair of a damaged joint (arthr/o means joint, and -plasty means surgical repair); however, this term has come to mean the surgical placement of an artificial joint. These procedures are named for the involved joint and the amount of the joint that is replaced.

- The joint replacement part is a prosthesis that this is commonly referred to as an implant.
- A total knee replacement (TKR) means that all of the parts of the knee were replaced. This procedure is also known as a total knee arthroplasty.
- A partial knee replacement (PKR) describes a procedure in which only part of the knee is replaced.
- A total hip replacement (THR), also known as a total hip arthroplasty, is performed to restore a damaged hip to full function. During the surgery, a plastic lining is fitted into the acetabulum to restore a smooth surface. The head of the femur is removed and replaced with a metal ball attached to a metal shaft that is fitted into the femur. These smooth surfaces restore the function of the hip joint.

- Bone-conserving hip resurfacing is an alternative to removing the head of the femur. Function is restored to the hip by placing a metal cap over the head of the femur to allow it to move smoothly over a metal lining in the acetabulum.
- Revision surgery is the replacement of a worn or failed implant.

Spinal Column
- A percutaneous diskectomy (per-kyou-TAY-nee-us dis-KECK-toh-mee) is performed to treat a herniated intervertebral disk. In this procedure, a thin tube is inserted through the skin of the back to suction out the ruptured disk or to vaporize it with a laser. Percutaneous means performed through the skin.
- A percutaneous vertebroplasty (per-kyou-TAY-nee-us VER-tee-broh-plas-tee) is performed to treat osteoporosis- related compression fractures (vertebr/o means vertebra, and -plasty means surgical repair). In this minimally invasive procedure, bone cement is injected to stabilize compression fractures within the spinal column.
- A laminectomy (lam-ih-NECK-toh-mee) is the surgical removal of a lamina, or posterior portion, of a vertebra (lamin means lamina, and -ectomy means surgical removal).
- Spinal fusion is a technique to immobilize part of the spine by joining together (fusing) two or more vertebrae. Fusion means to join together.

Bones
- A craniectomy (kray-nee-EK-toh-mee) is the surgical removal of a portion of the skull (crani means skull, and -ectomy means surgical removal). This procedure is performed to treat craniostenosis or to relieve increased intracranial pressure due to swelling of the brain. The term intracranial pressure describes the amount of pressure inside the skull.
- A craniotomy (kray-nee-OT-oh-mee) is a surgical incision or opening into the skull (crani means skull, and -otomy means a surgical incision). This procedure is performed to gain access to the brain to remove a tumor, to relieve intracranial pressure, or to obtain access for other surgical procedures.
- A cranioplasty (KRAY-nee-oh-plas-tee) is the surgical repair of the skull (crani/o means skull, and -plasty means surgical repair).
- Osteoclasis (oss-tee-OCK-lah-sis) is the surgical fracture of a bone to correct a deformity (oste/o means bone, and -clasis means to break).
- An ostectomy (oss-TECK-toh-mee) is the surgical removal of bone (ost means bone, and -ectomy means the surgical removal).
- Osteoplasty (OSS-tee-oh-plas-tee) is the surgical repair of a bone or bones (oste/o means bone, and -plasty means surgical repair).

- Osteorrhaphy (oss-tee-OR-ah-fee) is the surgical suturing, or wiring together, of bones (oste/o means bone, and -rrhaphy means surgical suturing).
- Osteotomy (oss-tee-OT-oh-mee) is a surgical incision or sectioning of a bone (oste means bone, and -otomy means a surgical incision).
- A periosteotomy (pehr-ee-oss-tee-OT-oh-mee) is an incision through the periosteum to the bone (perimeans surrounding, oste means bone, and -otomy means surgical incision).

Treatment of Fractures

- Closed reduction, also known as manipulation, is the attempted realignment of the bone involved in a fracture or joint dislocation. The affected bone is returned to its normal anatomic alignment by manually applied forces and then is usually immobilized to maintain the realigned position during healing.
- When a closed reduction is not practical, a surgical procedure known as an open reduction is required to realign the bone parts.
- Immobilization, also known as stabilization, is the act of holding, suturing, or fastening the bone in a fixed position with strapping or a cast.
- Traction is a pulling force exerted on a limb in a distal direction in an effort to return the bone or joint to normal alignment.

External and Internal Fixation

- External fixation is a fracture treatment procedure in which pins are placed through the soft tissues and bone so that an external appliance can be used to hold the pieces of bone firmly in place during healing. When healing is complete, the appliance is removed.
- Internal fixation, also known as open reduction internal fixation (ORIF), is a fracture treatment in which a plate or pins are placed directly into the bone to hold the broken pieces in place. This form of fixation is not usually removed after the fracture has healed.

Abbreviations Related To The Skeletal System

- bone density testing = BDT
- closed reduction = CR
- fracture = Fx
- osteoarthritis = OA
- osteoporosis = OP
- temporomandibular joint = TMJ
- total hip arthroplasty = THA
- total joint arthroplasty = TJA
- total knee arthroplasty = TKA

Note: To avoid errors or confusion, always be cautious when using abbreviations.

Critical Thinking Exercise

The following story and questions are designed to stimulate critical thinking through class discussion or as a brief essay response. There are no right or wrong answers to these questions.

Dr. Johnstone didn't like what he saw. The x-rays of Gladys Gwynn's hip showed a fracture of the femoral neck and severe osteoporosis of the hip. Mrs. Gwynn had been admitted to the orthopedic ward of Hamilton Hospital after a fall that morning at Sunny Meadows, an assisted-living facility.

The accident had occurred when Sheri Smith, a new aide, lost her grip while helping Mrs. Gwynn in the shower.

A frail but alert and cheerful woman of 85, Gladys Gwynn has osteoarthritis and osteoporosis that have forced her to rely on a walker. Although her finances were limited, she has been living at Sunny

Meadows since her husband's death 4 years ago. Dr. Johnstone knewthat she didn'thave any close relatives and he didnot think that she had signed a health care power of attorney designating someone to help with medical decisions like this.

A total hip replacement would be the logical treatment for a younger patient because it could restore some of her lost mobility. However, for a frail patient like Mrs. Gwynn, internal fixation of the fracture might be the treatment of choice. This would repair the break, but not improve her mobility.

Dr. Johnstone needs to make a decision soon, but he knows that Mrs. Gwynn is groggy from pain

medication. With one more look at the x-ray, Dr. Johnstone sighedand walked toward Mrs. Gwynn's room.

Suggested Discussion Topics

1. Because of the pain medication, Gladys Gwynn is unable to speak for herself. Since she has no relatives to help, is it appropriate for Dr. Johnstone to make the decision about surgery for her?
2. Under the circumstances, is it possible that when Gladys moved into Sunny Meadows they had her sign a Health Care Power of Attorney to someone at the facility?
3. Because the accident happened when Sheri Smith was helping Mrs. Gwynn, do you think Sheri should be held responsible for the accident? Given that Sheri is an employee of Sunny Meadows should that facility be held responsible?
4. The recovery time for internal fixation surgery is shorter than that following a total hip replacement. The surgery is also less expensive and has a less strenuous recovery period; however, Mrs. Gwynn probably will not be able to walk again. Given the patient's condition, and the limited dollars available for health care, which procedure should be performed?
5. Would you have answered question 3 differently if Mrs. Gwynn were your mother?

Scott J. Barnard

Medical Terminology for Health Professions 4.0

CHAPTER 4

THE MUSCULAR SYSTEM

This list contains essential word parts and medical terms for this chapter.

Word Parts

- bih -cele
- dysh fasci/o
- fibr/o
- -ia
- -ic
- kines/o, kinesi/o
- my/o
- -plegia
- -rrhexis
- tax/o
- ten/o, tend/o, tendin/o
- ton/o
- tri-

Medical Terms

- abduction (ab-DUCK-shun)
- adduction (ah-DUCK-shun)
- adhesion (ad-HEE-zhun)
- ataxia (ah-TACK-see-ah)
- atonic (ah-TON-ick)
- atrophy (AT-roh-fee)
- bradykinesia (brad-ee-kih-NEE-zee-ah)
- carpal tunnel syndrome (KAR-pul)
- chronic fatigue syndrome
- circumduction (ser-kum-DUCK-shun)
- contracture (kon-TRACK-chur)
- dorsiflexion (dor-sih-FLECK-shun)
- dyskinesia (dis-kih-NEE-zee-ah)
- dystaxia (dis-TACK-see-ah)

- dystonia (dis-TOH-nee-ah)
- electromyography (ee-leck-troh-my-OGrah-fee)
- electroneuromyography (ee-leck-troh-new-rohmy- OG-rah-fee)
- epicondylitis (ep-ih-kon-dih-LYE-tis)
- ergonomics (er-goh-NOM-icks)
- exercise physiologist (fiz-ee-OL-oh-jist)
- fasciitis (fas-ee-EYE-tis)
- fibromyalgia syndrome (figh-broh-my-ALjee- ah)
- ganglion cyst (GANG-glee-on SIST)
- heel spur
- hemiparesis (hem-ee-pah-REE-sis)
- hemiplegia (hem-ee-PLEE-jee-ah)
- hyperkinesia (high-per-kye-NEE-zee-ah)
- hypertonia (high-per-TOH-nee-ah)
- hypokinesia (high-poh-kye-NEE-zee-ah)
- hypotonia (high-poh-TOH-nee-ah)
- impingement syndrome (im-PINJ-ment SIN-drohm)
- intermittent claudication (klaw-dih- KAY-shun)
- muscular dystrophy (DIS-troh-fee)
- myasthenia gravis (my-as-THEE-nee-ah GRAH-vis)
- myocele (MY-oh-seel)
- myoclonus (my-oh-KLOH-nus)
- myofascial release (my-oh-FASH-ee-ahl)
- myolysis (my-OL-ih-sis)
- myoparesis (my-oh-PAR-eh-sis)
- myorrhaphy (my-OR-ah-fee)
- myotonia (my-oh-TOH-nee-ah)
- nocturnal myoclonus (nock-TER-nal my-oh-KLOH-nus)
- oblique (oh-BLEEK)
- paralysis (pah-RAL-ih-sis)
- paraplegia (par-ah-PLEE-jee-ah)
- physiatrist (fiz-ee-AT-rist)
- plantar fasciitis (PLAN-tar fas-ee-EYE-tis)
- polymyositis (pol-ee-my-oh-SIGH-tis)
- pronation (proh-NAY-shun)
- quadriplegia (kwad-rih-PLEE-jee-ah)
- sarcopenia (sar-koh-PEE-nee-ah)
- shin splint
- singultus (sing-GUL-tus)
- spasmodic torticollis (spaz-MOD-ick tor-tih- KOL-is)
- sphincter (SFINK-ter)
- sprain
- tenodesis (ten-ODD-eh-sis)
- tenodynia (ten-oh-DIN-ee-ah)

- tenolysis (ten-OL-ih-sis)
- tenorrhaphy (ten-OR-ah-fee)

Objectives

On completion of this chapter, you should be able to:
1. Describe the functions and structures of the muscular system including muscle fibers, fascia, tendons, and the three types of muscle.
2. Recognize, define, spell, and pronounce the terms related to muscle movements and explain how the muscles are named.
3. Recognize, define, pronounce, and spell the terms related to the pathology and the diagnostic and treatment procedures of the muscular system.

Structures Of The Muscular System

The body has more than 600 muscles, which make up about 40%–45% of the body's weight. Skeletal muscles are made up of fibers, are covered with fascia, and are attached to bones by tendons.

Muscle Fibers

Muscle fibers are the long, slender cells that make up muscles. Each muscle consists of a group of fibers that are held together by connective tissue and enclosed in a fibrous sheath.

Fascia

- Fascia (FASH-ee-ah) is the sheet of fibrous connective tissue that covers, supports, and separates muscles or groups of muscles (plural, fasciae or fascias). Fascia is flexible to allow muscle movements; however, it does not have elastic properties to accommodate the swelling of the enclosed tissues.
- Myofascial (my-oh-FASH-ee-ahl) means pertaining to muscle tissue and fascia (my/o means muscle, fasci means fascia, and -al means pertaining to).

Tendons

A tendon is a narrow band of nonelastic, dense, fibrous connective tissue that attaches a muscle to a bone. Do not confuse tendons with ligaments, which connect one bone to another bone. For example, the Achilles tendon attaches the gastrocnemius muscle (the major muscle of the calf of the leg) to the heel bone. An aponeurosis is a sheetlike fibrous connective tissue that resembles a flattened tendon that serves as a fascia to bind muscles together or as a means of connecting muscle to bone (plural, aponeuroses).

Types Of Muscle Tissue

The three types of muscle tissue are skeletal, smooth, and myocardial. These muscle types are described according to their appearance and function.

Skeletal Muscles

Skeletal muscles are attached to the bones of the skeleton and make body motions possible.

Skeletal muscles are also known as voluntary muscles because we have conscious (voluntary) control over these muscles.

Skeletal muscles are also known as striated muscles because under a microscope, the dark and light bands in the muscle fibers create a striped appearance. Striated means striped.

Smooth Muscles

Smooth muscles are located in the walls of internal organs such as the digestive tract, blood vessels, and ducts leading from glands. Their function is to move and control the flow of fluids through these structures. Smooth muscles are also known as involuntary muscles because they are under the control of the autonomic nervous system and are not under voluntary control.

Smooth muscles are also known as unstriated muscles because they do not have the dark and light bands that produce the striped appearance seen in striated muscles.

Smooth muscles are also known as visceral muscles because they are found in the large internal organs (except the heart) and in hollow structures such as those of the digestive and urinary systems. Visceral means relating to the internal organs.

Myocardial Muscle

Myocardial muscles (my-oh-KAR-dee-al), also known as myocardium or cardiac muscle, form the muscular walls of the heart (my/o means muscle, cardi means heart, and -al means pertaining to). Myocardial muscle is like striated skeletal muscle in appearance, but is similar to smooth muscle in that its action is involuntary. It is the constant contraction and relaxation of the myocardial muscle that causes the heartbeat.

Muscle Contraction And Relaxation

A wide range of muscle movements are made possible by the combination of specialized muscle types, muscle innervation, and organization into antagonistic muscle pairs.

Muscle Innervation

- Muscle innervation (in-err-VAY-shun) is the stimulation of a muscle by an impulse transmitted by a motor nerve. Motor nerves enable the brain to stimulate a muscle to contract. When the stimulation stops, the muscle relaxes. If the nerve impulse is disrupted because of injury or disease, the muscle will be unable to function properly or can be paralyzed and unable to contract.

- Neuromuscular (new-roh-MUS-kyou-lar) means pertaining to the relationship between nerve and muscle (neur/o means nerve, muscul means muscle, and -ar means pertaining to).

Antagonistic Muscle Pairs

All muscles are arranged in antagonistic pairs. The term antagonistic refers to working in opposition to each other. Muscles within each pair are made up of specialized cells that can change length or shape by contracting and relaxing. When one muscle of a pair contracts, the other muscle of the pair relaxes. It is these contrasting actions that make motion possible.

Contraction is the tightening of a muscle. As the muscle contracts, it becomes shorter, and thicker, causing the belly (center) of the muscle to enlarge.

Relaxation occurs when a muscle returns to its original form. As the muscle relaxes it becomes longer, and thinner, and the belly is no longer enlarged.

As an example, the triceps and biceps work as a pair to make movement of the arm possible.

Contrasting Muscle Motion

These muscle motions, which occur as pairs of opposites, are described in the following text.

Abduction and Adduction

Abduction (ab-DUCK-shun) is the movement of a limb away from the midline of the body (ab- means away from, duct means to lead, and -ion means action). An abductor is a muscle that moves a part away from the midline. In contrast, adduction (ah-DUCK-shun) is the movement of a limb toward the midline of the body (ad- means toward, duct means to lead, and -ion means action). An adductor is a muscle that moves a part toward the midline.

Flexion and Extension

Flexion (FLECK-shun) means decreasing the angle between two bones by bending a limb at a joint (flex means to bend, and -ion means action). A flexor is a muscle that bends a limb at a joint.

In contrast, extension means increasing the angle between two bones or the straightening of a limb (exmeans away from, tens means to stretch out, and -ion means action). An extensor is a muscle that straightens a limb at a joint.

Hyperextension is the extreme or overextension of a limb or body part beyond its normal limit. For example, movement of the head far backward or far forward beyond the normal range of motion causes hyperextension of the muscles of the neck.

Elevation and Depression

Elevation is the act of raising or lifting a body part, such as raising the ribs when breathing in. A levator is a muscle that raises a body part. In contrast, depression is the act of lowering a body part, such as lowering the ribs when breathing out. A depressor is a muscle that lowers a body part.

Abduction moves away from the midline. During abduction, the arm moves outward away from the side
of the body.
- Flexion decreases an angle, as in bending a joint. During flexion, the knee or elbow are bent.
- Extension increases an angle, as in straightening a joint. During extension, the knee or elbow are straightened.
- Elevation raises a body part. During elevation, the levator anguli oris raises the corner of the mouth in a smile.
- Depression lowers a body part. During depression, the depressor anguli oris lowers the corner of the mouth in a frown.
- Rotation turns a bone on its own axis. Circumduction is the circular movement at the far end of a limb.
- Supination turns the palm of the hand upward or forward.
- Pronation turns the palm of the hand downward or backward.
- Dorsiflexion bends the foot upward at the ankle. Plantar flexion bends the foot downward at the ankle.

Rotation and Circumduction

Rotation is a circular movement around an axis such as the shoulder joint. An axis is an imaginary line that runs lengthwise through the center of the body. In contrast, circumduction (ser-kum-DUCK-shun) is the circular movement of a limb at the far end. An example of circumduction is the swinging motion of the far end of the arm.
- A rotator muscle turns a body part on its axis. For example, the head of the humerus (the bone of the upper arm) rotates within the shoulder joint.
- The rotator cuff is the group of muscles and their tendons that hold the head of the humerus securely in place as it rotates within the shoulder joint.

Supination and Pronation

Supination (soo-pih-NAY-shun) is the act of rotating the arm or the leg so that the palm of the hand, or sole of the foot, is turned forward or upward.
- In contrast, pronation (proh-NAY-shun) is the act of rotating the arm or leg so that the palm of the hand or sole of the foot is turned downward or backward.

Dorsiflexion and Plantar Flexion

Dorsiflexion (dor-sih-FLECK-shun) is the movement that bends the foot upward at the ankle. Pointing the toes and foot upward decreases the angle between the top of the foot and the front of the leg.
In contrast, plantar flexion (PLAN-tar FLECK-shun) is the movement that bends the foot downward at the ankle. Plantar means pertaining to the sole of the foot.

Pointing the toes and foot downward increases the angle between the top of the foot and the front of the leg.

Muscles Named for Their Origin and Insertion

The movements of skeletal muscles are made possible by two points of attachment known as the origin and insertion. Some muscles are also named for these points.
- The origin, which is the less moveable attachment, is the place where the muscle begins. The origin is located nearest the midline of the body or on a less moveable part of the skeleton.
- The insertion, which is the more moveable attachment, is the place where the muscle ends by attaching to a bone or tendon. In contrast to the origin, this that is farthest from the midline of the body.
- For example, the sternocleidomastoid muscle, helps bend the neck and rotate the head. This muscle is named for its two points of origin and one point of insertion. The origins of this muscle are near the midline at the sternum (breastbone) and the clavicle (collar bone). The insertion of this muscle, which is away from the midline, is into the mastoid process of the temporal bone (located just behind the ear).

Muscles Named for Their Action

Some muscles are named for their action, such as flexion or extension.
For example, the flexor carpi muscles and the extensor carpi muscles are the pair of muscles that make flexion (bending) and extension (straightening) of the wrist possible. Carpi means wrist or wrist bones.

Muscles Named for Their Location

Some muscles are named for their location on the body or the organ they are near:
- For example, the pectoralis major is a thick, fanshaped muscle situated on the anterior chest wall. In the male, this muscle makes up the bulk of the chest muscles. In the female, this muscle lies under the breast. Pectoral means relating to the chest.
- Other muscles indicate their location by including the terms lateralis and medialis in their names. Lateralis means toward the side. Medialis means toward the midline. For example, the vastus lateralis and the vastus medialis. These muscles flex and extend the leg at the knee.
- Some muscles indicate their location by including external and internal in their names. External, or superficial mean near the surface and internal means deeper location. The external oblique and internal oblique flex and rotate the spinal column and compress the abdomen.

Muscles Named for Fiber Direction

Some muscles are named for the direction in which their fibers run.
- Oblique (oh-BLEEK) means slanted or at an angle. As an example, the external oblique and internal oblique muscles have a slanted alignment.

- Rectus (RECK-tus) means in straight alignment with the vertical axis of the body. As an example, the rectus abdominis muscle has a straight alignment.
- A sphincter (SFINK-ter) is a ring-like muscle that tightly constricts the opening of a passageway. A sphincter is named for the passage involved. As an example, the anal sphincter closes the anus.
- Transverse (trans-VERSE) means in a crosswise direction. An example is the transverse abdominis muscle, which has a crosswise alignment.

Muscles Named for Number of Divisions

Muscles may be named according to the number of divisions forming them.
- The biceps brachii (BRAY-kee-eye), also known as the biceps, is formed from two divisions (bi- means two, and -ceps means head). This muscle of the anterior upper arm flexes the elbow.
- The triceps brachii (BRAY-kee-eye), also known as the triceps, is formed from three divisions (tri- means three, and -ceps means head). This muscle of the posterior upper arm extends the elbow.

Muscles Named for Their Size or Shape

Some muscles are named because they are broad or narrow or large or small.
- For example, the gluteus maximus (GLOO-tee-us) is the largest muscle of the buttock.
- Other muscles are named because they are shaped like a familiar object. For example, the deltoid muscle is shaped like an inverted triangle or the Greek letter delta. The deltoid forms the muscular cap of the shoulder.

Muscles Named for Strange Reasons

Some muscles, such as the hamstrings, have seemingly strange names. The reason this group of muscles is so named is because these are the muscles by which a butcher hangs a slaughtered pig.

The hamstring group, located at the back of the upper leg, consists of three separate muscles: the biceps femoris, semitendinosus, and semimembranosus muscles. The primary functions of the hamstrings are knee flexion and hip extension.

Medical Specialties Related To The Muscular System

- An exercise physiologist (fiz-ee-OL-oh-jist) is a specialist who works under the supervision of a physician to develop, implement, and coordinate exercise programs, and administer medical tests to promote physical fitness.
- A neurologist (new-ROL-oh-jist) is a physician who specializes in treating the causes of paralysis and similar muscular disorders in which there is a loss of function.

- A physiatrist (fiz-ee-AT-rist) is a physician who specializes in physical medicine and rehabilitation with the focus on restoring function. Rehabilitation is restoration, following disease, illness, or injury, of the ability to function in a normal or near-normal manner.
- A rheumatologist (roo-mah-TOL-oh-jist) is a physician who specializes in the diagnosis and treatment of arthritis and disorders such as osteoporosis, fibromyalgia and tendonitis that are characterized by inflammation in the joints and connective tissues.
- A sports medicine physician specializes in treating sports-related injuries of the bones, joints, and muscles.

Pathology Of The Muscular System
Fibers, Fascia, and Tendons

- Fasciitis (fas-ee-EYE-tis), which is also spelled fascitis, is inflammation of a fascia (fasci means fascia, and -itis means inflammation).
- Fibromyalgia syndrome (figh-broh-my-AL-jee-ah) is a debilitating chronic condition characterized by fatigue, diffuse and or specific muscle, joint, or bone pain, and a wide range of other symptoms (fibr/o means fibrous connective tissue, my means muscle, and -algia means pain). Debilitating means a condition causing weakness. Contrast fibromyalgia syndrome with chronic fatigue syndrome.
- Tenodynia (ten-oh-DIN-ee-ah), also known as tenalgia, is pain in a tendon (ten/o means tendon, and -dynia means pain).
- Tendinitis (ten-dih-NIGH-tis) is an inflammation of the tendons caused by excessive or unusual use of the joint (tendon means tendon, and -itis means inflammation). The terms tendonitis, tenonitis, and tenontitis all have the same meaning.

Chronic Fatigue Syndrome

Chronic fatigue syndrome (CFS) is a disorder of unknown cause that affects many body systems. It is discussed in this chapter because many of the symptoms are similar to those of the fibromyalgia syndrome.
CFS is a debilitating and complex disorder characterized by profound fatigue that is not improved by bed
rest and may be made worse by physical or mental activity. Those with CFS often function at a much lower level of activity than they were capable of before the beginning of the illness. This persistent overwhelming fatigue lasts more than 2 months and does not improve with bed rest.

Muscle Disorders

- An adhesion (ad-HEE-zhun) is a band of fibrous tissue that holds structures together abnormally. Adhesions can form in muscles, or in internal organs, as the result of an injury or surgery.

- Atrophy (AT-roh-fee) means weakness or wearing away of body tissues and structures. Atrophy of a muscle or muscles can be caused by pathology or by disuse of the muscle over a long period of time.
- Myalgia (my-AL-jee-ah), also known as myodynia, is tenderness or pain in the muscles (my means muscle, and -algia means pain).
- A myocele (MY-oh-seel) is the herniation (protrusion) of muscle substance through a tear in the fascia surrounding it (my/o means muscle, and -cele means a hernia). A hernia is the protrusion of a part or structure through the tissues normally containing it.
- Myolysis (my-OL-ih-sis) is the degeneration of muscle tissue (my/o means muscle, and -lysis means destruction or breaking down in disease). Degeneration means deterioration or breaking down. Deterioration means the process of becoming worse.
- Myomalacia (my-oh-mah-LAY-shee-ah) is abnormal softening of muscle tissue (my/o means muscle, and -malacia means abnormal softening).
- Myorrhexis (my-oh-RECK-sis) is the rupture or tearing of a muscle (my/o means muscle, and -rrhexis means rupture).
- Polymyositis (pol-ee-my-oh-SIGH-tis) is a muscle disease characterized by the simultaneous inflammation and weakening of voluntary muscles in many parts of the body (poly- means many, myos means muscle, and -itis means inflammation). The affected muscles are typically those closest to the trunk or torso, and the resulting weakness can be severe.
- Sarcopenia (sar-koh-PEE-nee-ah) is the loss of muscle mass, strength, and function that comes with aging (sarc/o means flesh, and -penia means deficiency). A weight or resistance training program can significantly improve muscle mass and slow, but not stop this process.

Muscle Tone

Muscle tone, also known as tonus, is the state of balanced muscle tension (contraction and relaxation) that makes normal posture, coordination, and movement possible. As used here the term tonic means pertaining to muscle tone.
- Atonic (ah-TON-ick) means lacking normal muscle tone or strength (a- means without, ton means tone, and -ic means pertaining to).
- Dystonia (dis-TOH-nee-ah) is a condition of abnormal muscle tone that causes the impairment of voluntary muscle movement (dys- means bad, ton means tone, and -ia means condition).
- Hypertonia (high-per-TOH-nee-ah) is a condition of excessive tone of the skeletal muscles (hyper- means excessive, ton means tone, and -ia means condition). Hypertonia is the opposite of hypotonia.
- Hypotonia (high-poh-TOH-nee-ah) is a condition in which there is diminished tone of the skeletal muscles (hypo- means deficient, ton means tone, and -ia means condition). Hypotonia is the opposite of hypertonia.

- Myotonia (my-oh-TOH-nee-ah) is a neuromuscular disorder characterized by the slow relaxation of the muscles after a voluntary contraction (my/o means muscle, ton means tone, and -ia means condition).

Voluntary Muscle Movement

- Ataxia (ah-TACK-see-ah) is the inability to coordinate muscle activity during voluntary movement (a- means without, tax means coordination, and -ia means condition). These movements, which are often shaky and unsteady, are most frequently caused by abnormal activity in the cerebellum.
- Dystaxia (dis-TACK-see-ah), also known as partial ataxia, is a mild form of ataxia (dys- means bad, tax means coordination, and -ia means condition).
- A contracture (kon-TRACK-chur) is the permanent tightening of fascia, muscles, tendons, ligaments, or skin that occurs when normally elastic connective tissues are replaced with nonelastic fibrous tissues. The most common causes of contractures are scarring or the lack of use due to immobilization or inactivity.
- Intermittent claudication (klaw-dih-KAY-shun) is pain in the leg muscles that occurs during exercise and is relieved by rest. Intermittent means coming and going at intervals, and claudication means limping. This condition, which is due to poor circulation, is associated with peripheral vascular disease.
- A spasm is a sudden, violent, involuntary contraction of one or more muscles.
- A cramp is a localized muscle spasm named for its cause, such as a heat cramp or writer's cramp.
- Spasmodic torticollis (spaz-MOD-ick tor-tih-KOL-is), also known as wryneck, is a stiff neck due to spasmodic contraction of the neck muscles that pull the head toward the affected side. Spasmodic means relating to a spasm, and torticollis means a contraction, or shortening, of the muscles of the neck.

Muscle Function

- Bradykinesia (brad-ee-kih-NEE-zee-ah) is extreme slowness in movement (brady- means slow, kines means movement, and -ia means condition). This is one of the symptoms of Parkinson's disease.
- Dyskinesia (dis-kih-NEE-zee-ah) is the distortion or impairment of voluntary movement such as in a tic or spasm (dys- means bad, kines means movement, and -ia means condition). A tic is a spasmodic muscular contraction that often involves parts of the face. Although these movements appear purposeful, they are not under voluntary control.

- Hyperkinesia (high-per-kye-NEE-zee-ah), also known as hyperactivity, is abnormally increased muscle function or activity (hyper- means excessive, kines means movement, and -ia means condition). Hyperkinesia is the opposite of hypokinesia.
- Hypokinesia (high-poh-kye-NEE-zee-ah) is abnormally decreased muscle function or activity (hypomeans deficient, kines means movement, and -ia means condition). Hypokinesia is the opposite of hyperkinesia.

Myoclonus

Myoclonus (my-oh-KLOH-nus) is the sudden, involuntary jerking of a muscle or group of muscles (my/o means muscle, clon mean violent action, and -us is a singular noun ending).
- Nocturnal myoclonus (nock-TER-nal my-oh-KLOHnus) is jerking of the limbs that can occur normally as a person is falling asleep. Nocturnal means pertaining to night.
- Singultus (sing-GUL-tus), also known as hiccups, is myoclonus of the diaphragm that causes the characteristic hiccup sound with each spasm.

Myasthenia Gravis

Myasthenia gravis (my-as-THEE-nee-ah GRAH-vis) is a chronic autoimmune disease that affects the neuromuscular junction and produces serious weakness of voluntary muscles. Myasthenia means muscle weakness (my means muscle, and -asthenia means weakness or lack of strength). Gravis comes from the Latin meaning grave or serious.

Muscular Dystrophy

The condition commonly known as muscular dystrophy (DIS-troh-fee) is properly referred to as muscular dystrophies. This general term describes a group of more than 30 genetic diseases that are characterized by progressive weakness and degeneration of the skeletal muscles that control movement, without affecting the nervous system. There is no specific treatment to stop or reverse any form of muscular dystrophy. Three of the most common forms are described below.
- Duchenne muscular dystrophy (DMD) is the most common form of muscular dystrophy. This condition affects primarily boys with onset between the ages of 3 and 5 years. The disorder progresses rapidly so that most of these boys are unable to walk by age 12 and later need a respirator to breathe.
- Becker muscular dystrophy (BMD) is very similar to, but less severe than, Duchenne muscular dystrophy.

Repetitive Stress Disorders

Repetitive stress disorders, also known as repetitive motion disorders, are a variety of muscular conditions that result from repeated motions performed in the course of normal work, daily activities, or recreation such as sports. The symptoms caused by these frequently repeated motions involve muscles, tendons, nerves, and joints.

- Compartment syndrome involves the compression of nerves and blood vessels due to swelling within the enclosed space created by the fascia that separates groups of muscles. This syndrome can be caused by trauma, tight bandages or casts, or by repetitive activities such as running.
- Overuse injuries are minor tissue injuries that have not been given time to heal. Such injuries can be caused by spending hours at the computer keyboard or by lengthy sports training sessions.
- Overuse tendinitis (ten-dih-NIGH-tis), also known as overuse tendinosis, is inflammation of tendons caused by excessive or unusual use of a joint (tendin- means tendon, and -itis means inflammation).
- Stress fractures, which are also overuse injuries.

Myofascial Pain Syndrome

Myofascial pain syndrome is a chronic pain disorder that affects muscles and fascia throughout the body. This condition, which is caused by the development of trigger points, produces local and referred muscle pain. Trigger points are tender areas that most commonly develop where the fascia comes into contact with a muscle. Referred pain describes pain that originates in one area of the body, but felt in another.

Rotator Cuff Injuries

- Impingement syndrome (im-PINJ-ment) occurs when inflamed and swollen tendons are caught in the narrow space between the bones within the shoulder joint. A common sign of impingement syndrome is discomfort when raising your arm above your head.
- Rotator cuff tendinitis (ten-dih-NIGH-tis) is an inflammation of the tendons of the rotator cuff. This condition is often named for the cause, such as tennis shoulder or pitcher's shoulder.
- A ruptured rotator cuff develops when rotator cuff tendinitis is left untreated or if the overuse continues. This occurs as the irritated tendon weakens and tears.

Carpal Tunnel Syndrome

The carpal tunnel is a narrow, bony passage under the carpal ligament that is located one-fourth of an inch below the inner surface of the wrist. Carpal means pertaining to the wrist. The median nerve, and the tendons that bend the fingers, pass through this tunnel. Carpal tunnel syndrome symptoms occur when the tendons that pass through the carpal tunnel are chronically overused and become inflamed and swollen.

- This swelling creates pressure on the median nerve as it passes through the carpal tunnel.
- This pressure causes pain, burning, and paresthesia in the thumb, index finger, and middle finger. The ring finger and little finger are not affected because these fingers are innervated by a different nerve.

Paresthesia is an abnormal sensation such as burning, tingling, or numbness.
- Carpal tunnel release is the surgical enlargement of the carpal tunnel or cutting of the carpal ligament to relieve nerve pressure. This treatment is used to relieve the pressure on tendons and nerves in severe cases of carpal tunnel syndrome.

Ganglion Cyst

A ganglion cyst (GANG-glee-on SIST) is a harmless fluidfilled swelling that occurs most commonly on the outer surface of the wrist. This condition, which can be caused by repeated minor injuries, is usually painless and does not require treatment. (Do not confuse this use of the term ganglion here with the nerve ganglions.

Epicondylitis

Epicondylitis (ep-ih-kon-dih-LYE-tis) is inflammation of the tissues surrounding the elbow (epi- means on, condyl means condyle, and -itis means inflammation).
- Lateral epicondylitis, also known as tennis elbow, is characterized by pain on the outer side of the forearm.
- Medial epicondylitis, also known as golfer's elbow, is characterized by pain on the palm-side of the forearm.

Ankle and Foot Problems
- A heel spur is a calcium deposit in the plantar fascia near its attachment to the calcaneus (heel) bone that can be one of the causes of plantar fasciitis.
- Plantar fasciitis (PLAN-tar fas-ee-EYE-tis) is an inflammation of the plantar fascia on the sole of the foot. This condition causes foot or heel pain when walking or running.

Sports Injuries

The following injuries are frequently associated with sports overuse; however, some may also be caused by other forms of trauma.
- A sprain is an injury to a joint, such as ankle, knee, or wrist that usually involves a stretched or torn ligament.
- A strain is an injury to the body of the muscle or to the attachment of a tendon. Strains usually are associated with overuse injuries that involve a stretched or torn muscle or tendon attachment.
- A shin splint is a painful condition caused by the muscle tearing away from the tibia (shin bone). Shin splints can develop in the anterolateral (front and side) muscles or in the posteromedial (back and middle) muscles of the lower leg. This type of injury is usually caused by repeated stress to the lower leg, such as running on hard surfaces.
- A hamstring injury can be a strain or tear on any of the three hamstring muscles that straighten the hip and bend the knee. When these muscles

contract too quickly, an injury can occur that is characterized by sudden and severe pain in the back of the thigh.
- Achilles tendinitis (ten-dih-NIGH-tis) is a painful inflammation of the Achilles tendon caused by excessive stress being placed on that tendon.

Spinal Cord Injuries

The spinal cord is surrounded and protected by the bony vertebrae. This protection is essential because the spinal cord is soft, with the consistency of toothpaste.
- The type of paralysis caused by a spinal cord injury (SCI) is determined by the level of the vertebra closest to the injury. The higher on the spinal cord the injury occurs, the greater the area of the body that may be affected.
- An injury occurs when a vertebra is broken and a piece of the broken bone is pressing into the spinal cord. The cord can also be injured if the vertebrae are pushed or pulled out of alignment.
- When the spinal cord is injured, the ability of the brain to communicate with the body below the level of the injury may be reduced or lost altogether. When that happens, the affected parts of the body will not function normally.
- An incomplete injury means that the person has some function below the level of the injury, even though that function isn't normal.
- A complete injury means that there is complete loss of sensation and muscle control below the level of the injury; however, a complete injury does not mean that there is no hope of any improvement.

Types of Paralysis

Paralysis (pah-RAL-ih-sis) is the loss of sensation and voluntary muscle movements in a muscle through disease or injury to its nerve supply. Damage can be either temporary or permanent (plural, paralyses).
- Myoparesis (my-oh-PAR-eh-sis) is a weakness or slight muscular paralysis (my/o means muscle, and -paresis means partial or incomplete paralysis).
- Hemiparesis (hem-ee-pah-REE-sis) is slight paralysis or weakness affecting one side of the body (hemimeans half, and -paresis means partial or incomplete paralysis). Contrast hemiparesis with hemiplegia.
- Hemiplegia (hem-ee-PLEE-jee-ah) is total paralysis affecting only one side of the body (hemi- means half, and -plegia means paralysis). This form of paralysis is usually associated with a stroke or brain damage. Damage to one side of the brain causes paralysis on the opposite side of the body. An individual affected with hemiplegia is known as a hemiplegic. Contrast with hemiparesis.
- Paraplegia (par-ah-PLEE-jee-ah) is the paralysis of both legs and the lower part of the body. An individual affected with paraplegia is known as a paraplegic.

- quadriplegia (kwad-rih-PLEE-jee-ah) is paralysis of all four extremities (quadr/i means four, and -plegia means paralysis). An individual affected with quadriplegia is known as a quadriplegic.
- Cardioplegia (kar-dee-oh-PLEE-jee-ah), also known as cardiac arrest, is paralysis of heart muscle (cardi/o means heart, and -plegia means paralysis). This can be caused by a direct blow or trauma. Temporary stopping of cardiac activity can be induced by using drugs.

Diagnostic Procedures Of The Muscular System

- Deep tendon reflexes (DTR) are tested with a reflex hammer that is used to strike a tendon. A reflex is an involuntary response to a stimulus. No response, or an abnormal response, can indicate a disruption of the nerve supply to the involved muscles. Reflexes also are lost in deep coma or because of medication such as heavy sedation.
- Range of motion testing (ROM) is a diagnostic procedure to evaluate joint mobility and muscle strength. Range of motion exercises are used to increase strength, flexibility, and mobility.
- Electromyography (ee-leck-troh-my-OG-rah-fee) is a diagnostic test that measures the electrical activity within muscle fibers in response to nerve stimulation (electr/o means electricity, my/o means muscle, and -graphy means the process of producing a picture or record). The resulting record is called an electromyogram. Electromyography is most frequently used when people have symptoms of weakness, and examination shows impaired muscle strength.
- Electroneuromyography (ee-leck-troh-new-roh-my- OG-rah-fee), also known as nerve conduction studies, is a diagnostic procedure for testing and recording neuromuscular activity by the electric stimulation of the nerve trunk that carries fibers to and from the muscle (electr/o means electricity, neur/o means nerve, my/o means muscle, and -graphy means the process of producing a picture or record). The primary goal of this examination is to determine the site of a nerve lesion or of muscle pathology.

Treatment Procedures Of The Muscular System

Medications

- An antispasmodic, also known as an anticholingeric, is administered to suppress smooth muscle contractions of the stomach, intestine, or bladder. For example, atropine is an antispasmodic that can be administered preoperatively to relax smooth muscles during surgery.
- A skeletal muscle relaxant is administered to relax certain muscles and to relieve the stiffness, pain, and discomfort caused by strains, sprains, or other muscle injuries. These medications act on the central nervous system and may have a negative interaction with alcohol and some antidepressants.

- A neuromuscular blocker, also known as a neuromuscular blocking agent, is a drug that causes temporary paralysis by blocking the transmission of nerve stimuli to the muscles. These drugs are used as an adjunct to anesthesia during surgery to cause skeletal muscles to relax. As used here, adjunct means in addition to.

Ergonomics

- Ergonomics (er-goh-NOM-icks) is the study of the human factors that affect the design and operation of tools and the work environment. This term is usually applied to the design of equipment and workspaces, with the goal of reducing injuries, strain and stress.

Occupational and Physical Therapy

Occupational therapy consists of activities to promote recovery and rehabilitation to assist patients in normalizing their ability to perform the activities of daily living (ADL). These activities include bathing, grooming, brushing teeth, eating, and dressing. Physical therapy is treatment to prevent disability or to restore functioning through the use of exercise, heat, massage, and other methods to improve circulation, flexibility, and muscle strength.

- Myofascial release is a specialized soft tissue manipulation technique used to ease the pain of conditions such as fibromyalgia, myofascial pain syndrome, movement restrictions, temporomandibular joint disorders (TMJ), and carpal tunnel syndrome.
- Therapeutic ultrasound utilizes high-frequency sound waves to treat muscle injuries by generating heat deep within muscle tissue. This heat eases pain, reduces muscle spasms, and accelerates healing by increasing the flow of blood into the target tissues.

Rice

The most common first aid treatment of muscular injuries is known by the acronym RICE. These letters stand for Rest, Ice, Compression, and Elevation. Rest and ice are recommended for the first few days after the injury to ease pain. Compression, such as wrapping with a stretch bandage, and elevation help to minimize swelling. After the first few days, as the pain decreases, using heat, accompanied by stretching and light exercises, helps to bring blood to the injured area to speed healing.

Fascia

- A fasciotomy (fash-ee-OT-oh-mee) is a surgical incision through the fascia to relieve tension or pressure (fasci means fascia, and -otomy means a surgical incision). Without this procedure, the pressure causes a loss of circulation that damages the affected tissues.
- Fascioplasty (FASH-ee-oh-plas-tee) is the surgical repair of fascia (fasci/o means fascia, and -plasty means surgical repair).

Tendons

- Tenodesis (ten-ODD-eh-sis) is the surgical suturing of the end of a tendon to a bone (ten/o means tendon, and -desis means to bind or tie together). Tenodesis is the opposite of tenolysis.
- Tenolysis (ten-OL-ih-sis), also known as tendolysis, is the release of a tendon from adhesions (ten/o means tendon, and -lysis means to set free). Tenolysis is the opposite of tenodesis.
- A tenectomy (teh-NECK-toh-mee), also known as a tenonectomy, is the surgical resection of a portion of a tendon or tendon sheath (ten means tendon, and -ectomy means surgical removal). The term resection describes the removal of tissue or part or all of an organ by surgery.
- Tenoplasty (TEN-oh-plas-tee), also known as tendinoplasty, is the surgical repair of a tendon (ten/o means tendon, and -plasty means surgical repair).
- Tenorrhaphy (ten-OR-ah-fee) is surgical suturing together of the divided ends of a tendon (ten/o means tendon, and -rrhaphy means surgical suturing).
- A tenotomy (teh-NOT-oh-mee), also known as a tendotomy, is the surgical division of a tendon for relief of a deformity caused by the abnormal shortening of a muscle, such as strabismus (ten means tendon, and -otomy means surgical incision).

Muscles

- A myectomy (my-ECK-toh-mee) is the surgical excision of a portion of a muscle (my means muscle, and -ectomy means surgical removal). Excision means cutting out or removal.
- Myoplasty (MY-oh-plas-tee) is the surgical repair of a muscle (my/o means muscle, and -plasty means surgical repair).
- Myorrhaphy (my-OR-ah-fee) is the surgical suturing a muscle wound (my/o means muscle, and -rrhaphy means surgical suturing).
- A myotomy (my-OT-oh-mee) is a surgical incision into a muscle (my means muscle, and -otomy means surgical incision).

Abbreviations Related To The Muscular System

- carpal tunnel syndrome = CTS
- electromyography = EMG
- fibromyalgia syndrome = FMS
- hemiplegia = hemi
- impingement syndrome = IS
- intermittent claudication = IC
- muscular dystrophy = MD
- myasthenia gravis = MG
- polymyositis = PM
- quadriplegia, quadriplegic = quad

- repetitive stress disorder = RSD

Note: To avoid errors or confusion, always be cautious when using abbreviations.

Critical Thinking Exercise

The following story and questions are designed to stimulate critical thinking through class discussion or as a brief essay response. There are no right or wrong answers to these questions.

"Leg muscles save back muscles ... Mandatory OSHA meeting Tuesday at noon. Bring lunch," states the company memo. Sandor Padilla, a 28-year-old cargo loader, sighs. "Third meeting this year and its not even June yet!" He has only 2 minutes to reach the tarmac. "Oh well, cargo waits for no man," he thinks as he jogs off to work.

Sandor enjoys his job. It keeps him fit, but lets his mind follow more creative avenues. Today, his thoughts stray to his daughter Reina's fifth birthday party, just 2 weeks away. "A pony or a clown?

Hot dogs or tacos?" he muses. Single parenting has its moments. As he is busy thinking of other

things, the heavy crate slips, driving him into a squatting position that injures his thigh muscles. His cry of pain brings Janet Wilson, his supervisor, running to help. The first aid station ices his leg to reduce swelling and pain. After the supervisor completes the

incident report, Sandor is taken to the emergency room. Dr. Basra, the orthopedic specialist on call, diagnoses myorrhexis of the left rectus femoris. A myorrhaphy is required to treat this injury. After several days in the hospital, Sandor is sent home with a Vicodin prescription for pain and orders for physical therapy sessions three times a week. He is not expected to return to work for at least 90 days.

AirFreight Systems receives the first report of injury and compares it with the supervisor's incident report. Ruling: Safety Violation. No Liability. Return to work in 30 days or dismissal.

Suggested Discussion Topics

1. On what basis do you think AirFreight determined that this was a safety violation? Use lay terms to explain Sandor's injury and the treatment that was required.
2. He attends the meetings; however on the day of the accident, he was busy thinking about his daughter's birthday party and not about his work. Could the responsibility for this accident be considered negligence on Sandor's part? Do you think Sandor should be held responsible, or blameless, is in this situation? If you think he was responsible, what did he do wrong?
3. It was determined that AirFreight was not responsible for the accident. Therefore do you think the company can take away Sandor's job if he does not return in 30 calendar days?

Scott J. Barnard

CHAPTER 5

THE CARDIOVASCULAR SYSTEM

This list contains essential word parts and medical terms for this chapter.

Word Parts
- angi/o
- aort/o
- arteri/o
- ather/o
- bradyh cardi/o
- -crasia
- -emia
- erythr/o
- hem/o, hemat/o
- leuk/o
- phleb/o
- tachyh thromb/o
- ven/o

Medical Terms
- ACE inhibitor
- anemia (ah-NEE-mee-ah)
- aneurysm (AN-you-rizm)
- angina (an-JIH-nuh)
- angioplasty (AN-jee-oh-plas-tee)
- anticoagulant (an-tih-koh-AG-you-lant)
- aplastic anemia (ay-PLAS-tick ah-NEE-mee-ah)
- arrhythmia (ah-RITH-mee-ah)
- atherectomy (ath-er-ECK-toh-mee)
- atheroma (ath-er-OH-mah)
- atherosclerosis (ath-er-oh-skleh-ROH-sis)
- atrial fibrillation
- automatedexternal defibrillator (dee-fih-brih-LAY-ter)
- beta-blocker

- blood dyscrasia (dis-KRAY-zee-ah)
- bradycardia (brad-ee-KAR-dee-ah)
- cardiac arrest
- cardiac catheterization (KAR-dee-ack kath-eh-tereye- ZAY-shun)
- cardiomyopathy (kar-dee-oh-my-OP-pah-thee)
- carotid endarterectomy (kah-ROT-id end-ar-ter- ECK-toh-mee)
- cholesterol (koh-LES-ter-ol)
- chronic venous insufficiency
- coronary thrombosis (KOR-uh-nerr-ee throm- BOH-sis)
- defibrillation (dee-fih-brih-LAY-shun)
- diuretic (dye-you-RET-ick)
- electrocardiogram (ee-leck-troh-KAR-dee-oh-gram)
- embolism (EM-boh-lizm)
- embolus (EM-boh-lus)
- endocarditis (en-doh-kar-DYE-tis)
- erythrocytes (eh-RITH-roh-sights)
- hemoglobin (hee-moh-GLOH-bin)
- hemolytic anemia (hee-moh-LIT-ick ah-NEE-mee-ah)
- hemostasis (hee-moh-STAY-sis)
- ischemic heart disease (iss-KEE-mick)
- leukemia (loo-KEE-mee-ah)
- leukocytes (LOO-koh-sites)
- leukopenia (loo-koh-PEE-nee-ah)
- megaloblastic anemia (MEG-ah-loh-blas-tick ah- NEE-mee-ah)
- myelodysplastic syndrome (my-eh-loh-dis-PLAStick SIN-drohm)
- myocardial infarction (my-oh-KAR-dee-al in- FARK-shun)
- orthostatic hypotension (or-thoh-STAT-ick highpoh- TEN-shun)
- paroxysmal atrial tachycardia (par-ock-SIZ-mal tack-ee-KAR-dee-ah)
- pericardium (pehr-ih-KAR-dee-um)
- pernicious anemia (per-NISH-us ah-NEE-mee-ah)
- phlebitis (fleh-BYE-tis)
- Raynaud's phenomenon (ray-NOHZ)
- septicemia (sep-tih-SEE-mee-ah)
- sickle cell anemia
- tachycardia (tack-ee-KAR-dee-ah)
- thallium stress test (THAL-ee-um)
- thrombocytopenia (throm-boh-sigh-toh-PEE-nee-ah)
- thrombolytic (throm-boh-LIT-ick)
- thrombosis (throm-BOH-sis)
- thrombotic occlusion (throm-BOT-ick ah-KLOOzhun)
- thrombus (THROM-bus)
- transfusion reaction
- valvulitis (val-view-LYE-tis)
- varicose veins (VAR-ih-kohs VAYNS)

- ventricular fibrillation (ven-TRICK-you-ler fihbrih- LAY-shun)
- ventricular tachycardia (ven-TRICK-you-ler tackee-KAR-dee-ah)

Objectives

On completion of this chapter, you should be able to:
1. Describe the heart in terms of chambers, valves, blood flow, heartbeat, and blood supply.
2. 2. Differentiate among the three different types of blood vessels and describe the major function of each.
3. Identify the major components of blood and the major functions of each component.
4. State the difference between pulmonary and systemic circulation.
5. Recognize, define, spell, and pronounce the terms related to the pathology and the diagnostic and treatment procedures of the cardiovascular system.

Functions Of The Cardiovascular System

The cardiovascularsystem consists of the heart, blood vessels, and blood. The term cardiovascular means pertaining to the heart and blood vessels (cardi/o means heart, vascul means blood vessels, and -ar means pertaining to). These structures work together to efficiently pump blood to all body tissues.
- Blood is a fluid tissue that transports oxygen and nutrients to the other body tissues.
- Blood returns some waste products from these tissues to the kidneys and carries carbon dioxide back to the lungs.
- Blood cells also play important roles in the immune system.

Structures Of The Cardiovascular System

The major structures of the cardiovascular system are the heart, blood vessels, and blood.

The Heart

The heart is a hollow, muscular organ located between the lungs. It is a very effective pump that furnishes the power to maintain the blood flow needed throughout the entire body. The pointed lower end of the heart is known as the apex.

The Pericardium

The pericardium (pehr-ih-KAR-dee-um), also known as the pericardial sac, is the double-walledmembranous sac that encloses the heart (peri- means surrounding, cardi means heart, and -um is a singular noun ending). Membranous means pertaining to membrane, which is a thin layer of pliable tissue that covers or encloses a body part.
- The parietal pericardium is the tough outer layer that forms a fibrous sac that surrounds and protects the heart.

- The visceral pericardium, which is the inner layer of the pericardium, also forms the outer layer of the heart. When referred to as the outer layer of the heart, it is known as the epicardium.
- Pericardial fluid is found between these two layers, where it acts as a lubricant to prevent friction when the heart beats.

The Walls of the Heart

The walls of the heart are made up of three layers: the epicardium, myocardium, and endocardium.
- The epicardium (ep-ih-KAR-dee-um) is the external layer of the heart and the inner layer of the pericardium (epi- means upon, cardi means heart, and -um is a singular noun ending).
- The myocardium (my-oh-KAR-dee-um), also known as myocardial muscle, is the middle and thickest of the heart's three layers and consists of specialized cardiac muscle tissue (my/o means muscle, cardi means heart, and -um is a singular noun ending). The constant contraction and relaxation of this muscle creates the pumping movement that maintains the flow of blood throughout the body.
- The endocardium (en-doh-KAR-dee-um), which consists of epithelial tissue, is the inner lining of the heart (endo- means within, cardi means heart, and - um is a singular noun ending). This surface comes into direct contact with the blood as it is being pumped through the heart.

Blood Supply to the Myocardium

The myocardium, which beats constantly, must have a continuous supply of oxygen and nutrients plus prompt waste removal in order to survive. If for any reason this blood supply is disrupted, the myocardiumin the affected area dies. The coronary arteries (KOR-uh-nerr-ee), which supply oxygen-rich blood to the myocardium. The veins, which are shown here in blue, remove waste products from the myocardium.

The Chambers of the Heart

The heart is divided into left and right sides. Each side is subdivided to form the four chambers of the heart.
- The atria (AY-tree-ah) are the two upper chambers of the heart. They are the receiving chambers, and all blood vessels coming into the heart enter here (singular, atrium).
- The atria are separated by the interatrial septum. A septum is a wall that separates two chambers.
- The ventricles (VEN-trih-kuhls) are the two lower chambers of the heart. They are the pumping chambers, and all blood vessels leaving the heart emerge from the ventricles. A ventricle is defined as a normal hollow chamber of the heart or the brain.

- The ventricles of the heart, which are separated by the interventricular septum, are the pumping chambers (inter- means between, ventricul means ventricle, and -ar means pertaining to). The walls of the ventricles are thicker than those of the atria because the ventricles must pump blood throughout the body.

The Valves of the Heart

The flow of blood through the heart is controlled by four valves: the tricuspid, pulmonary semilunar, mitral, and aortic semilunar valves. If any of these valves is not working correctly, blood does not flow properly through the heart and cannot be pumped effectively to all parts of the body.
- The tricuspid valve (try-KUS-pid) controls the opening between the right atrium and the right ventricle. Tricuspid means having three cusps (points), which describes the shape of this valve.
- The pulmonary semilunar valve (sem-ee-LOO-nar) is located between the right ventricle and the pulmonary artery. Pulmonary means pertaining to the lungs, and semilunar means half-moon; this valve is shaped like a half-moon.
- The mitral valve (MY-tral), also known as the bicuspid valve, is located between the left atrium and left ventricle. Mitral means shaped like a bishop's miter (hat). Bicuspid means having two cusps (points), which describes the shape of this valve.
- The aortic semilunar valve (ay-OR-tick sem-ee-LOOnar) is located between the left ventricle and the aorta. Aortic means pertaining to the aorta, and semilunar means half-moon.

Systemic and Pulmonary Circulation

Blood is pumped through the systemic and pulmonary circulation systems. Together these systems allow blood to bring oxygen to the cells and to remove waste products.

Pulmonary Circulation

Pulmonary circulation is the flow of blood only between
the heart and lungs.
- The pulmonary arteries carry deoxygenated blood out of the right ventricle and into the lungs. This is the only place in the body where deoxygenated blood is carried by arteries instead of veins.
- In the lungs, carbon dioxide from the body is exchanged for oxygen from the inhaled air.
- The pulmonary veins carry the oxygenated blood from the lungs into the left atrium of the heart. This is the only place in the body where veins carry oxygenated blood.

Systemic Circulation

Systemic circulation includes the flow of blood to all parts of the body except the lungs.
- Oxygenated blood flows out of the left ventricle and into arterial circulation.
- The veins carry deoxygenated blood into the right atrium.
- From here, the blood flows into the pulmonary circulation before being pumped out of the heart into the arteries again.

The Sinoatrial Node

- The sinoatrial node (sigh-noh-AY-tree-ahl), which is often referred to as the SA node, is located in the posterior wall of the right atrium near the entrance of the superior vena cava.
- The SA node establishes the basic rhythm and rate of the heartbeat. For this reason, it is known as the natural pacemaker of the heart.
- Electrical impulses from the SA node start each wave of muscle contraction in the heart.
- The impulse in the right atrium spreads over the muscles of both atria, causing them to contract simultaneously. This contraction forces blood into the ventricles.

The Atrioventricular Node

- The impulses from the SA node also travel to the atrioventricular node (ay-tree-oh-ven-TRICK-youlahr), which is also known as the AV node.
- The AV node is located on the floor of the right atrium near the interatrial septum. From here, it transmits the electrical impulses onward to the bundle of His.

The Bundle of His

- The bundle of His (HISS) is a group of fibers located within the interventricular septum. These fibers carry an electrical impulse to ensure the sequence of the heart contractions. These electrical impulses travel onward to the right and left ventricles and the Purkinje fibers.
- Purkinje fibers (per-KIN-jee) are specialized conductive fibers located within the walls of the ventricles. These fibers relay the electrical impulses to the cells of the ventricles, and it is this stimulation that causes the ventricles to contract. This contraction of the ventricles forces blood out of the heart and into the aorta and pulmonary arteries.

Electrical Waves

The activities of the electrical conduction system of the heart can be visualized as wave movements on a monitor or an electrocardiogram. The P wave is due to the stimulation (contraction) of the atria. The qRS complex shows the stimulation (contraction) of the ventricles. The atria relax as the ventricles contract.

The Blood Vessels

There are three major types of blood vessels: arteries, capillaries, and veins. These vessels form the arterial and venous circulatory systems.

Arteries

- The arteries are large blood vessels that carry blood away from the heart to all regions of the body.
- The walls of the arteries are composed of three layers. This structure makes them muscular and elastic so they can expand and contract with the pumping beat of the heart. The term endarterial means pertaining to the inner portion of an artery or within an artery.
- Arterial blood is bright red in color because it is oxygen-rich. It is the pumping action of the heart that causes blood to spurt out when an artery is cut.
- The aorta (ay-OR-tah), which is the largest blood vessel in the body, is the main trunk of the arterial system and begins from the left ventricle of the heart.
- The carotid arteries (kah-ROT-id) are the major arteries that carry blood upward to the head. The common carotid located on each side of the neck divides into the internal carotid, which brings oxygen-rich blood to the brain, and the external carotid, which brings blood to the face. Any disruption in this flow of blood can result in a stroke or other brain damage.
- The arterioles (ar-TEE-ree-ohlz) are the smaller, thinner branches of arteries that carry blood to the capillaries.

Veins

Veins form a low-pressure collecting system to return oxygen-poor blood to the heart.

- The walls of the veins are thinner and less elastic than those of the arteries.
- Veins have valves that enable blood to flow only toward the heart and prevent it from flowing away from the heart.
- Venules (VEN-youls) are smallest veins that join to form the larger veins.
- Superficial veins are located near the body surface. Deep veins are located within the tissues and away from the body surface.

The Venae Cavae

- The venae cavae (VEE-nee KAY-vee) are the two largest veins in the body. These are the veins that return blood into the heart (singular, vena cava).
- The superior vena cava transports blood from the upper portion of the body to the heart.
- The inferior vena cava transports blood from the lower portion of the body to the heart.

Capillaries

Capillaries, which are only one epithelial cell in thickness, are the smallest blood vessels in the body. The capillaries form networks of expanded vascular beds that have the important role of delivering oxygen and nutrients to the cells of the tissues. Vascular means pertaining to blood vessels.
- Arterioles deliver blood to the capillaries. Here the rate of flow of arterial blood slows as it enters one end of the bed.
- The capillaries further slow the flow of blood to allow plasma to flow into the tissues for the exchange of oxygen, nutrients, and waste materials with the surrounding cells.
- Ninety percent of this fluid, which is now oxygen-poor, leaves the opposite end of the capillary bed through the venules, and it continues to flow as venous blood that increases in speed as it begins its return journey to the heart. The remaining 10% of this fluid is left behind in the tissues and becomes lymph.

Pulse and Blood Pressure
- The pulse is the rhythmic pressure against the walls of an artery caused by the contraction of the heart.
- Blood pressure is the measurement of the amount of systolic and diastolic pressure exerted against the walls of the arteries.
- Systolic pressure (sis-TOL-ick), which occurs when the ventricles contract, is the highest pressure against the walls of an artery. The term systole means contraction of the heart, and systolic means pertaining to this contraction phase.
- Diastolic pressure (dye-ah-STOL-ick), which occurs when the ventricles are relaxed, is the lowest pressure against the walls of an artery. The term diastole means relaxation of the heart, and diastolic means pertaining to this relaxation phase.

Blood

Blood is the fluid tissue in the body. It is composed of 55% liquid plasma and 45% formed elements.

Plasma

Plasma (PLAZ-mah) is a straw-colored fluid that contains nutrients, hormones, and waste products. Plasma is 91% water. The remaining 9% consists mainly of proteins, including the clotting proteins.
- Fibrinogen (figh-BRIN-oh-jen) and prothrombin (proh-THROM-bin) are the clotting proteins found in plasma. They have an important role in clot formation to control bleeding.
- Serum (SEER-um) is plasma fluid after the blood cells and the clotting proteins have been removed.

Formed Elements of the Blood

The formed elements of the blood include the erythrocytes, leukocytes, and thrombocytes.

Erythrocytes

Erythrocytes (eh-RITH-roh-sights), also known as red blood cells (RBC), are mature red blood cells produced by the red bone marrow (erythr/o means red, and -cytes means cells). The primary role of these cells is to transport oxygen to the tissues. This oxygen is transported by the hemoglobin (hee-moh-GLOH-bin), which is the iron-containing pigment of the erythrocytes.

Leukocytes

Leukocytes (LOO-koh-sites), also known as white blood cells (WBC), are the blood cells involved in defending the body against infective organisms and foreign substances (leuk/o means white, and -cytes means cells). The following are the major groups of leukocytes:

- Neutrophils (NEW-troh-fills), which are formed in red bone marrow, are the most common type of WBC. Through phagocytosis, neutrophils play a major role in the immune system's defense against pathogens including bacteria, viruses, and fungi. Phagocytosis is the process of destroying pathogens by surrounding and swallowing them.
- Basophils (BAY-soh-fills), which are formed in red bone marrow, are the least common type of WBC. Basophils are responsible for the symptoms of allergies.
- Eosinophils (ee-oh-SIN-oh-fills) are formed in red bone marrow and then migrate to tissues throughout the body. Eosinophils destroy parasitic organisms and play a major role in allergic reactions.
- Lymphocytes (LIM-foh-sights) are formed in red bone marrow, lymph nodes, and the spleen (lymph/o means lymph, and -cytes means cells). Lymphocytes identify foreign substances and germs (bacteria or viruses) in the body and produce antibodies that specifically target them. Lymphocytes are discussed further in Chapter 6.
- Monocytes (MON-oh-sights) are formed in red bone marrow, lymph nodes, and the spleen. Through phagocytosis, monocytes provide immunological defenses against many infectious organisms.

Thrombocytes

- Thrombocytes (THROM-boh-sights), also known as platelets, are the smallest formed elements of the blood (thromb/o means clot, and -cytes means cells). The thrombocytes play an important role in the clotting of blood.
- When a blood vessel is damaged, the thrombocytes are activated and become sticky.
- This action causes the thrombocytes to clump together to form a clot that stops the bleeding.

Blood Types

Blood types are classified according to the presence, or absence, of certain antigens. An antigen is any substance that the body regards as being foreign. The four major blood types are A, AB, B, and O. The A, AB, and B groups are based on the presence of the A and/or B antigens on the red blood cells. In type O blood, both antigens are absent.

The Rh Factor

The Rh factor refers to the presence, or absence of the Rh antigen on red blood cells. Because this antigen was first found in Rhesus monkeys, this factor was named for them.
- About 85% of Americans are Rh positive (Rh+). This means that these individuals have the Rh antigen.
- The remaining 15% are Rh negative (Rh−). This means that these individuals do not have the Rh antigen.
- The Rh factor is an important consideration in crossmatching blood for transfusions.
- The Rh factor can cause difficulties when an Rhpositive infant is born to an Rh-negative mother.

Blood Gases

Blood gases are gases that are normally dissolved in the liquid portion of blood. The major blood gases are oxygen (O2), carbon dioxide (CO2), and nitrogen (N2).

MEDICAL SPECIALTIES RELATED TO THE CARDIOVASCULAR SYSTEM
- A cardiologist (kar-dee-OL-oh-jist) is a physician who specializes in diagnosing and treating abnormalities, diseases, and disorders of the heart (cardi means heart, and -ologist means specialist).
- A hematologist (hee-mah-TOL-oh-jist) is a physician who specializes in diagnosing and treating abnormalities, diseases, and disorders of the blood and bloodforming tissues (hemat means blood, and -ologist means specialist).
- A vascular surgeon is a physician who specializes in the diagnosis, medical management, and surgical treatment of disorders of the blood vessels.

Pathology Of The Cardiovascular System

Disorders of the heart can be present from before birth or develop at any time throughout life.

Congenital Heart Defects

Congenital heart defects are structural abnormalities caused by the failure of the heart to develop normally before birth.

Congenital means present at birth. Some congenital heart defects are apparent at birth, whereas others may not be detected until later in life.

Coronary Artery Disease

Coronary artery disease is atherosclerosis of the coronary arteries that reduces the blood supply to the heart muscle. This creates an insufficient supply of oxygen that can cause angina (pain), a myocardial infarction (heart attack), or death. End-stage coronary artery disease is characterized by unrelenting angina pain and a severely limited lifestyle.

Atherosclerosis

- Atherosclerosis (ath-er-oh-skleh-ROH-sis) is hardening and narrowing of the arteries caused by a buildup of cholesterol plaque on the interior walls of the arteries (ather/o means plaque or fatty substance, and -sclerosis means abnormal hardening).
- This type of plaque (PLACK), which is found within the lumen of an artery, is a fatty deposit that is similar to the buildup of rust inside a pipe. (This substance is not the same as dental plaque.)
- The plaque can protrude outward into the lumen of the vessel or protrude inward into the wall of the vessel. The lumen is the opening within these vessels through which the blood flows.
- An atheroma (ath-er-OH-mah), which is a characteristic of atherosclerosis, is a deposit of plaque on or within the arterial wall (ather means plaque, and -oma means tumor).

Ischemic Heart Disease

- Ischemic heart disease (iss-KEE-mick) is a group of cardiac disabilities resulting from an insufficient supply of oxygenated blood to the heart. These diseases are usually associated with coronary artery disease. Ischemic means pertaining to the disruption of the blood supply.
- Ischemia (iss-KEE-mee-ah) is a condition in which there is an insufficient oxygen supply due to a restricted blood flow by to a part of the body (isch means to hold back, and -emia means blood). For example, cardiac ischemia is the lack of blood flow and oxygen to the heart muscle.

Angina

- Angina (an-JIH-nuh), also known as angina pectoris, is a condition of episodes of severe chest pain due to inadequate blood flow to the myocardium. These episodes are due to ischemia of the heart muscle.

Myocardial Infarction

- A myocardial infarction (my-oh-KAR-dee-al in-FARKshun), also known as a heart attack, is the occlusion of one or more coronary arteries caused by plaque buildup. As used here, occlusion means total blockage.
- Infarction means a sudden insufficiency of blood. An infarct is a localized area of dead tissue caused by a lack of blood.

- This damage to the myocardium impairs the heart's ability to pump blood throughout the body.
- The most frequently recognized symptoms of a myocardial infarction include pain in the middle of the chest that may spread to the back, jaw, or left arm. Many individuals having a heart attack have mild symptoms or none at all.

Heart Failure

Heart failure, which is also referred to as congestive heart failure, occurs most commonly in the elderly. This is a chronic condition in which the heart is unable to pump out all of the blood that it receives. The decreased pumping action causes congestion. Congestion means a fluid buildup.
- Left-sided heart failure, which is also known as pulmonary edema, causes an accumulation of fluid in the lungs. This occurs because the left side of the heart is not efficiently pumping blood to and from the lungs.
- Right-sided heart failure causes fluid buildup beginning with the feet and legs. This swelling can also affect the liver, gastrointestinal tract, or arms. This occurs because the right side of the heart is not efficiently pumping blood to and from the rest of the body, with the exception of the lungs.
- Cardiomegaly (kar-dee-oh-MEG-ah-lee) is the abnormal enlargement of the heart that is frequently associated with heart failure when the heart enlarges in an effort to compensate for the loss of its pumping ability (cardi/o means heart, and -megaly means abnormal enlargement).

Carditis

Carditis (kar-DYE-tis) is an inflammation of the heart (card means heart, and -itis means inflammation). Note the spelling of carditis: In this term, the word root (combining form) card/o is used to avoid having a double i when it is joined with the suffix -itis.
- Endocarditis (en-doh-kar-DYE-tis) is an inflammation of the inner lining of the heart (endo- means within, card means heart, and -itis means inflammation).
- Bacterial endocarditis is an inflammation of the lining or valves of the heart caused by the presence of bacteria in the bloodstream. One cause of this condition is bleeding during dental surgery because it allows bacteria from the mouth to enter the bloodstream.
- Myocarditis (my-oh-kar-DYE-tis) is an inflammation of themyocardium(my/omeansmuscle, cardmeans heart, and -itis means inflammation). This uncommon condition can develop as a complication of a viral infection.
- Pericarditis (pehr-ih-kar-DYE-tis) is an inflammation of the pericardium that causes an accumulation of fluid within the pericardial sac (peri- means surrounding, card means heart, and -itis means inflammation).

This fluid restricts the beating of the heart and reduces the ability of the heart to pump blood throughout the body.

Diseases of the Myocardium

- Cardiomyopathy (kar-dee-oh-my-OP-pah-thee) is the term used to describe all diseases of the heart muscle (cardi/o means heart, my/o means muscle, and -pathy means disease).
- Dilated cardiomyopathy is a disease of the heart muscle that causes the heart to become enlarged, and to pump less strongly. The progression of this condition is usually slow and only presents with symptoms when quite advanced. Dilated means the expansion of a hollow structure.

Heart Valves

- A heart murmur is an abnormal sound heard when listening to the heart or neighboring large blood vessels. Heart murmurs are most often caused by defective heart valves.
- Valvulitis (val-view-LYE-tis) is an inflammation of a heart valve (valvul means valve, and -itis means inflammation).
- Valvular prolapse (VAL-voo-lar proh-LAPS) is the abnormal protrusion of a heart valve that results in the inability of the valve to close completely (valvul means valve, and -ar means pertaining to). Prolapse means the falling or dropping down of an organ or internal part. This condition is named for the affected valve, such as a mitral valve prolapse.
- Valvular stenosis (steh-NOH-sis) is a condition in which there is narrowing, stiffening, thickening, or blockage of one or more valves of the heart. Stenosis is the abnormal narrowing of an opening. These conditions are named for the affected valve, such as aortic valve stenosis.

Cardiac Arrest and Arrhythmias

Cardiac arrest is an event in which the heart abruptly stops or develops a very abnormal arrhythmia that prevents it from pumping blood. Sudden cardiac death results if treatment is not provided within a few minutes.

- The term arrhythmia (ah-RITH-mee-ah) describes an abnormality, or the loss of the normal rhythm, of the heartbeat.
- Bradycardia (brad-ee-KAR-dee-ah) is an abnormally slow resting heart rate (brady- means slow, card means heart, and -ia means abnormal condition). This term is usually applied to rates less than 60 beats per minute. Bradycardia is the opposite of tachycardia.
- Tachycardia (tack-ee-KAR-dee-ah) is an abnormally rapid resting heart rate (tachy- means rapid, card means heart, and -ia means abnormal condition). This term is usually applied to rates greater than 100 beats per minute. Tachycardia is the opposite of bradycardia.
- Palpitation (pal-pih-TAY-shun) is a pounding or racing heart with or without irregularity in rhythm. This is associated with certain heart

disorders; however, it also occur as part of a panic attack Atrial and Ventricular Fibrillation
- Atrial fibrillation, also known as A fib, occurs when the normal rhythmic contractions of the atria are replaced by rapid irregular twitching of the muscular heart wall. This condition causes an irregular and quivering action of the atria. The term fibrillation means a fast, uncontrolled heart beat.
- Paroxysmal atrial tachycardia (par-ock-SIZ-mal tack-ee-KAR-dee-ah), also known as PAT, is an episode that begins and ends abruptly during which there are very rapid and regular heartbeats that originate in the atrium. PAT is caused by an abnormality in the body's electrical system. Paroxysmal means pertaining to sudden occurrence. Compare with ventricular tachycardia.
- Ventricular fibrillation (ven-TRICK-you-ler fih-brih- LAY-shun), also known as V fib, is the rapid, irregular, and useless contractions of the ventricles. Instead of pumping strongly, the heart muscle quivers ineffectively. This condition is the cause of many sudden cardiac deaths.
- Ventricular tachycardia, also known as V tach, a very rapid heart beat that begins within the ventricles. This condition is potentially fatal because the heart is beating so rapidly that it is unable to adequately pump blood through the body. For some patients, this condition can be controlled with an implantable cardioverter defibrillator. Compare with paroxysmal atrial tachycardia.

Blood Vessels
- Angiitis (an-jee-EYE-tis), also known as vasculitis, is the inflammation of a blood or lymph vessel (angi means vessel, and -itis means inflammation). Note: This term is also spelled angitis.
- Angiostenosis (AN-jee-oh-steh-NOH-sis) is the abnormal narrowing of a blood vessel (angi/o means vessel, and -stenosis means abnormal narrowing).
- A hemangioma (hee-man-jee-OH-mah) is a benign tumor made up of newly formed blood vessels (hem means blood, angi means blood or lymph vessel, and -oma means tumor).
- Hypoperfusion(high-poh-per-FYOU-zhun) is a deficiency of blood passing through an organ or body part. Perfusion is the flow of blood through the vessels of an organ.
- Polyarteritis (pol-ee-ar-teh-RYE-tis), also known as polyarteritis nodosa, is a form of angiitis involving several medium and small arteries at the same time (poly- means many, arter means artery, and -itis mean inflammation). Polyarteritis is a serious blood vessel disease that occurs when certain immune cells attack the affected arteries.

Peripheral Vascular Disease

The term peripheral vascular disease refers to disorders of the blood vessels located outside the heart and brain. These disorders usually involve narrowing of the vessels that carry blood to the legs, arms, stomach, or kidneys.

- Peripheral arterial occlusive disease, also known as peripheral artery disease, is an example of a peripheral vascular disease caused by atherosclerosis. It is a common, and serious, problem affecting more than 20% of patients over 70 years of age. Impaired circulation to the extremities and vital organs causes changes in the skin color and temperature, plus intermittent claudication.
- Raynaud's phenomenon (ray-NOHZ) is a peripheral arterial occlusive disease in which intermittent attacks are triggered by cold or stress. The symptoms, which are due to constricted circulation, include pallor the fingers and toes.

Arteries

- An aneurysm (AN-you-rizm) is a localized weak spot, or balloon-like enlargement, of the wall of an artery. The rupture of an aneurysm can be fatal because of the rapid loss of blood. Aneurysms are named for the artery involved such as aortic aneurysms, abdominal aortic aneurysms, and popliteal aneurysms.
- Arteriosclerosis (ar-tee-ree-oh-skleh-ROH-sis), also known as hardening of the arteries, is any of a group of diseases characterized by thickening and the loss of elasticity of arterial walls (arteri/o means artery, and -sclerosis mean abnormal hardening).

Veins

- Chronic venous insufficiency, also known as venous insufficiency, is a condition in which venous circulation is inadequate due to partial vein blockage or leakage of venous valves. This condition primarily affects the feet and ankles, and the leakage of venous blood into the tissues causes discoloration of the skin.
- Phlebitis (fleh-BYE-tis) is the inflammation of a vein (phleb means vein, and -itis mean inflammation). This usually occurs in a superficial vein.
- Varicose veins (VAR-ih-kohs VAYNS) are abnormally swollen veins, usually occurring in the superficial veins of the legs. Varicose veins occur when the valves in the veins malfunction and allow blood to pool in these veins, causing them to enlarge.

Thromboses and Embolisms

Thromboses and embolisms are both serious conditions that can result in the blockage of a blood vessel.

Thrombosis

A thrombosis (throm-BOH-sis) is the abnormal condition of having a thrombus (thromb means clot, and -osis means abnormal condition or disease) (plural, thromboses).

- A thrombus (THROM-bus) is a blood clot attached to the interior wall of an artery or vein (thromb means clot, and -us is a singular noun ending) (plural, thrombi).
- A thrombotic occlusion (throm-BOT-ick ah-KLOOzhun) is the blocking of an artery by a thrombus. Thrombotic means caused by a thrombus. As used here, occlusion means blockage.
- A coronary thrombosis (KOR-uh-nerr-ee throm- BOH-sis) is damage to the heart muscle caused by a thrombus blocking a coronary artery (coron means crown, and -ary means pertaining to; thromb means clot, and -osis means abnormal condition).
- A deep vein thrombosis (DVT), also known as a deep venous thrombosis, is the condition of having a thrombus attached to the wall of a deep vein. Sometimes such a blockage forms in the legs of a bedridden patient or in someone who has remained seated too long on an airplane. The danger is that the thrombus will break loose and travel to a lung where it can be fatal.

Embolism

An embolism (EM-boh-lizm) is the sudden blockage of a blood vessel by an embolus (embol means something inserted, and -ism means condition). The embolism is often named for the causative factor, such as an air embolism or a fat embolism.

- An embolus (EM-boh-lus) is a foreign object, such as a blood clot, quantity of air or gas, or a bit of tissue or tumor that is circulating in the blood (embol means something inserted, and -us is a singular noun ending) (plural, emboli).

Blood Disorders

- Blood dyscrasia (dis-KRAY-zee-ah) is any pathologic condition of the cellular elements of the blood (dysmeans bad, and -crasia means a mixture or blending).
- Hemochromatosis (hee-moh-kroh-mah-TOH-sis), also known as iron overload disease, is a genetic disorder in which the intestines absorb too much iron (hem/o means blood, chromat means color, and -osis means abnormal condition or disease). The excess iron that is absorbed enters the bloodstream and accumulates in organs where it causes damage.
- The term leukopenia (loo-koh-PEE-nee-ah) describes any situation in which the total number of leukocytes in the circulating blood is less than normal (leuk/o means white, and -penia means deficiency). Since these cells combat infection, this condition can place patients at an increased of risk.

- Polycythemia (pol-ee-sy-THEE-mee-ah) is an abnormal increase in the number of red cells in the blood due to excess production of these cells by the bone marrow.
- Septicemia (sep-tih-SEE-mee-ah), formerly known as blood poisoning, is a systemic condition caused by the spread of microorganisms and their toxins via the circulating blood.
- Thrombocytopenia (throm-boh-sigh-toh-PEE-neeah) is a condition in which there is an abnormally small number of platelets circulating in the blood (thromb/o means thrombus, cyt/o means cell and -penia means deficiency). Because these cells help the blood to clot, this condition is sometimes associated with abnormal bleeding.
- Thrombocytosis (throm-boh-sigh-TOH-sis) is an abnormal increase in the number of platelets in the circulating blood (thromb/o means thrombus, cyt means cell, and -osis means abnormal condition).
- A hemorrhage (HEM-or-idj) is the loss of a large amount of blood in a short time. This term also means to bleed.
- A transfusion reaction is a serious, and potentially fatal, complication of a blood transfusion in which a severe immune response occurs because the patient's blood and the donated blood do not match.

Cholesterol

- Cholesterol (koh-LES-ter-ol) is a fatty substance that travels through the blood and is found in all parts of the body. It aids in the production of cell membranes, some hormones, and vitamin D. Some cholesterol comes from dietary sources, and some is created by the liver. Excessively high levels of certain types of cholesterol can lead to heart disease.
- Hyperlipidemia (high-per-lip-ih-DEE-mee-ah), also known as hyperlipemia, is the general term used to described elevated levels of cholesterol and other fatty substances in the blood (hyper- means excessive, lipid means fat, and -emia means blood condition).

Leukemia

- Myelodysplastic syndrome (my-eh-loh-dis-PLAStick), previously known as preleukemia, is a group of bone marrow disorders that are characterized by the insufficient production of one or more types of blood cells due to dysfunction of the bone marrow.
- Leukemia (loo-KEE-mee-ah) is a type of cancer characterized by a progressive increase in the number of abnormal leukocytes (white blood cells) found in blood forming tissues, other organs, and in the circulating blood (leuk means white, and -emia means blood condition).

Anemias

- Anemia (ah-NEE-mee-ah) is a lower than normal number of erythrocytes (red blood cells) in the blood (an- means without or less than, and -emia means blood condition). The severity of this condition is usually measured by a decrease in the amount of hemoglobin in the blood. When inadequate hemoglobin is present, all parts of the body receive less oxygen and have less energy than is needed to function properly.

- Aplastic anemia (ay-PLAS-tick ah-NEE-mee-ah) is characterized by an absence of all formed blood elements caused by the failure of blood cell production in the bone marrow (a- means without, plast means growth, and -ic means pertaining to). Anemia, a low red blood cell count, leads to fatigue and weakness. Leukopenia, a low white blood cell count, causes an increased risk of infection. Thrombocytopenia, a low platelet count, results in bleeding especially from mucus membranes and skin.
- Hemolytic anemia (hee-moh-LIT-ick ah-NEE-meeah) is a condition of an inadequate number of circulating red blood cells due to the premature destruction of red blood cells by the spleen (hem/o means relating to blood, and -lytic means to destroy). Hemolytic means pertaining to breaking down of red blood cells.
- Iron-deficiency anemia is the most common form of anemia. Iron, an essential component of hemoglobin, is normally obtained through food diet and by recycling iron from old red blood cells. Without sufficient iron to help create hemoglobin, blood cannot carry oxygen effectively.
- Megaloblastic anemia (MEG-ah-loh-blas-tick ah- NEE-mee-ah) is a blood disorder characterized by anemia in which the red blood cells are larger than normal. This condition usually results from a deficiency of folic acid or of vitamin B12.
- Pernicious anemia (per-NISH-us ah-NEE-mee-ah) is caused by a lack of the protein intrinsic factor (IF) that helps the body absorb vitamin B12 from the gastrointestinal tract. Vitamin B12 is necessary for the formation of red blood cells.
- Sickle cell anemia is a genetic disorder that causes abnormal hemoglobin, resulting in some red blood cells assuming an abnormal sickle shape. This sickle shape interferes with normal blood flow, resulting in damage to most of the body systems.
- Thalassemia (thal-ah-SEE-mee-ah) is an inherited blood disorder that causes mild or severe anemia due to reduced hemoglobin and fewer red blood cells than normal. Cooley's anemia is the name that is sometimes is used to refer to any type of thalassemia that requires treatment with regular blood transfusions.

Hypertension

Hypertension, commonly known as high blood pressure, is the elevation of arterial blood pressure to a level that is likely to cause damage to the cardiovascular system. Hypertension is the opposite of hypotension.

- Essential hypertension, also known as primary or idiopathic hypertension, is consistently elevated blood pressure of unknown cause. Idiopathic means a disease of unknown cause.

- Secondary hypertension is caused by a different medical problem, such as a kidney disorder or a tumor on the adrenal glands. When the other problem is cured, the secondary hypertension is usually resolved.
- Malignant hypertension is characterized by very high blood pressure. This condition, which can be fatal, is usually accompanied by damage to the organs, the brain, and optic nerves, or failure of the heart and kidneys.

Hypotension

- Hypotension (high-poh-TEN-shun) is lower than normal arterial blood pressure. Symptoms can include dizziness, lightheadedness, or fainting. Hypotension is the opposite of hypertension.
- Orthostatic hypotension (or-thoh-STAT-ick highpoh- TEN-shun), also known as postural hypotension, is low blood pressure that occurs upon standing up. Orthostatic means relating to an upright or standing position.

Diagnostic Procedures Of The Cardiovascular System

- Angiography (an-jee-OG-rah-fee) is a radiographic (x-ray) study of the blood vessels after the injection of a contrast medium (angi/o means blood vessel, and -graphy means the process of recording). The resulting film is an angiogram.
- Cardiac catheterization (KAR-dee-ack kath-eh-tereye- ZAY-shun) is a diagnostic procedure in which a catheter is passed into a vein or artery and then guided into the heart. When the catheter is in place, a contrast medium is introduced to produce an angiogram to determine how well the heart is working. This procedure is also used during treatment. See the section on clearing blocked arteries later in this chapter.
- Digital subtraction angiography (DSA) combines angiography with computerized components to clarify the view of the area of interest by removing the soft tissue and bones from the images.
- Duplex ultrasound is a diagnostic procedure to image the structures of the blood vessels and the flow of blood n Phlebography (fleh-BOG-rah-fee), also known as venography, is a radiographic test that provides an image of the leg veins after a contrast dye is injected into a vein in the patient's foot (phleb/o means vein, and -graphy means the process of recording). The resulting film is a phlebogram. This is a very accurate test for detecting deep vein thrombosis.

Electrocardiography

Electrocardiography (ee-leck-troh-kar-dee-OG-rah-fee) is the noninvasive process of recording the electrical activity of the myocardium (electr/o means electric, cardi/o means heart, and graphy means the process of recording a picture or record). A noninvasive procedure does not require the insertion of an instrument or device through the skin or a body opening for diagnosis or treatment.

- An electrocardiogram (ee-leck-troh-KAR-dee-ohgram) is a record of the electrical activity of the myocardium (electr/o means electric, cardi/o means heart, and -gram means picture or record)..
- A Holter monitor is a portable electrocardiograph that is worn by an ambulatory patient to continuously monitor the heart rates and rhythms over a 24-hour period.
- A stress test is performed to assess cardiovascular health and function during and after stress. This involves monitoring with an electrocardiogram while the patient exercises on a treadmill.
- A thallium stress test (THAL-ee-um) is performed to evaluate how well blood flows through the coronary arteries of the heart muscle during exercise.

Treatment Procedures Of The Cardiovascular System

Medications

Many heart conditions are controlled with medications; however, successful treatment depends on patient compliance. Compliance is the accuracy and consistency with which the patient follows the physician's instructions.

Antihypertensives

- An antihypertensive (an-tih-high-per-TEN-siv) is a medication administered to lower blood pressure. Some of these drugs are also used to treat other heart conditions.
- An ACE inhibitor (Angiotensin-Converting Enzyme) blocks the action of the enzyme that causes the blood vessels to contract resulting in hypertension. When this enzyme is blocked, the blood vessels are able to dilate (enlarge), and this reduces the blood pressure. These medications are used primarily to treat hypertension and heart failure.
- A beta-blocker reduces the workload of the heart by slowing the rate of the heart beat. They are commonly prescribed to lower blood pressure, relieve angina, or to treat heart failure.
- Calcium channel blocker agents cause the heart and blood vessels to relax by decreasing the movement of calcium into the cells of these structures. This relaxation reduces the workload of the heart by increasing the supply of blood and oxygen. Some calcium channel blocking agents are used to treat hypertension or to relieve and control angina.
- A diuretic (dye-you-RET-ick) is administered to stimulate the kidneys to increase the secretion of urine to rid the body of excess sodium and water. These medications are administered to treat hypertension and heart failure by reducing the amount of fluid circulating in the blood.

Additional Medications

- An antiarrhythmic (an-tih-ah-RITH-mick) is a medication administered to control irregularities of the heartbeat.

- An anticoagulant (an-tih-koh-AG-you-lant) slows coagulation and prevents new clots from forming. Coagulation is the process of clotting blood (see Coumadin).
- Aspirin in very small daily dose, such as an 81 mg baby aspirin, may be recommended to reduce the risk of a heart attack or stroke by slightly reducing the ability of the blood to clot.
- Cholesterol-lowering drugs, such as statins, are used to combat hyperlipidemia by reducing the undesirable cholesterol levels in the blood.
- Coumadin, which is the brand name for warfarin, is an anticoagulant administered to prevent blood clots from forming or growing larger. This medication is often prescribed for patients with clotting difficulties, certain types of heartbeat irregularities, or after a heart attack or after heart valve replacement surgery.
- Digitalis (dij-ih-TAL-is), also known as digoxin, strengthens the contraction of the heart muscle, slows the heart rate, and helps eliminate fluid from body tissues. It is often used to treat heart failure or certain types of arrhythmias.
- A thrombolytic (throm-boh-LIT-ick), also known as a clot-busting drug, dissolves or causes a thrombus to break up (thromb/o means clot, and -lytic means to destroy).
- Tissue plasminogen activator (plaz-MIN-oh-jen) is a thrombolytic that is administered to some patients having a heart attack or stroke. If administered within a few hours after symptoms begin, this medication can dissolve the damaging blood clots.
- A vasoconstrictor (vas-oh-kon-STRICK-tor) causes blood vessels to narrow. Examples of uses of these medications include antihistamines and decongestants. A vasoconstrictor is the opposite of a vasodilator.
- A vasodilator (vas-oh-dye-LAYT-or) causes blood vessels to expand. A vasodilator is the opposite of a vasoconstrictor.
- Nitroglycerin is a vasodilator that is prescribed to prevent or relieve the pain of angina by dilating the blood vessels to the heart. This increases the blood flow and oxygen supply to the heart. Nitroglycerin can be administered sublingually (under the tongue), transdermally (through the skin), or orally as a spray.

Clearing Blocked Arteries

- Percutaneous transluminal coronary angioplasty (PTCA), commonly referred to simply as angioplasty (AN-jee-oh-plas-tee), is also known as a balloon angioplasty. This is a procedure in which a small balloon on the end of a catheter is used to open a partially blocked coronary artery by flattening the plaque deposit and stretching the lumen.
- A stent is a wire-mesh tube that is commonly placed after the artery has been opened. This provides support to the arterial wall, keeps the plaque from expanding again, and prevents restenosis.

- Restenosis describes the condition when an artery that has been opened by angioplasty closes again (re means again, and -stenosis means narrowing).
- An atherectomy (ath-er-ECK-toh-mee) is the surgical removal of plaque buildup from the interior of an artery (ather means plaque, and -ectomy means surgical removal). A stent may be put in place after the atherectomy to prevent the artery from becoming blocked again.
- A carotid endarterectomy (kah-ROT-id end-ar-ter- ECK-toh-mee) is the surgical removal of the lining of a portion of a clogged carotid artery leading to the brain. This procedure is performed to reduce the risk of a stroke caused by a disruption of the blood flow to the brain.

Coronary Artery Bypass Graft

- Coronary artery bypass graft (CABG) is also known as bypass surgery. In this surgery, which requires opening the chest, a piece of vein from the leg or chest is implanted on the heart to replace a blocked coronary artery and to improve the flow of blood to the heart.
- A minimally invasive coronary artery bypass, also known as a keyhole bypass or a buttonhole bypass, is an alternative technique for some bypass patients. This procedure is performed with the aid of a fiber optic camera through small openings between the ribs.

Treatment of Cardiac Arrhythmias

- Defibrillation (dee-fih-brih-LAY-shun), also known as cardioversion, is the use of electrical shock to restore the heart's normal rhythm. This shock is provided by a device known as a defibrillator.
- An automated external defibrillator (AED) is designed for use by nonprofessionals in emergency situations when defibrillation is required. This piece of equipment automatically samples the electrical rhythms of the heart and, if necessary, externally shocks the heart to restore a normal cardiac rhythm.
- An artificial pacemaker is used primarily as treatment for bradycardia or atrial fibrillation. This electronic device can be attached externally or implanted under the skin with connections leading into the heart to regulate the heartbeat.
- An implantable cardioverter defibrillator (KAR-deeoh- ver-ter dee-fib-rih-LAY-ter) is a double-action pacemaker. (1) It constantly regulates the heartbeat to ensure that the heart does not beat too slowly. (2) If a dangerous disruption of the heart's rhythm occurs, it acts as an automatic defibrillator.
- Valvoplasty (VAL-voh-plas-tee), also known as valvuloplasty, is the surgical repair or replacement of a heart valve (valv/o means valve, and -plasty means surgical repair).
- Cardiopulmonary resuscitation, commonly known as CPR, is an emergency procedure for life support consisting of artificial respiration

and manual external cardiac compression. Cardiopulmonary means pertaining to the heart and lungs.

Blood Vessels, Blood, and Bleeding

- An aneurysmectomy (an-you-riz-MECK-toh-mee) is the surgical removal of an aneurysm (aneurysm means aneurysm, and -ectomy means surgical removal).
- An aneurysmorrhaphy (an-you-riz-MOR-ah-fee), also known as aneurysmoplasty, is the surgical suturing of an aneurysm (aneurysm/o means aneurysm, and -rrhaphy means surgical suturing).
- An arteriectomy (ar-teh-ree-ECK-toh-mee) is the surgical removal of part of an artery (arteri means artery, and -ectomy means surgical removal).
- Hemostasis (hee-moh-STAY-sis) means to stop or control bleeding (hem/o means blood, and -stasis means stopping or controlling). This could be accomplished by the formation of a blood clot by the body or through the external application of pressure to block the flow of blood.
- Plasmapheresis (plaz-mah-feh-REE-sis) is the removal of whole blood from the body and separation of the blood's cellular elements. The red blood cells and platelets are suspended in saline or a plasma substitute and returned to the circulatory system. For blood donors, this makes more frequent donations possible. Patients with certain autoimmune disorders receive their own red blood cells and platelets back cleansed of antibodies.

Abbreviations Related To The Cardiovascular System

- anticoagulant = AC
- atrial fibrillation = AF
- cardiac catheterization = card cath, CC
- cholesterol = C
- chronic venous insufficiency = CVI
- coronary artery disease = CAD
- Electrocardiogram = EKG, ECG
- ischemic heart disease = IHD
- MIDCAB = minimally invasive direct coronary artery bypass
- myocardial infarction = MI
- peripheral artery disease = PAD
- peripheral vascular disease = PVD
- tissue plasminogen activator = tPA
- ventricular fibrillation = VF

Critical Thinking Exercise

The following story and questions are designed to stimulate critical thinking through class discussion or as a brief essay response. There are no right or wrong answers to these questions.

Randi Marchant, a 42-year-old waitress, was vacuuming the family room when she felt that painful squeezing in her chest again. Third time today, but this one really hurt. She sat down to catch her breath and stubbed out the cigarette she had left smoldering in the half-filled ashtray by the couch. Randi's husband, Jimmy and stepdaughter Melonie had pestered her until she finally had taken time off work to see her doctor. Dr. Harris found that her blood pressure was 158/88—probably owing to the noon rush stress at work, she rationalized. At least her cholesterol test was only 30 points above average this time. It had been slowly coming down, even though she cheated on her diet. Another wave of pain tightened its icy fingers around her heart, and the pain moved up into both sides of her jaw. Randi thought, "Probably just a little heartburn. Since the pain doesn't radiate down my left arm, it couldn't be my heart, could it?"

"Don't think about the pain," she told herself. "Think of something else. Melonie's prom dress needs altering." Randi fell to the floor, clutching her chest, just as Melonie walked in. She saw her stepmother slumped on the floor and screamed, "Oh my God! Help, somebody, help!"

Suggested Discussion Topics
1. What information in the story indicates that Randi might be a candidate for heart disease?
2. Discuss why Randi thought this was not a heart attack.
3. What can Melonie do immediately to try to save Randi's life?
4. Assuming that Randi is having a heart attack, discuss why it is important that she receive appropriate treatment quickly.

CHAPTER 6

THE LYMPHATIC AND IMMUNE SYSTEMS

This list contains essential word parts and medical terms for this chapter.

Word Parts
- antih carcin/o
- immun/o
- lymph/o
- lymphaden/o
- lymphangi/o
- neo-, ne/o
- -oma
- onc/o
- phag/o
- -plasm
- sarc/o
- splen/o
- -tic tox/o

Medical Terms
- acquired immunodeficiency syndrome (im-younoh- deh-FISH-en-see)
- allergen (AL-er-jen)
- anaphylaxis (an-ah-fih-LACK-sis)
- antibiotic
- antibody (AN-tih-bod-ee)
- antifungal (an-tih-FUNG-gul)
- antigen (AN-tih-jen)
- antigen-antibody reaction
- autoimmune disorder (aw-toh-ih-MYOUN)
- bacilli (bah-SILL-eye)
- bacteria (back-TEER-ree-ah)
- carcinoma (kar-sih-NOH-mah)

- carcinoma in situ (kar-sih-NOH-mah in SIGH-too)
- complement (KOM-pleh-ment)
- cytomegalovirus (sigh-toh-meg-ah-loh-VYE-rus)
- cytotoxic drug (sigh-toh-TOK-sick)
- ductal carcinoma in situ
- hemolytic (hee-moh-LIT-ick)
- herpes zoster (HER-peez ZOS-ter)
- Hodgkin's lymphoma (HODJ-kinz lim-FOH-mah)
- human immunodeficiency virus (im-you-nohdeh- FISH-en-see)
- immunodeficiency disorder (im-you-noh-deh- FISH-en-see)
- immunoglobulins (im-you-noh-GLOB-you-lins)
- immunosuppressant (im-you-noh-soo-PRES-ant)
- immunotherapy (ih-myou-noh-THER-ah-pee)
- infectious mononucleosis (mon-oh-new-klee- OH-sis)
- infiltrating ductal carcinoma (in-FILL-trate-ng DUK-tal kar-sih-NOH-mah)
- interferon (in-ter-FEAR-on)
- lymphadenitis (lim-fad-eh-NIGH-tis)
- lymphadenopathy (lim-fad-eh-NOP-ah-thee)
- lymphangioma (lim-fan-jee-OH-mah)
- lymphedema (lim-feh-DEE-mah)
- lymphocytes (LIM-foh-sights)
- lymphokines (LIM-foh-kyens)
- lymphoma (lim-FOH-mah)
- lymphoscintigraphy (lim-foh-sin-TIH-grah-fee)
- macrophage (MACK-roh-fayj)
- malaria (mah-LAY-ree-ah)
- mammography (mam-OG-rah-fee)
- metastasis (meh-TAS-tah-sis)
- metastasize (meh-TAS-tah-sighz)
- myoma (my-OH-mah)
- myosarcoma (my-oh-sahr-KOH-mah)
- non-Hodgkin's lymphoma (non-HODJ-kinz lim- FOH-mah)
- opportunistic infection (op-ur-too-NIHS-tick)
- osteosarcoma (oss-tee-oh-sar-KOH-mah)
- parasite (PAR-ah-sight)
- pathogen (PATH-oh-jen)
- rabies (RAY-beez)
- rickettsia (rih-KET-see-ah)
- rubella (roo-BELL-ah)
- sarcoma (sar-KOH-mah)
- spirochetes (SPY-roh-keets)
- splenomegaly (splee-noh-MEG-ah-lee)
- staphylococci (staf-ih-loh-KOCK-sigh)
- streptococci (strep-toh-KOCK-sigh)

- teletherapy (tel-eh-THER-ah-pee)
- tetanus (TET-ah-nus)
- toxoplasmosis (tock-soh-laz-MOH-sis)
- varicella (var-ih-SEL-ah)

Objectives

On completion of this chapter, you should be able to:
1. Identify the medical specialists who treat disorders of the lymphatic and immune systems.
2. Describe the major functions and structures of the lymphatic and immune systems.
3. Recognize, define, spell, and pronounce the major terms related to the pathology, diagnostic, and treatment procedures of the lymphatic and immune systems.
4. Recognize, define, spell, and pronounce terms related to oncology.

Medical Specialties Related To The Lymphatic And Immune Systems

- An allergist (AL-er-jist) specializes in diagnosing and treating conditions of altered immunologic reactivity, such as allergic reactions.
- An immunologist (im-you-NOL-oh-jist) specializes in diagnosing and treating disorders of the immune system (immunmeans protected, and -ologistmeans specialist).
- An oncologist (ong-KOL-oh-jist) is a physician who specializes in diagnosing and treating malignant disorders such as tumors and cancer (onc means tumor, and -ologist means specialist).

Functions Of The Lymphatic System

The lymphatic system performs three primary functions in cooperation with other body systems. These are:
- Absorbing fats and fat-soluble vitamins from the small intestine.
- Removing waste from the tissues.
- Providing aid to the immune system.

Absorption of Fats and Fat-Soluble Vitamins

Food is digested in the small intestine. From here, the nutrients, fats, and fat-soluble vitamins are absorbed for use throughout the body.
- The villi are small finger-like projections that line the small intestine. These structures contain blood vessels and lacteals (LACK-tee-ahls), which are specialized structures of the lymphatic system.
- The blood vessels in the villi absorb most of the nutrients from the digested food directly into the bloodstream.
- Fats and fat-soluble vitamins that cannot be absorbed directly into the bloodstream are absorbed and transported by the lacteals of the lymphatic system.

Waste Removal from the Tissues

The lymphatic system removes waste products and excess fluids created by the cells. It also destroys pathogens and takes away foreign substances that are present in the tissues.

Cooperating with the Immune System

The lymph nodes play an active role in cooperation with the immune system to protect the body against invading microorganisms and diseases. These functions are described in the discussion of the immune system.

Structures Of The Lymphatic System

The major structures of the lymphatic system are lymph, lymphatic vessels and ducts, and lymph nodes. Additional structures include the tonsils, thymus, spleen, lacteals,
Peyer's patches, the vermiform appendix, and lymphocytes. Lymphocytes, which are specialized white blood cells, have roles in both the lymphatic and immune systems and are discussed under the heading of "Specialized Cells of the Antigen-Antibody Reaction."

Lymphatic Circulation

Lymphatic circulation transports lymph from tissues throughout the body and eventually returns this fluid to the venous circulation. Lymph is a clear, watery fluid that transports waste products and proteins out of the spaces between the cells of the body tissues. It also destroys bacteria or other pathogens that are present in the tissues.
Because the lymphatic vessels are closely aligned with those of the cardiovascular system, the lymphatic system is sometimes referred to as the secondary circulatory
system.
Despite the similarities, there are major differences between these two circulatory systems. While studying this section.
- Blood circulates throughout the entire body. Lymph flows in only one direction, from its point of origin until its return to the venous circulation in the region of the neck.
- Blood flows in an open system in which it leaves, and re-enters, the blood vessels through the capillaries. Lymphatic circulation is a closed system. From the time lymph enters the lymphatic capillaries, it does not leave the lymphatic vessels again until it returns to the venous circulation.
- Blood is pumped throughout the body by the heart. The lymphatic system does not have a pump-like organ. Instead, lymph must depend on help from the movements of nearby muscles and blood vessels to aid in its flow.
- The color of blood makes the arteries and veins readily visible. Lymph is a clear fluid, and the lymphatic vessels are not readily visible.

- Blood is filtered by the kidneys, and waste products are excreted by the urinary system. Lymph is filtered by lymph nodes located along the lymphatic vessels throughout the body.

Interstitial Fluid and Lymph Creation

Interstitial fluid (in-ter-STISH-al), also known as intercellular or tissue fluid, is plasma from arterial blood that flows out of the capillaries and into the spaces between the cells. This interstitial fluid transports food, oxygen, and hormones to the cells.
- About 90% of this fluid is reabsorbed by the capillaries and returned to the venous circulation. Reabsorbed means to be taken up again by the body.
- The remaining 10% of the interstitial fluid that was not reabsorbed becomes lymph. It is transported by the lymphatic vessels and is filtered by lymph nodes located along these vessels.

Lymphatic Capillaries

Lymphatic capillaries are microscopic, blind-ended tubes located near the surface of the body. The capillary walls are only one cell in thickness. These cells separate briefly to allow lymph to enter the capillary, and the action of the cells as they close forces the lymph to flow forward.

Lymphatic Vessels and Ducts

Lymph flows from the lymphatic capillaries into the progressively larger lymphatic vessels, which are located deeper within the tissues. Like veins, lymphatic vessels have valves to prevent the backward flow of lymph. The larger lymphatic vessels eventually join together to form two ducts. Each duct drains a specific part of the body and returns the lymph to the venous circulation.
- The right lymphatic duct collects lymph from the right side of the head and neck, the upper right quadrant of the body and the right arm. The right lymphatic duct empties into the right subclavian vein.
- The thoracic duct, which is the largest lymphatic vessel in the body, collects lymph from the left side of the head and neck, the upper left quadrant of the trunk, the left arm, and the entire lower portion of the trunk and both legs. The thoracic duct empties into the left subclavian vein.

Lymph Nodes

Each small, bean-shaped lymph node contains specialized lymphocytes that are capable of destroying pathogens. Unfiltered lymph flows into the nodes, and here the lymphocytes destroy harmful substances such as bacteria, viruses, and malignant cells. Additional structures within the node filter the lymph to remove additional impurities. After these processes are complete, the lymph leaves the node and continues its journey to again become part of the venous circulation.

There are between 400 and 700 lymph nodes located along the larger lymphatic vessels, and approximately half of these nodes are in the abdomen. Most of the others nodes are positioned on the branches of the larger lymphatic vessels throughout the body. The exceptions are the three major groups of lymph nodes that are named for their locations.

- Cervical lymph nodes (SER-vih-kal) are located along the sides of the neck (cervic means neck, and -al means pertaining to).
- Axillary lymph nodes (AK-sih-lar-ee) are located under the arms in the area known as the armpits (axill means armpit, and -ary means pertaining to).
- Inguinal lymph nodes (ING-gwih-nal) are located in the inguinal (groin) area of the lower abdomen (inguin means groin, and -al means pertaining to).

Additional Structures of the Lymphatic System

The remaining structures of this body system are made up of lymphoid tissue. The term lymphoid means pertaining to the lymphatic system or resembling lymph or lymphatic tissue. Although these structures consist of lymphoid tissue, their primary roles are in conjunction with the immune system.

The Tonsils

- The tonsils (TON-sils) are three masses of lymphoid tissue that form a protective ring around the back of the nose and the upper throat. These structures play an important role in the immune system by preventing pathogens from entering the body through the nose and mouth.
- The adenoids (AD-eh-noids), also known as the nasopharyngeal tonsils, are located in the nasopharynx.
- The palatine tonsils (PAL-ah-tine) are located on the left and right sides of the throat in the area that is visible through the mouth. Palatine means referring to the hard and soft palates.
- The lingual tonsils (LING-gwal) are located at the base of the tongue. Lingual means pertaining to the tongue.

The Thymus

The thymus (THIGH-mus) is located superior to (above) the heart. Although it is composed largely of lymphoid tissue, the thymus is an endocrine gland that assists the immune system.

Peyer's Patches and the Vermiform Appendix

These structures, which consist of lymphoid tissue, work with the immune system to protect against the entry of pathogens through the digestive system.

- Peyer's patches (PIE-erz) are located on the walls of the ileum. The ileum is last section of the small intestine.
- The vermiform appendix hangs fromthe lower portion of the cecum. The cecum is the first section of the large intestine. Recent research

indicates that the appendix plays an important role in the immune system.

The Spleen

The spleen is a saclike mass of lymphoid tissue located in the left upper quadrant of the abdomen, just inferior to (below) the diaphragm and posterior to (behind) the stomach.

- The spleen filters microorganisms and other foreign material from the blood.
- The spleen forms lymphocytes and monocytes, which are specialized white blood cells with roles in the immune system.
- The spleen has the hemolytic (hee-moh-LIT-ick) function of destroying worn-out red blood cells and releasing their hemoglobin for reuse (hem/o means blood, and -lytic means to destroy).
- The spleen also stores extra erythrocytes (red blood cells) and maintains the appropriate balance between these cells and the plasma of the blood.

Pathology and Diagnostic Procedures of the Lymphatic System

- Lymphadenitis (lim-fad-eh-NIGH-tis), also known as swollen glands, is an inflammation of the lymph nodes (lymphaden means lymph node, and -itis means inflammation). The terms lymph nodes and lymph glands are sometimes used interchangeably. Swelling of the lymph nodes is frequently an indication of the presence of an infection.
- Lymphadenopathy (lim-fad-eh-NOP-ah-thee) is any disease process affecting a lymph node or nodes (lymphaden/o means lymph node, and -pathy means disease).
- A lymphangioma (lim-fan-jee-OH-mah) is a benign tumor formed by an abnormal collection of lymphatic vessels due to a congenital malformation of the lymphatic system (lymphangi means lymph vessel, and -oma means tumor).
- Splenomegaly (splee-noh-MEG-ah-lee) is an abnormal enlargement of the spleen (splen/o means spleen, and -megaly means abnormal enlargement). This condition can be due to bleeding caused by an injury, an infectious disease such as mononucleosis, or abnormal functioning of the immune system.
- Splenorrhagia (splee-noh-RAY-jee-ah) is bleeding from the spleen (splen/o means spleen, and -rrhagia means bleeding).
- Lymphoscintigraphy (lim-foh-sin-TIH-grah-fee) is a diagnostic test that is performed to detect damage or malformations of the lymphatic vessels.

Lymphedema

- Lymphedema (lim-feh-DEE-mah) is swelling due to an abnormal accumulation of lymph fluid within the tissues (lymph means lymph, and -edema means swelling).

- Primary lymphedema is a hereditary disorder due to malformation of the lymphatic system. This condition, which can appear at any time in life, most commonly produces swelling in the feet and legs.
- Secondary lymphedema is caused by damage to the lymphatic system that most commonly produces swelling in the limb nearest to the damaged lymphatic vessels. Cancer treatment (surgery, chemotherapy, and/or radiation) and trauma (burns, injuries, and scarring) are the most frequent causes of this condition.

The Antigen-Antibody Reaction

An antigen-antibody reaction, also known as the immune reaction, involves binding antigens to antibodies. This reaction labels a potentially dangerous antigen so it can be recognized, and destroyed, by other cells of the immune system.
- An antigen (AN-tih-jen) is any substance that the body regards as being foreign, and includes viruses, bacteria, toxins, and transplanted tissues. The immune system immediately responds to the presence of any antigen.
- An allergen (AL-er-jen) is a substance that produces an allergic reaction in an individual.
- An antibody (AN-tih-bod-ee) is a disease-fighting protein created by the immune system in response to the presence of a specific antigen (the prefix antimeans against). The terms antibody and immunoglobulin are often used interchangeably.

Immunoglobulins

Immunoglobulins (im-you-noh-GLOB-you-lins) bind with specific antigens in the antigen-antibody response. The five primary types of immunoglobulins, which are secreted by plasma cells, are also known as antibodies. Plasma cells are specialized white blood cells that produce antibodies coded to destroy specific antigens.

Lymphocytes

Lymphocytes (LIM-foh-sights) are white blood cells that are formed in bone marrow as stem cells (lymph/o means lymph, and -cytes means cells). These cells undergo further maturation and differentiation in lymphoid tissues throughout the body.

These changes enable these lymphocytes to act as specialized antibodies that are capable of attacking specific antigens. Maturation means the process of becoming mature. Differentiation means to be modified to perform a specific function.

B Cells

B cells, also known as B lymphocytes, are specialized lymphocytes that produce and secrete antibodies. Each lymphocyte makes a specific antibody that is capable of destroying a specific antigen.

- B cells are most effective against viruses and bacteria circulating in the blood.
- When a B cell is confronted with the antigen that it is coded to destroy, that B cell is transformed into a plasma B cell. These cells are capable of producing and secreting antibodies that are coded to destroy a specific antigen.

Dendritic Cells

Dendritic cells (den-DRIT-ic) are specialized white blood cells that patrol the body searching for antigens that produce infections. When such a cell is found the dendritic cells grab, swallow, and internally break apart the captured antigen. Fragments of the destroyed antigen are then moved to the surface of the cell where these fragments are displayed on tentacle-like extensions of the dendritic cell. The purpose of this display is to alert, and activate, T cells to protect against this specific antigen.

T Cells

T cells, also known as T lymphocytes, are small lymphocytes that mature in the thymus as a result of exposure to the hormone thymosin, which is secreted by the thymus.
- T cells contribute to the immune defense by coordinating immune defenses and by killing infected cells on contact.
- Interferon (in-ter-FEAR-on) is a family of proteins produced by the T cells whose specialty is fighting viruses by slowing or stopping their multiplication.
- Lymphokines (LIM-foh-kyens), which are produced by the T cells, direct the antigen-antibody response by signaling between the cells of the immune system. Lymphokines attract macrophages to the infected site and prepare them to attack the invaders.
- A macrophage (MACK-roh-fayj) is a type of white blood cell that surrounds and kills invading cells (macro- means large, and -phage means a cell that eats). Macrophages also remove dead cells and stimulate the action of other immune cells.

n A phagocyte (FAG-oh-sight) is a large white blood cell that can destroy substances such as cell debris, dust, pollen, and pathogens by the process of phagocytosis (phag/o means to eat or swallow, and -cyte means cell). Phagocytosis is the process of destroying pathogens by surrounding and swallowing them.

Complement

Complement (KOM-pleh-ment) is a group of proteins that normally circulate in the blood in an inactive form and are activated by contact with nonspecific antigens such as foreign blood cells or bacteria. Complement then marks these foreign invaders and attracts phagocytes to destroy these antigens.

Immunity

Immunity is the state of being resistant to a specific disease.
- Natural immunity is passed from the mother to her fetus (developing child) before birth. This immunity lasts only a short time.
- Passive immunity is passed from the mother to her child after birth through breast milk.
- Acquired immunity, also known as active immunity, is the production of antibodies against a specific antigen by the immune system either by contracting an infectious disease such as chickenpox, or by vaccination against a disease such as poliomyelitis (polio).
- Vaccination, also known as immunization, is providing protection for susceptible individuals from communicable diseases by the administration of a vaccine to provide acquired immunity against a specific disease. A vaccine is a preparation containing an antigen, consisting of whole or partial diseasecausing organisms, which have been killed or weakened.

Pathology and Diagnostic Procedures of the Immune System

The effectiveness of the immune system depends upon the individual's
- General health: If the immune system is compromised by poor health, it cannot be fully effective.
- Age: Older individuals usually have more acquired immunity; however, their immune systems tend to respond less quickly and effectively to new challenges. Babies and very young children do not yet have as much acquired immunity, and their bodies sometimes have difficulty resisting challenges to the immune system.
- Heredity: Genes and genetic disorders affect the individual's general health and the functioning of his or her immune system.

Allergic Reactions

- An allergic reaction occurs when the body's immune system reacts to a harmless allergen such as pollen, food, or animal dander as if it were a dangerous invader.
- An allergy, also known as hypersensitivity, is an overreaction by the body to a particular antigen.
- A localized allergic response, also known as a cellular response, includes redness, itching, and burning where the skin has come into contact with an allergen. For example, contact with poison ivy can cause a localized allergic response in the form of an itchy rash.

Although the body reacts mildly the first time it is exposed to the allergen, sensitivity is established, and future contacts can cause much more-severe symptoms.
- A systemic reaction, which is also described as anaphylaxis (an-ah-fih-LACK-sis) or as anaphylactic shock, is a severe response to an allergen.

The symptoms of this response develop quickly. Without medical aid, the patient can die within a few minutes.
- A scratch test is a diagnostic test to identify commonly troublesome allergens such as tree pollen and ragweed. Swelling and itching indicate an allergic reaction.
- Antihistamines are medications administered to relieve or prevent the symptoms of hay fever, which is a common allergy to wind-borne pollens, and other types of allergies. Antihistamines work by preventing the effects of histamine, which is a substance produced by the body that causes the itching, sneezing, runny nose, and watery eyes of an allergic reaction.

Autoimmune Disorders

An autoimmune disorder (aw-toh-ih-MYOUN), also known as an autoimmune disease, is any of a large group of diseases characterized by a condition in which the immune system produces antibodies against its own tissues. This abnormal functioning of the immune system appears to be genetically transmitted and predominantly occurs in women during the childbearing years. Autoimmune disorders affect most body systems.

Immunodeficiency Disorders

An immunodeficiency disorder (im-you-noh-deh-FISHen- see) occurs when the immune response is compromised. Compromised means weakened, reduced, absent, or not functioning properly.

The Human Immunodeficiency Virus

The human immunodeficiency virus (im-you-noh-deh- FISH-en-see), commonly known as HIV, is a bloodborne infection in which the virus damages or kills the cells of the immune system, causing it to progressively fail, thus leaving the body at risk of developing many lifethreatening opportunistic infections. In the early stages of HIV, medical intervention can prolong the patient's life.
- An opportunistic infection (op-ur-too-NIHS-tick) is caused by a pathogen that does not normally produce an illness in healthy humans. However, when the host is debilitated, these pathogens are able to cause an infection. Debilitated means weakened by another condition. Because the immune systems of patients with HIV or AIDS are weakened, many opportunistic infections can develop.
- Acquired immunodeficiency syndrome, commonly known as AIDS, is the most advanced, and fatal, stage of an HIV infection.
- Kaposi's sarcoma (KAP-oh-seez sar-KOH-mah) is an example of an opportunistic infection that is frequently associated with HIV. This cancer causes patches of abnormal tissue to grow under the skin, in the lining of the mouth, nose, and throat, or in other organs.
- ELISA, which is the acronym for enzyme-linked immunosorbent assay, is a blood test used to screen for the presence of HIV antibodies.

- A Western blot test is a blood test that produces more accurate results than the ELISA test. The Western blot test is performed to confirm the diagnosis when the results of the ELISA test are positive. This is necessary because the ELISA test sometimes produces a false positive result in which the test erroneously indicates the presence of HIV.

Treatment of the Immune System

A variety of treatment procedures are used to correct or control the symptoms of disorders of the immune system.

Immunotherapy

- Immunotherapy (ih-myou-noh-THER-ah-pee) is a disease treatment that involves either stimulating or repressing the immune response (immun/o means immune, and -therapy means treatment).
- In the treatment of cancers, immunotherapy is used to stimulate the immune response to fight the malignancy. Stimulate means to cause greater activity.
- In the treatment of allergies, immunotherapy is used to repress the body's sensitivity to a particular allergen. Repress means to decrease, slow, or stop a normal response. This treatment is also known as allergy desensitization.

Antibody Therapy

- Synthetic immunoglobulins, also known as immune serum, are used as a postexposure preventive measure against certain viruses, including rabies and some types of hepatitis. Postexposure means that the patient has been exposed to the virus, for example, has been bitten by an animal with rabies. The goal of this treatment is to prevent the disease from developing.
- Synthetic interferon is used in the treatment of multiple sclerosis, hepatitis C, and some cancers.
- Monoclonal antibodies are any of a class of antibodies produced in the laboratory by identical offspring of a clone of specific cells. These artificially produced antibodies are used to enhance the patient's immune response to certain malignancies, including some non-Hodgkin's lymphoma, melanoma, breast cancer and colon cancer. Monoclonal means pertains to a single clone of cells. As used here, a clone is an exact replica of a group of bacteria.

Immunosuppression

- Immunosuppression (im-you-noh-sup-PRESH-un) is treatment to repress or interfere with the ability of the immune system to respond to stimulation by antigens.

- An immunosuppressant (im-you-noh-soo-PRES-ant) is a substance that prevents or reduces the body's normal immune response. This medication is administered to prevent the rejection of donor tissue and to depress autoimmune disorders.
- A corticosteroid drug (kor-tih-koh-STEHR-oid) is a hormone-like preparation administered primarily as an anti-inflammatory and as an immunosuppressant.
- A cytotoxic drug (sigh-toh-TOK-sick) is a medication that kills or damages cells (cyt/o means cell, tox means poison, and -ic means pertaining to). These drugs are

used as immunosuppressants or as antineoplastics.
Antineoplastics are discussed under "Chemotherapy" later in this chapter.

Pathogenic Organisms

A pathogen (PATH-oh-jen) is a microorganism that causes a disease in humans. A microorganism is a living organism that is so small it can be seen only with the aid of a microscope. Pathogenic means capable of producing disease.

Bacteria

- Bacteria (back-TEER-ree-ah) are one-celled microscopic organisms (singular, bacterium). Most bacteria are not harmful to humans. Bacteria that are pathogenic in humans include bacilli, rickettsia, spirochetes, staphylococci, and streptococci.
- Bacilli (bah-SILL-eye) are rod-shaped spore-forming bacteria (singular, bacillus). Tetanus (TET-ah-nus) is caused by the bacillus Clostridium tetani, and is transmitted through a cut or wound. Tetanus is commonly known as lockjaw because it produces muscle spasms that are so severe a patient cannot open his or her mouth or swallow.
- A rickettsia (rih-KET-see-ah) is a small bacterium that lives in lice, fleas, ticks, and mites (plural, rickettsiae). Rocky Mountain spotted fever, which is caused by Rickettsia rickettsii, is transmitted to humans by the bite of an infected tick. The signs and symptoms of this serious disease include a fever of sudden onset, headache, and muscle pain followed by the development of a rash.
- Spirochetes (SPY-roh-keets) are spiral-shaped bacteria that have flexible walls and are capable of movement. Lyme disease, which is caused by the spirochete Borrelia burgdorferi, is transmitted to humans by the bite of an infected deer tick. Symptoms include fever, headache, fatigue, and a characteristic skin rash. If left untreated, this infection can spread to the joints, heart, and nervous system.
- Staphylococci (staf-ih-loh-KOCK-sigh) are a group of about 30 species of bacteria that form irregular groups or clusters resembling grapes (singular, staphylococcus). Most staphylococci are harmless and reside normally on the skin and mucous membranes of humans and other

organisms; however, others are capable of producing very serious infections.
- Staphylococcus aureus (staf-ih-loh-KOCK-us OR-eeus), also known as staph aureus, is a form of staphylococci that commonly infects wounds and causes serious problems such as toxic shock syndrome or produces food poisoning. Toxic shock syndrome is a rare but potentially fatal disease caused by bacterial toxins.
- Streptococci (strep-toh-KOCK-sigh) are bacteria that forma chain (singular, streptococcus). Many streptococcal species are harmless; however, other members of this group are responsible for illnesses including strep throat, meningitis, endocarditis, and necrotizing fasciitis.

Septic Shock

Septic shock is a serious condition that occurs when an overwhelming bacterial infection affects the body. Toxins released by these pathogens can produce direct tissue damage resulting in low blood pressure. This damage causes vital organs (the brain, heart, kidneys, and liver) to not function properly or to fail completely. Septic shock occurs most often in the very old and the very young. It also occurs in those with underlying or debilitating illnesses.

Antibiotic Resistant Bacteria

- Antibiotic resistant bacteria, also known as superbugs, develop when an antibiotic fails to kill all of the bacteria it targets. When this occurs the surviving bacteria become resistant to that particular drug. When more and more bacteria become resistant to first-line treatments, the consequences are severe, as illnesses last longer, and the risks of complications and death increase.
- Methicillin-resistant Staphylococcus aureus, commonly known as MRSA, is resistant to most antibiotics. The first symptom of MRSA looks like small, red bumps with a black top. These bumps soon become red-hot abscesses that require immediate care. MRSA infections are serious, difficult to treat, and can be fatal. Originally these infections were nosocomial (hospital acquired); however, MRSA infections are increasingly present in the general population.

Fungus, Yeast, and Parasites

- A fungus (FUNG-gus) is a simple parasitic organism (plural, fungi). Some of these fungi are harmless to humans, others are pathogenic. Tinea pedis, commonly known as athlete's foot, is a fungal infection that commonly develops between the toes and on the feet.
- Yeast is a type of fungus. Candidiasis (kan-dih-DYEah- sis), formerly known as moniliasis, is now also known as a yeast infection or thrush. These infections, which are caused by the pathogenic yeast Candida albicans, occur on the skin or mucous membranes in the warm, moist areas such as the vagina or the mouth.

- A parasite (PAR-ah-sight) is a plant or animal that lives on, or within, another living organism at the expense of that organism. For example, malaria (mah-LAY-ree-ah) is a disease caused by a parasite that lives in certain mosquitoes that is transferred to humans by the bite of an infected mosquito. Symptoms develop from 7 days to 4 weeks after being infected and include fever, shaking chills, headache, muscle aches, and tiredness.
- Another parasite is toxoplasmosis (tock-soh-plaz- MOH-sis) which is most commonly transmitted from animals (pets) to humans by contact with contaminated feces. If a woman contracts this condition during pregnancy, it can result in abnormalities in the developing child such as microcephalus or hydrocephalus. Microcephalus is an abnormally small head and underdeveloped brain. Hydrocephalus is a condition in which excess cerebrospinal fluid accumulates in the ventricles of the brain. For this reason, it is recommended that pregnant women not perform tasks such as cleaning a kitty-litter box.

Viruses

Viruses (VYE-rus-ez) are very small infectious agents that live only by invading other cells (singular, virus). After invading the cell, the virus reproduces and then breaks the cell wall to release the newly formed viruses. These viruses spread to other cells and repeat the process.

Viral Infections

- Herpes zoster (HER-peez ZOS-ter), which is also known as shingles, is an acute viral infection characterized by painful skin eruptions that follow the underlying route of an inflamed nerve. This inflammation occurs when the dormant varicella (chickenpox) virus is reactivated later in life. A vaccine is available to prevent such a reoccurance.
- Infectious mononucleosis (mon-oh-new-klee-OHsis), also known as mono, is caused by the Epstein-Barr virus (EBV). This condition is characterized by fever, a sore throat, and enlarged lymph nodes. Swelling of the spleen or liver involvement can also develop.
- Measles is an acute, highly contagious infection caused by the rubeola virus and transmitted by respiratory droplets. Symptoms include a high fever, a runny nose, coughing, photophobia, and a red, itchy rash over the entire body. Photophobia means sensitivity to light. Complications of measles can be serious.
- Mumps is an acute viral disease characterized by the swelling of the parotid glands, which are the salivary glands located just in front of the ears. In adults, mumps can also cause painful swelling of the ovaries or testicles.
- Rubella (roo-BELL-ah), also known as German measles or 3-day measles, is a viral infection characterized by a low-grade fever, swollen glands, inflamed eyes, and a fine, pink rash. Although not usually severe or long

- lasting, rubella is serious in a woman during early pregnancy because of its ability to cause defects in a developing fetus. Measles and rubella share similar symptoms, and in fact the term "German" measles comes from the Latin word "germanus," meaning similar.
- The measles, mumps, and rubella vaccination (MMR) can prevent these three viral conditions.
- Rabies (RAY-beez) is an acute viral infection that is most commonly transmitted to humans by the bite or saliva of an infected animal. In humans, signs and symptoms of rabies usually occur 30–90 days after the bite. Once symptoms develop, rabies is almost always fatal. If at risk, it is necessary to undergo testing immediately so that postexposure treatment can be started as quickly as possible.
- Varicella (var-ih-SEL-ah), also known as chickenpox, is caused by the herpes virus Varicella zoster and is highly contagious. This condition is characterized by a fever and a rash consisting of hundreds of itchy, fluidfilled blisters that burst and form crusts.
- West Nile virus is spread to humans by the bite of an infected mosquito. A mild form of this condition has flu-like symptoms. A more severe variety spreads to the spinal cord and brain.

Cytomegalovirus

- Cytomegalovirus (sigh-toh-meg-ah-loh-VYE-rus) (CMV) is a member of the herpesvirus family that cause a variety of diseases (cyt/o means cell, megal/o means large, vir means virus, and -us is a singular noun ending).
- CMV is found in most body fluids and can be present as a silent infection in which the individual has no signs or symptoms of the infection.
- CMV can potentially cause a serious illness when the individual has a weakened immune system. CMV can be transmitted from the mother to her unborn child. This transmission can cause serious congenital disabilities in the child.

Medications to Control Infections

- Antibiotics are medications that are capable of inhibiting growth, or killing pathogenic bacterial microorganisms (anti- means against, bio means life, and -tic means pertaining to). Inhibit means to slow the growth or development. Antibiotics are not effective against viral infections.
- A bactericide is a substance that causes the death of bacteria (bacteri means bacteria, and -cide means causing death). This group of antibiotics includes penicillins and cephalosporins. A bacteriostatic is an agent that slows or stops the growth of bacteria (bacteri means bacteria, and -static means causing control). This group of antibiotics includes tetracycline, sulfonamide, and erythromycin.
- An antifungal (an-tih-FUNG-gul) is an agent that destroys or inhibits the growth of fungi (anti- means against, fung means fungus, and -al means

pertaining to). Lotrimin is an example of a topical antifungal that is applied to treat, or prevent, athlete's foot. This type of medication is also known as an antimycotic.
- An antiviral drug (an-tih-VYE-ral), such as acyclovir, is used to treat viral infections or to provide temporary immunity (anti- means against, vir means virus, and -al means pertaining to).

Oncology

Oncology (ong-KOL-oh-jee) is the study of the prevention, causes, and treatment of tumors and cancer (onc means tumor, and -ology means study of). Most cancers are named for the part of the body where the cancer originated. Cancer can attack all body systems and is the second leading cause of death in the United States after heart conditions.

Tumors

A tumor, which is also known as a neoplasm, is a growth of tissue that forms an abnormal mass. Within this mass, the multiplication of cells is uncontrolled, abnormally rapid, and progressive (neo- means new or strange, and -plasm means formation).
- A tumor can be benign (not life-threatening) or malignant (harmful, capable of spreading, and potentially life-threatening).
- A benign tumor is a noncancerous growth; however, these tumors can cause problems by placing pressure on adjacent structures. For example, a myoma (my- OH-mah) is a benign tumor made up of muscle tissue (my means muscle, and -oma means tumor).
- A malignant tumor is harmful, capable of spreading to distant body sites including other body system, can become progressively worse, and is progressively lifethreatening. For example, a myosarcoma (my-oh-sahr-KOH-mah) is a malignant tumor derived from muscle tissue (myo means muscle, sarc means flesh, and -oma means tumor).
- Angiogenesis (an-jee-oh-JEN-eh-sis) is the process through which the tumor supports its growth by creating its own blood supply (angi/o means vessel, and -genesis means reproduction). Angiogenesis is the opposite of antiangiogenesis.
- Antiangiogenesis is a form of treatment that disrupts this blood supply to the tumor (anti- means against, angi/o means vessel, and -genesis means reproduction). Antiangiogenesis is the opposite of angiogenesis.

Cancer

Cancer is a class of diseases characterized by the uncontrolled division of cells and the ability of these cells to invade other tissues, either by invasion through direct growth into adjacent tissue or by spreading into distant sites by metastasizing.
- To metastasize (meh-TAS-tah-sighz) is the process by which cancer spreads from one place to another. The cancer moves from the primary site and metastasizes (spreads) to a secondary site.

- A metastasis (meh-TAS-tah-sis) is a new cancer site that results from the spreading process (meta- means beyond, and -stasismeans stopping). Themetastasis can be within the same body system or within another body system at a distance from the primary site (plural, metastases).

Carcinomas

- A carcinoma (kar-sih-NOH-mah) is a malignant tumor that occurs in epithelial tissue (carcin means cancer, and -oma means tumor). Epithelial tissue forms the protective covering for all of the internal and external surfaces of the body.
- Carcinomas tend to infiltrate and produce metastases that can affect any organ or part of the body.
- Carcinoma in situ (kar-sih-NOH-mah in SIGH-too) describes a malignant tumor in its original position that has not yet disturbed or invaded the surrounding tissues. In situ means in the place where the cancer first occurred.
- For example, an adenocarcinoma (ad-eh-noh-karsih- NOH-mah) is any one of a large group of carcinomas derived from glandular tissue (aden/o means gland, carcin means cancer, and -oma means tumor).

Sarcomas

- A sarcoma (sar-KOH-mah) is a malignant tumor that arises from connective tissues, including hard tissues, soft tissues, and liquid tissues (sarc means flesh, and -oma means tumor) (plural, sarcomas or sarcomata).
- Hard tissue sarcomas arise from bone or cartilage. For example, an osteosarcoma (oss-tee-ohsar- KOH-mah) is a malignant tumor usually involving the upper shaft of long bones, the pelvis, or knee (oste/o means bone, sarc means flesh, and -oma means tumor).
- Soft tissue sarcomas arise from tissues such as muscle, connective tissues such as tendons, blood and lymphatic vessels, nerves, and fat. For example, a synovial sarcoma (sih-NOH-vee-al sar-KOH-mah) is a malignant tumor of the tissue surrounding a synovial joint. The most common locations are the knee, ankle, shoulder, and hip.
- Liquid tissue sarcomas arise from blood and lymph. One example is leukemia (loo-KEE-mee-ah), which affects the blood,

Staging

Staging is the process of classifying tumors with respect to how far the disease has progressed, the potential for its responding to therapy, and the patient's prognosis. Specific staging systems are used for different types of cancer.

Lymphomas

- Lymphoma (lim-FOH-mah) is a general term applied to malignancies affecting lymphoid tissues (lymph means lymph, and -oma means

tumor). This includes lymph nodes, the spleen, liver, and bone marrow. The two most common types of lymphomas are Hodgkin's lymphoma and non-Hodgkin's lymphoma.
- Hodgkin's lymphoma (HODJ-kinz lim-FOH-mah), also known as Hodgkin's disease, is distinguished from other lymphomas by the presence of large, cancerous lymphocytes known as Reed-Sternberg cells.
- Non-Hodgkin's lymphoma is the term used to describe all lymphomas other than Hodgkin's lymphoma. There are many different types of non-Hodgkin's lymphoma, some aggressive (fast-growing) and some indolent (slow-growing).

Breast Cancer

Breast cancer is a carcinoma that develops from the cells of the breast and can spread to adjacent lymph nodes and other body sites. There are several types of breast cancer named for their location or amount of spreading.
- Ductal carcinoma in situ is breast cancer at its earliest stage before the cancer has broken through the wall of the milk duct. At this stage, the cure rate is nearly 100%.
- Infiltrating ductal carcinoma (in-FILL-trate-ng DUKtal kar-sih-NOH-mah), also known as invasive ductal carcinoma, starts in the milk duct, breaks through the wall of that duct, and invades the fatty breast tissue. This form of cancer accounts for the majority of all breast cancers. Infiltrating and invasive are terms used to describe cancer that has spread beyond the layer of tissue in which it developed and the cancer is now growing into surrounding, healthy tissues.
- Infiltrating lobular carcinoma, also known as invasive lobular carcinoma, is cancer that starts in the milk glands (lobules), breaks through the wall of the gland, and invades the fatty tissue of the breast. Once this cancer reaches the lymph nodes, it can rapidly spread to distant parts of the body.
- Inflammatory breast cancer (IBC) is the most aggressive and least common form of breast cancer. IBC grows rapidly, and symptoms include pain, rapid increase in the breast size, redness or a rash on the breast, and the swelling of nearby lymph nodes. IBC can be detected by magnetic resonance imaging (MRI); however, it is not detected by mammography or ultrasound.
- Male breast cancer can occur in the small amount of breast tissue that is normally present in men. The types of cancers are similar to those occurring in women.

Detection of Breast Cancer

Early detection of breast cancer is very important and utilizes the following techniques.

- Breast self-examination is an essential self-care procedure for the early detection of breast cancer. The focus of this self-examination is checking for a new lump or for changes in an existing lump, shape of the nipple, or the skin covering the breast.
- Professional palpation of the breast is performed to feel the texture, size, and consistency of the breast.
- Mammography (mam-OG-rah-fee) is a radiographic examination of the breasts to detect the presence of tumors or precancerous cells (mammo/o means breast, and -graphy means the process of producing a picture or record). The resulting record is a mammogram.
- Ultrasound is used as an initial follow-up test when an abnormality is found by mammography.
- A surgical biopsy (BYE-op-see) is the removal of a small piece of tissue for examination to confirm or establish a diagnosis (bi- means pertaining to life, and -opsy means view of). After a diagnosis has been established, treatment is then based on the stage of the cancer.
- A needle breast biopsy is a technique in which an x-ray-guided needle is used to remove small samples of tissue from the breast. It is less painful and disfiguring than a surgical biopsy.
- In a sentinel-node biopsy, after the sentinel lymph node has been identified, only this and the other affected nodes are removed for biopsy. If the cancer has not spread, this spares the remaining nodes in that group. The sentinel node is the first lymph node to come into contact with cancer cells as they leave the organ of origination and start spreading into the rest of the body.
- Lymph node dissection is a surgical procedure in which all of the lymph nodes in a major group are removed to determine or slow the spread of cancer. For example, an axillary lymph node dissection (ALND) is sometimes performed as part of the surgical treatment of the breast.

Surgical Treatment of Breast Cancer

- A lumpectomy is the surgical removal of only the cancerous tissue and a surrounding margin of normal tissue.
- A mastectomy (mas-TECK-toh-mee) is the surgical removal of the entire breast and nipple (mast means breast, and -ectomy means surgical removal). Although simply described as a mastectomy, this procedure often includes the removal of axillary lymph nodes under the adjacent arm.
- A modified radical mastectomy is the surgical removal of the entire breast and all of the axillary lymph nodes under the adjacent arm.
- A radical mastectomy is the surgical removal of an entire breast and many of the surrounding tissues.

Cancer Treatments

The most common forms of cancer treatments are surgery, chemotherapy, and radiation therapy.

Surgery

Most commonly cancer surgery involves removing the malignancy plus a margin of normal surrounding tissue. It may also involve the removal of one or more nearby lymph nodes to detect whether the cancer has stated to spread.

Chemotherapy

Chemotherapy is the use of chemical agents and drugs in combinations selected to destroy malignant cells and tissues.

- Chemoprevention is the use of natural or synthetic substances such as drugs or vitamins to reduce the risk of developing cancer, or to reduce the chance that cancer will recur. Chemoprevention may also be used to reduce the size or slow the development of an existing tumor.
- An antineoplastic (an-tih-nee-oh-PLAS-tick) is medication that blocks the development, growth, or proliferation of malignant cells (anti- means against, ne/o means new, plast means growth or formation, and -ic means pertaining to). Proliferation means to increase rapidly.
- Cytotoxic drugs, which are also used for both immunosuppression and chemotherapy, are discussed earlier in this chapter.

Radiation Therapy

Radiation therapy is used in the treatment of some cancers, with the goal of destroying the cancer while sparing healthy tissues.

- Brachytherapy (brack-ee-THER-ah-pee) is the use of radioactive materials in contact with, or implanted into, the tissues to be treated (brachy- means short, and -therapy means treatment).
- Teletherapy (tel-eh-THER-ah-pee) is radiation therapy administered at a distance from the body (telemeans distant, and -therapy means treatment). With the assistance of three-dimensional computer imaging, it is possible to aim doses more precisely.

Additional Therapies

- Adjuvant therapy (AD-jeh-vant) is used after the primary treatments have been completed to decrease the chance that a cancer will recur. The term adjuvant refers to an agent intended to increase the effectiveness of a drug; however, adjuvant treatments for cancer can also include chemotherapy, hormone therapy, radiation, immunotherapy, or targeted therapy.
- Targeted therapy is a developing form of anti-cancer drug therapy that uses drugs or other substances to identify and attack specific cancer cells without harming normal cells. A monoclonal antibody is a type of targeted therapy.

Abbreviations Related To The Lymphatic And Immune Systems
- antibody = A, Ab
- antigen = AG, Ag
- carcinoma = CA, Ca
- carcinoma in situ = CIS
- ductal carcinoma in situ = DCIS
- herpes zoster = HZ
- Hodgkin's lymphoma = HL
- immunoglobulin = IG
- lymphedema = LE
- metastasis = MET
- metastasize = met
- non-Hodgkin's lymphoma = NHL
- rickettsia = Rick
- varicella = VSZ

Critical Thinking Exercise

The following story and questions are designed to stimulate critical thinking through class discussion or as a brief essay response. There are no right or wrong answers to these questions.

Hernani Fermin, a 35-year-old married father, was diagnosed HIV positive 2 years ago. He is a sales representative for a nationally recognized pharmaceutical company, and his hectic travel schedule was beginning to take a toll on his health. A few weeks ago, his doctor suggested he rethink his career goals. "You know, stress and this disease don't mix," Dr. Wettstein reminded him. "Why don't you look for something closer to home?"

That evening over lasagna, his wife Emily suggested teaching. Hernani had enjoyed sharing the challenging concepts of math and science with seventh graders during the 6 years he had taught in a rural school upstate. It was only the financial demands of Kim and Kili's birth 7 years ago that had tempted him into the better paying field of pharmaceuticals.

Hernani sent out resumes for the next 5 weeks. Finally, one was well received by South Hills Middle School. They had an opening in their math department, plus a need for someone to coach afterschool athletics, and they wanted to meet with him. He hadn't interviewed since the twins were born. He thought about the questions normally asked—would there be some questions about his health? Being HIV positive shouldn't have any bearing on his ability to teach, but parents might be concerned about having him coach. And it might disqualify him for the school's health insurance policy. Hernani believed in honesty, but what would happen if he revealed his HIV status?

Suggested Discussion Topics

1. Do you think Hernani should reveal his HIV status to South Hills Middle School? If so, why? If not, why not?

2. Do you think South Hills Middle School would hire Hernani for a coaching job if they knew he was HIV positive? Why or why not? Would the possibility of a team or coaching injury, and the bloodborne transmission of HIV, affect their decision?
3. If South Hills Middle School decided that Hernani was not suitable for a coaching job, would they consider him for a different teaching position?
4. How would you feel if your child were in a class Hernani was teaching or on one of the teams he was coaching? Why?

Scott J. Barnard

Medical Terminology for Health Professions 4.0

CHAPTER 7

THE RESPIRATORY SYSTEM

This list contains essential word parts and medical terms for this chapter.

Word Parts
- bronch/o, bronchi/o
- cyan/o
- laryng/o
- ox/i, ox/o, ox/y
- pharyng/o
- phon/o
- pleur/o
- -pnea
- pneum/o, pneumon/o, pneuh pulm/o, pulmon/o
- somn/o
- spir/o
- tachyh thorac/o, -thorax
- trache/o

Medical Terms
- anoxia (ah-NOCK-see-ah)
- anthracosis (an-thrah-KOH-sis)
- antitussive (an-tih-TUSS-iv)
- aphonia (ah-FOH-nee-ah)
- apnea (AP-nee-ah)
- asbestosis (ass-beh-STOH-sis)
- asphyxia (ass-FICK-see-ah)
- asphyxiation (ass-fick-see-AY-shun)
- aspiration pneumonia (ass-pih-RAY-shun)
- asthma (AZ-mah)
- atelectasis (at-ee-LEK-tah-sis)
- bradypnea (brad-ihp-NEE-ah)
- bronchodilator (brong-koh-dye-LAY-tor)
- bronchorrhea (brong-koh-REE-ah)

- bronchoscopy (brong-KOS-koh-pee)
- bronchospasm (brong-koh-spazm)
- Cheyne-Stokes respiration (CHAYN-STOHKS)
- croup (KROOP)
- cystic fibrosis (SIS-tick figh-BROH-sis)
- diphtheria (dif-THEE-ree-ah)
- dysphonia (dis-FOH-nee-ah)
- dyspnea (DISP-nee-ah)
- emphysema (em-fih-SEE-mah)
- empyema (em-pye-EE-mah)
- endotracheal intubation (en-doh-TRAY-kee-al in-too-BAY-shun)
- epistaxis (ep-ih-STACK-sis)
- hemoptysis (hee-MOP-tih-sis)
- hemothorax (hee-moh-THOH-racks)
- hypercapnia (high-per-KAP-nee-ah)
- hyperpnea (high-perp-NEE-ah)
- hypopnea (high-poh-NEE-ah)
- hypoxemia (high-pock-SEE-mee-ah)
- hypoxia (high-POCK-see-ah)
- laryngectomy (lar-in-JECK-toh-mee)
- laryngitis (lar-in-JIGH-tis)
- laryngoplegia (lar-ing-goh-PLEE-jee-ah)
- laryngoscopy (lar-ing-GOS-koh-pee)
- mediastinum (mee-dee-as-TYE-num)
- nebulizer (NEB-you-lye-zer)
- otolaryngologist (oh-toh-lar-in-GOL-oh-jist)
- pertussis (per-TUS-is)
- pharyngitis (fah-rin-JIGH-tis)
- pharyngoplasty (fah-RING-goh-plas-tee)
- pleurectomy (ploor-ECK-toh-mee)
- pleurisy (PLOOR-ih-see)
- pleurodynia (ploor-oh-DIN-ee-ah)
- pneumoconiosis (new-moh-koh-nee-OH-sis)
- pneumonectomy (new-moh-NECK-toh-mee)
- pneumothorax (new-moh-THOR-racks)
- polysomnography (pol-ee-som-NOG-rah-fee)
- pulmonologist (pull-mah-NOL-oh-jist)
- pulse oximeter (ock-SIM-eh-ter)
- pyothorax (pye-oh-THOH-racks)
- sinusitis (sigh-nuh-SIGH-tis)
- tachypnea (tack-ihp-NEE-ah)
- thoracentesis (thoh-rah-sen-TEE-sis)
- thoracostomy (thoh-rah-KOS-toh-mee)
- tracheostomy (tray-kee-OS-toh-mee)

- tracheotomy (tray-kee-OT-oh-mee)
- tuberculosis (too-ber-kew-LOH-sis)

Objectives

On completion of this chapter, you should be able to:
1. Identify and describe the major structures and functions of the respiratory system.
2. Recognize, define, spell, and pronounce terms related to the pathology and the diagnostic and treatment procedures of the respiratory system.

Structures Of The Respiratory System

The respiratory system brings oxygen into the body for transportation to the cells. It also removes carbon dioxide and some water waste from the body. For descriptive purposes, the respiratory system is divided into upper and lower respiratory tracts.

The upper respiratory tract consists of the nose, mouth, pharynx, epiglottis, larynx, and trachea.

The lower respiratory tract consists of the bronchial tree and lungs. These structures are located within, and protected by, the thoracic cavity which is also known as the rib cage.

The Nose

Air enters the body through the nose and passes through the nasal cavity, which is the interior portion of the nose.

- The nasal septum (NAY-zal SEP-tum) is a wall of cartilage that divides the nose into two equal sections. A septum is a wall that separates two chambers.
- Cilia (SIL-ee-ah), the thin hairs located just inside the nostrils, filter incoming air to remove debris.
- Mucous membranes (MYOU-kus) are the specialized tissues that line the respiratory, digestive, reproductive, and urinary systems.
- Mucus (MYOU-kus), which is secreted by the mucous membranes, protects and lubricates these tissues. In the nose mucus helps to moisten, warm, and filter the air as it enters. Notice the different spellings; however, they have the same pronunciation. Mucous is the name of the tissue; mucus is the secretion that flows from the tissue.
- The olfactory receptors (ol-FACK-toh-ree) are nerve endings that act as the receptors for the sense of smell. They are also important to the sense of taste. These receptors are located in the mucous membrane in the upper part of the nasal cavity.

The Tonsils

The tonsils form a protective circle of lymphatic tissue around the entrance to the respiratory system.

The Paranasal Sinuses

The paranasal sinuses, which are air-filled cavities lined with mucous membrane, are located in the bones of the skull. These sinuses are connected to the nasal cavity via short ducts (para- means near, nas means nose, and -al means pertaining to).

The functions of these sinuses are (1) to make the bones of the skull lighter, (2) to help produce sound by giving resonance to the voice, and (3) to produce mucus to provide lubrication for the tissues of the nasal cavity. The four paired sinuses are located on either side of the nose and are named for the bones in which they are located.

- The frontal sinuses are located in the frontal bone just above the eyebrows. An infection here can cause severe pain in this area.
- The sphenoid sinuses, which are located in the sphenoid bone, are close to the optic nerves and an infection here can damage vision.
- The maxillary sinuses, which are the largest of the paranasal sinuses, are located in the maxillary bones. An infection in these sinuses can cause pain in the posterior maxillary teeth.
- The ethmoid sinuses, which are located in the ethmoid bones, are irregularly shaped air cells that are separated from the orbital (eye) cavity by only a thin layer of bone.

The Pharynx

The pharynx (FAR-inks), which is commonly known as the throat, receives the air after it passes through the nose. The pharynx is made up of three divisions.

- The nasopharynx (nay-zoh-FAR-inks), which is the first division, is posterior to the nasal cavity and continues downward to behind the mouth (nas/o means nose, and -pharynx means throat). This portion of the pharynx is used only by the respiratory system for the transport of air and opens into the oropharynx.
- The oropharynx (oh-roh-FAR-inks), which is the second division, is the portion that is visible when looking into the mouth (or/o means mouth, and -pharynx means throat). The oropharynx is shared by the respiratory and digestive systems and transports air, food, and fluids downward to the laryngopharynx.
- The laryngopharynx (lah-ring-goh-FAR-inks), which is the third division, is also shared by both the respiratory and digestive systems (laryng/o means larynx, and -pharynx means throat). Air, food, and fluids continue downward to the openings of the esophagus and trachea where air enters the trachea and food and fluids flow into the esophagus.

The Larynx

- The larynx (LAR-inks), also known as the voice box, is a triangular chamber located between the pharynx and the trachea.

- The larynx is protected and supported by a series of nine separate cartilages. The thyroid cartilage is the largest, and when enlarged, it is commonly known as the Adam's apple.
- The larynx contains the vocal cords. During breathing, the cords are separated to let air pass. During speech, they close together, and sound is produced as air is expelled from the lungs, causing the cords to vibrate against each other.

Protective Swallowing Mechanisms

The respiratory and digestive systems share part of the pharynx. During swallowing, there is the risk of a blocked airway or pneumonia caused by food or water going into the trachea and entering the lungs instead of traveling into the esophagus. Two protective mechanisms act automatically during swallowing to ensure that only air goes into the lungs.
- During swallowing, the soft palate, which is the muscular posterior portion of the roof of the mouth, moves up and backward to close off the nasopharynx. This movement prevents food or liquid from going up into the nose.
- At the same time, the epiglottis (ep-ih-GLOT-is), which is a lid-like structure located at the base of the tongue, swings downward and closes off the laryngopharynx so that food does not enter the trachea and the lungs.

The Trachea
- The trachea (TRAY-kee-ah), commonly known as the windpipe, is the tube located directly in front of the esophagus that extends from the neck to the chest. Its role is to transport air to, and from, the lungs.
- The trachea is held open by a series of C-shaped cartilage rings. The wall between these rings is flexible, and this feature makes it possible for the trachea to adjust to different body positions.
- Within the lung, each primary bronchus divides and subdivides into increasingly smaller bronchioles (BRONG-kee-ohlz), which are the smallest branches of the bronchi.

The Alveoli
- Alveoli (al-VEE-oh-lye), also known as air sacs, are the very small grape-like clusters found at the end of each bronchiole (singular, alveolus). Each lung contains millions of alveoli that are filled with air from the bronchioles.
- A network of microscopic pulmonary capillaries surrounds the thin, elastic walls of the alveoli.
- During respiration, the exchange of oxygen and carbon dioxide between the alveolar air and the pulmonary capillary blood occurs through the walls of the alveoli.

The Lungs
The lungs, which are the organs of respiration, are divided into lobes. A lobe is a subdivision or part of an organ.
- The right lung has three lobes: the superior, middle, and inferior.
-
- The left lung has only two lobes: the superior and inferior. It is slightly smaller than the right lung because of the space taken up by the heart.
- The lungs produce a detergent-like substance, known as a surfactant, which reduces the surface tension of the lungs. This allows air to flow over the lungs and be absorbed more easily.

The Mediastinum
- The mediastinum (mee-dee-as-TYE-num) is the cavity located between the lungs. This cavity contains connective tissue and organs, including the heart and its veins and arteries, the esophagus, trachea, bronchi, the thymus gland, and lymph nodes.

The Pleura
- The pleura (PLOOR-ah) is a thin, moist, and slippery membrane that covers the outer surface of the lungs and lines the inner surface of the rib cage.
- The parietal pleura (pah-RYE-eh-tal) is the outer layer of the pleura that lines the walls of the thoracic cavity, covers the diaphragm, and forms the sac containing each lung. Parietal means relating to the walls of a cavity.
- The visceral pleura (VIS-er-al) is the inner layer of pleura that surrounds each lung. Visceral means relating to the internal organs.
- The pleural cavity, also known as the pleural space, is the airtight area between the layers of the pleural membranes. This space contains a thin layer of fluid that allows the membranes to slide easily during breathing.

The Diaphragm
The diaphragm (DYE-ah-fram) is the muscle that separates the thoracic cavity from the abdomen. It is the contraction and relaxation of this muscle that makes breathing possible. The phrenic nerves (FREN-ick) stimulate the diaphragm and cause it to contract.

Respiration
Respiration is the exchange of oxygen and carbon dioxide that is essential to life. A single respiration consists of one inhalation and one exhalation.

Inhalation and Exhalation
- Inhalation (in-hah-LAY-shun) is the act of taking in air as the diaphragm contracts and pulls downward. This action causes the thoracic cavity to

expand. This produces a vacuum within the thoracic cavity that draws air into the lungs.
- Exhalation (ecks-hah-LAY-shun) is the act of breathing out. As the diaphragm relaxes, it moves upward, causing the thoracic cavity to become narrower. This action forces air out of the lungs.

External Respiration
- External respiration is the act of bringing air into and out of the lungs and exchanging gases from this air.
- As air is inhaled into the alveoli, oxygen immediately passes into the surrounding capillaries and is carried by the erythrocytes (red blood cells) to all body cells.
- At the same time, the waste product carbon dioxide that has passed into the bloodstream is transported into the airspaces of the lungs to be exhaled.

Internal Respiration
- Internal respiration is the exchange of gases within the cells of the body organs, cells, and tissues.
- In this process, oxygen passes from the bloodstream into the cells.
- The cells give off the waste product carbon dioxide, and this passes into the bloodstream.
- The bloodstream transports the carbon dioxide to the lungs where it is expelled during exhalation.

Medical Specialties Related To The Respiratory System
- An otolaryngologist (oh-toh-lar-in-GOL-oh-jist), also known as an ENT, is a physician with specialized training in the diagnosis and treatment of diseases and disorders of the ears, nose, throat, and related structures of the head and neck (ot/o means ear, laryng/o means larynx, and -ologist means specialist).
- A pulmonologist (pull-mah-NOL-oh-jist) is a physician who specializes in diagnosing and treating diseases and disorders of the lungs and associated tissues (pulmon means lung, and -ologist means specialist).

Pathology Of The Respiratory System

Chronic Obstructive Pulmonary Diseases
Chronic obstructive pulmonary disease, also known as COPD, is a lung disease in which it is hard to breathe. In this condition, damage to the bronchi partially obstructs them, making it difficult to get air in and out. Most people with COPD, who are usually smokers or former smokers, also have both chronic bronchitis and emphysema.

Chronic Bronchitis

In chronic bronchitis (brong-KYE-tis), the airways have become inflamed and thickened, and there is an increase in the number and size of mucus-producing cells (bronch means bronchus, and -itis means inflammation). This results in excessive mucus production, which in turn causes coughing and difficulty getting air in and out of the lungs.

Emphysema

Emphysema (em-fih-SEE-mah) is the progressive loss of lung function that is characterized by (1) a decrease in the total number of alveoli, (2) the enlargement of the remaining alveoli, and (3) the progressive destruction of the walls of the remaining alveoli.

As the alveoli are destroyed, breathing becomes increasingly rapid, shallow, and difficult. In an effort to compensate for the loss of capacity, the lungs expand, and the chest sometimes assumes an enlarged barrel shape.

Asthma

- Asthma (AZ-mah) is a chronic allergic disorder characterized by episodes of severe breathing difficulty, coughing, and wheezing. These episodes are known as asthmatic attacks. Wheezing is a breathing sound caused by a partially obstructed airway. The frequency and severity of asthmatic attacks is influenced by a variety of factors including allergens, environmental agents, exercise, or infection.
- Airway inflammation is the swelling and clogging of the airways with mucus. This usually occurs after the airway has been exposed to inhaled allergens.
- A bronchospasm (brong-koh-spazm) is a contraction of the smooth muscle in the walls of the bronchi and bronchioles that tighten and squeeze the airway shut (bronch/o means bronchi, and -spasm means involuntary contraction).
- Exercise-induced bronchospasms (EIB) are the narrowing of the airways that develops after 5–15 minutes of physical exertion. This also can be due to cold weather or allergies.

Asthma Treatment

Most asthmatics take two kinds of medicines. Controller medicines, such as inhaled corticosteroids, are taken daily to prevent attacks. These medications help to control inflammation and to stop the airways from reacting to the factors that trigger the asthma. quick-relief, or rescue medicines, are taken at the first sign of an attack to dilate the airways and make breathing easier. These medications are known as bronchodilators and are discussed later in this chapter under medications.

Upper Respiratory Diseases

- Upper respiratory infections and acute nasopharyngitis are among the terms used to describe the common cold. An upper respiratory infection can be caused by any one of 200 different viruses.
- Allergic rhinitis (rye-NIGH-tis), commonly referred to as an allergy, is an allergic reaction to airborne allergens that causes an increased flow of mucus (rhin means nose, and -itis means inflammation).
- Croup (KROOP) is an acute respiratory syndrome in children and infants characterized by obstruction of the larynx, hoarseness, and a barking cough.
- Diphtheria (dif-THEE-ree-ah), now largely prevented through immunization, is an acute bacterial infection of the throat and upper respiratory tract. The diphtheria bacteria produce toxins that can damage the heart muscle and peripheral nerves.
- Epistaxis (ep-ih-STACK-sis), also known as a nosebleed, is bleeding from the nose that is usually caused by an injury, excessive use of blood thinners, or bleeding disorders.
- Influenza (in-flew-EN-zah), also known as the flu, is an acute, highly contagious viral respiratory infection that is spread by respiratory droplets and occurs most commonly in epidemics during the colder months. There are many strains of the influenza virus. Some strains can be prevented by annual immunization.
- Pertussis (per-TUS-is), also known as whooping cough, is a contagious bacterial infection of the upper respiratory tract that is characterized by recurrent bouts of a paroxysmal cough, followed by breathlessness, and a noisy inspiration. Paroxysmal means sudden or spasm-like.
- Rhinorrhea (rye-noh-REE-ah), also known as a runny nose, is the watery flow of mucus from the nose (rhin/o means nose, and -rrhea means abnormal discharge).
- Sinusitis (sigh-nuh-SIGH-tis) is an inflammation of the sinuses (sinus means sinus, and -itis means inflammation).

Pharynx and Larynx

- Pharyngitis (fah-rin-JIGH-tis), also known as a sore throat, is an inflammation of the pharynx (pharyng means pharynx, and -itis means inflammation).
- Laryngoplegia (lar-ing-goh-PLEE-jee-ah) is paralysis of the larynx (laryng/o means larynx, and -plegia means paralysis).
- A laryngospasm (lah-RING-goh-spazm) is the sudden spasmodic closure of the larynx (laryng/o means larynx, and -spasm means a sudden involuntary contraction).

Voice Disorders

- Aphonia (ah-FOH-nee-ah) is the loss of the ability of the larynx to produce normal speech sounds (a- means without, phon means voice or sound, and -ia means abnormal condition).
- Dysphonia (dis-FOH-nee-ah) is any change in vocal quality, including hoarseness, weakness, or the cracking of a boy's voice during puberty (dys- means bad, phon means voice or sound, and -ia means abnormal condition).
- Laryngitis (lar-in-JIGH-tis) is an inflammation of the larynx (laryng means larynx, and -itis means inflammation This term is also commonly used to describe voice loss that is caused by this inflammation.

Trachea and Bronchi

- Tracheorrhagia (tray-kee-oh-RAY-jee-ah) is bleeding from the mucous membranes of the trachea (trache/o means trachea, and -rrhagia means bleeding).
- Bronchorrhea (brong-koh-REE-ah) is an excessive discharge of mucus from the bronchi (bronch/o means bronchus, and -rrhea means abnormal flow).

Pleural Cavity

- Pleurisy (PLOOR-ih-see), also known as pleuritis, is an inflammation of the pleura that produces sharp chest pain with each breath. Pleurisy can be caused by influenza or by damage to the lung beneath the pleura (pleur means pleura, and -isy is a noun ending).
- Pleurodynia (ploor-oh-DIN-ee-ah) is pain in the pleura that occurs in relation to breathing movements (pleur/o means pleura, and -dynia means pain).
- A pneumothorax (new-moh-THOR-racks) is the accumulation of air in the pleural space causing a pressure imbalance that prevents the lung from fully expanding or can cause it to collapse (pneum/o means lung or air, and -thorax means chest). This can have an external cause such as a stab wound through the chest wall. It can be caused internally by a rupture in the pleura that allows air to leak into the pleural space.
- Pleural effusion (eh-FEW-zhun) is the abnormal accumulation of fluid in the pleural space. This produces a feeling of breathlessness because it prevents the lung from fully expanding. Effusion is the escape of fluid from blood or lymphatic vessels into the tissues or into a body cavity.
- Hemothorax (hee-moh-THOH-racks) is a collection of blood in the pleural cavity (hem/o means blood, and -thorax means chest). This condition often results from chest trauma, such as a stab wound, or it can be caused by disease or surgery.
- Hemoptysis (hee-MOP-tih-sis) is coughing up of blood or bloodstained sputum derived from the lungs or bronchial tubes as the result of a

pulmonary or bronchial hemorrhage (hem/o means blood, and -ptysis means spitting).
- Pyothorax (pye-oh-THOH-racks) is the presence of pus in the pleural cavity between the layers of the pleural membrane (py/o means pus, and -thorax means chest). This condition is also known as empyema of the pleural cavity. An empyema (em-pye-EE-mah) is a collection of pus within a body cavity.

Lungs

- Acute respiratory distress syndrome (ARDS) is not a specific disease. Instead, it is a form of the sudden onset of severe lung dysfunction affecting both lungs, making breathing extremely difficult. This syndrome is caused by trauma (injury), sepsis (systemic infection), diffuse (wide spread) pneumonia, or shock.
- Atelectasis (at-ee-LEK-tah-sis) is the collapse of part or all of a lung by blockage of the air passages or by very shallow breathing (atel means incomplete, and -ectasis means stretching or enlargement).
- A collapsed lung is unable to expand to receive air due to a pneumothorax or atelectasis.
- Pulmonary edema (eh-DEE-mah) is an accumulation of fluid in lung tissues. Edema means swelling.
- Pneumorrhagia (new-moh-RAY-jee-ah) is bleeding from the lungs (pneum/o means lungs, and -rrhagia means bleeding).

Tuberculosis

- Tuberculosis (too-ber-kew-LOH-sis) (TB), which is an infectious disease caused by Mycobacterium tuberculosis, usually attacks the lungs; however, it can also affect other parts of the body.
- TB occurs most commonly in individuals whose immune systems are weakened by another condition. A healthy individual can carry TB without showing symptoms of the disease.
- Multidrug-resistant tuberculosis is a dangerous form of tuberculosis because the germs have become resistant to the effect of the primary TB drugs.

Pneumonia Named for the Affected Lung Tissue

Pneumonia (new-MOH-nee-ah) is a serious infection or inflammation of the lungs in which the smallest bronchioles and alveoli fill with pus and other liquid (pneumon means lung, and -ia means abnormal condition). There are two types of pneumonia named for the parts of the lungs affected. These are:
- Bronchopneumonia (brong-koh-new-MOH-nee-ah) is a localized form of pneumonia that often affects the bronchioles and surrounding alveoli (bronch/o means bronchial tubes, pneumon means lung, and -ia means abnormal condition).

- Lobar pneumonia affects larger areas of the lungs, often including one or more sections, or lobes, of a lung. Double pneumonia is lobar pneumonia involving both lungs, and is usually a form of bacterial pneumonia.

Pneumonia Named for the Causative Agent

As many as 30 causes of pneumonia have been identified; however, the most common causative agents are inhaled substances, bacteria, fungi, and viruses.

- Aspiration pneumonia (ass-pih-RAY-shun) can occur when a foreign substance, such as vomit, is inhaled into the lungs. As used here, aspiration means inhaling or drawing a foreign substance into the upper respiratory tract.
- Bacterial pneumonia, which is often caused by Streptococcus pneumoniae, is the only form of pneumonia that can be prevented through vaccination.
- Mycoplasma pneumonia (my-koh-PLAZ-mah new- MOH-nee-ah) is a milder but longer lasting form of the disease caused by the bacteria Mycoplasma pneumoniae. It is sometimes referred to as walking pneumonia because often the patient is not bedridden.
- Pneumocystis carinii pneumonia (new-moh-SIS-tis kah-RYE-nee-eye new-MOH-nee-ah) is an opportunistic infection caused by the fungus Pneumocystis carinii.
- Viral pneumonia, which is caused by several different types of viruses, accounts for approximately half of all pneumonias.

Interstitial Lung Diseases

- Interstitial lung diseases (in-ter-STISH-al) are a group of almost 200 diseases that cause inflammation and scarring of the alveoli and their supporting structures. Interstitial means pertaining to between, but not within, the parts of a tissue. These lung conditions lead to a reduction of oxygen being transferred to the blood.
- Interstitial fibrosis is another name for the inflammation and thickening of the walls of the alveoli. Fibrosis is a condition in which normal tissue is replaced by fibrotic (hardened) tissue.
- Many connective tissue diseases such as rheumatoid arthritis, scleroderma, and lupus can cause interstitial lung disease. These conditions are also caused by environmental and occupational toxins that are inhaled.

Environmental and Occupational Lung Diseases

- Pneumoconiosis (new-moh-koh-nee-OH-sis) is fibrosis of the lung tissues caused by dust in the lungs that usually develops after prolonged environmental or occupational contact (pneum/o means lung, coni means dust, and -osis means abnormal condition or disease).

- Anthracosis (an-thrah-KOH-sis), also known as coal miner's pneumoconiosis or black lung disease, is caused by coal dust in the lungs (anthrac means coal dust, and -osis means abnormal condition or disease).
- Asbestosis (ass-beh-STOH-sis) is caused by asbestos particles in the lungs and usually occurs after working with asbestos (asbest means asbestos, and -osis means abnormal condition or disease).
- Byssinosis (biss-ih-NOH-sis), also known as brown lung disease, is caused by inhaling cotton dust into the lungs and usually occurs after working in a textile factory (byssin means cotton dust, and -osis means abnormal condition or disease).
- Silicosis (sill-ih-KOH-sis) is caused by inhaling silica dust in the lungs and usually occurs after working in occupations including foundry work, quarrying, ceramics, glass work, and sandblasting (silic means glass, and -osis means abnormal condition or disease).

Pulmonary Fibrosis

Pulmonary fibrosis (figh-BROH-sis) is the formation of scar tissue in the lung, resulting in decreased lung capacity and increased difficulty in breathing. This condition can be caused by autoimmune disorders, infections, dust, gases, toxins, and some drugs.

Cystic Fibrosis

Cystic fibrosis (SIS-tick figh-BROH-sis) is a genetic disorder in which the lungs and pancreas are clogged with large quantities of abnormally thick mucus. Treatment for cystic fibrosis includes:
- Digestive enzymes are administered to aid the digestive system.
- Antibiotics are administered to control lung infections.
- Postural drainage is performed with the patient positioned at various angles to allow gravity to help drain secretions from the lungs.
- Chest percussion is also performed to remove excess mucus from the lungs.

Breathing Disorders

The general term breathing disorders describes abnormal changes in the rate or depth of breathing. Specific terms describe in greater detail the changes that are occurring.
- Eupnea (youp-NEE-ah) is easy or normal breathing (eu- means good, and -pnea means breathing). This is the baseline for judging some breathing disorders. Eupnea is the opposite of apnea.
- Apnea (AP-nee-ah) is the absence of spontaneous respiration (a- means without and -pnea means breathing). Apnea is the opposite of eupnea.
- Sleep apnea syndromes are a group of potentially fatal disorders in which breathing repeatedly stops during sleep for long-enough periods to cause a measurable decrease in blood oxygen levels. Snoring, which

- can be a symptom of sleep apnea, is noisy breathing caused by vibration of the soft palate during sleep.
- Bradypnea (brad-ihp-NEE-ah) is an abnormally slow rate of respiration usually of less than 10 breaths per minute (brady- means slow, and -pnea means breathing). Bradypnea is the opposite of tachypnea.
- Tachypnea (tack-ihp-NEE-ah) is an abnormally rapid rate of respiration usually of more than 20 breaths per minute (tachy-means rapid, and -pneameans breathing). Tachypnea is the opposite of bradypnea.
- Cheyne-Stokes respiration (CHAYN-STOHKS) is a pattern of alternating periods of hypopnea or apnea, followed by hyperpnea.
- Dyspnea (DISP-nee-ah), also known as shortness of breath (SOB), is difficult or labored breathing (dysmeans painful, and -pnea means breathing). Shortness of breath is frequently one of the first symptoms of heart failure. It can also be caused by strenuous physical exertion or can be due to lung damage that produces dyspnea even at rest.
- Hyperpnea (high-perp-NEE-ah), which is commonly associated with exertion, is breathing that is deeper and more rapid than is normal at rest (hyper- means excessive, and -pnea means breathing). Hyperpnea is the opposite of hypopnea.
- Hypopnea (high-poh-NEE-ah) is shallow or slow respiration (hypo- means decreased, and -pnea means breathing). Hypopnea is the opposite of hyperpnea.
- Hyperventilation (high-per-ven-tih-LAY-shun) is an abnormally rapid rate of deep respiration that is usually associated with anxiety (hyper- means excessive, and -ventilation means breathing). This causes changes in the blood gas levels due to a decrease in carbon dioxide at the cellular level.

Lack of Oxygen

- Airway obstruction, commonly known as choking, occurs when food or a foreign object blocks the airway and prevents air from entering or leaving the lungs. This is a life-threatening emergency requiring immediate action by performing the abdominal thrust maneuver. This is also known as the Heimlich maneuver.
- Anoxia (ah-NOCK-see-ah) is the absence of oxygen from the body's gases, blood, or tissues (an- means without, ox means oxygen, and -ia means abnormal condition). If anoxia continues for more than 4–6 minutes, irreversible brain damage can occur.
- Asphyxia (ass-FICK-see-ah) is the condition that occurs when the body cannot get the air it needs to function. In this life-threatening condition, oxygen levels in the blood drop quickly, carbon dioxide levels rise, and unless the patient's breathing is restored within a few minutes, death or serious brain damage follows.
- Asphyxiation (ass-fick-see-AY-shun), also known as suffocation, is any interruption of normal breathing resulting in asphyxia. Asphyxiation can

be caused by an airway obstruction, drowning, smothering, choking, or inhaling gases such as carbon monoxide instead of air.
- Cyanosis (sigh-ah-NOH-sis) is a bluish discoloration of the skin caused by a lack of adequate oxygen (cyan means blue, and -osis means abnormal condition or disease).
- Hypercapnia (high-per-KAP-nee-ah) is the abnormal buildup of carbon dioxide in the blood (hyper- means excessive, capn means carbon dioxide, and -ia means abnormal condition).
- Hypoxemia (high-pock-SEE-mee-ah) is a condition of having below-normal oxygen level in the blood (hypmeans deficient, ox means oxygen, and -emia means blood). This condition is less severe than anoxia. Compare with hypoxia.
- Hypoxia (high-POCK-see-ah) is the condition of having below-normal oxygen levels in the body tissues and cells; however, it is less severe than anoxia (hyp- means deficient, ox means oxygen, and -ia means abnormal condition). Compare with hypoxemia.
- Altitude hypoxia, also known as altitude sickness, is a condition that can be brought on by the decreased oxygen in the air at higher altitudes, usually above 8,000 feet.
- Respiratory failure (RF), also known as respiratory acidosis, is a condition in which the level of oxygen in the blood becomes dangerously low or the level of carbon dioxide becomes dangerously high.
- Smoke inhalation is damage to the lungs in which particles from a fire coat the alveoli and prevent the normal exchange of gases.

Diagnostic Procedures Of The Respiratory System

- Bronchoscopy (brong-KOS-koh-pee) is the visual examination of the bronchi using a bronchoscope (bronch/o means bronchus, and -scopy means direct visual examination). A bronchoscope is a flexible, fiber optic device that is passed through the nose and down the airways. It can also be used for operative procedures, such as tissue repair, or the removal of a foreign object.
- Chest imaging, also known as a chest x-ray, is a valuable tool for diagnosing pneumonia, lung tumors, pneumothorax, pleural effusion, tuberculosis, and emphysema.
- Laryngoscopy (lar-ing-GOS-koh-pee) is the visual examination of the larynx using a laryngoscope inserted through the mouth and placed into the pharynx to examine the larynx (laryng/o means larynx, and -scopy means a direct visual examination). Mirror laryngoscopy is a simpler version of this test in which the larynx is viewed by shining a light on an angled mirror held at the back of the soft palate.
- A peak flow meter is a handheld device often used to test those with asthma to measure how quickly the patient can expel air.
- Polysomnography (pol-ee-som-NOG-rah-fee), also known as a sleep apnea study, measures physiological activity during sleep and is most

- often performed to detect nocturnal defects in breathing associated with sleep apnea (poly- means many, somn/o means sleep, and -graphy means the process of recording).
- Pulmonary function tests (PFT) are a group of tests that measure volume and flow of air by utilizing a spirometer. These tests are measured against a norm for the individual's age, height, and sex.
- A spirometer (spih-ROM-eh-ter) is a recording device that measures the amount of air inhaled or exhaled (volume) and the length of time required for each breath (spir/o means to breathe, and -meter means to measure).
- A pulse oximeter (ock-SIM-eh-ter) is an external monitor placed on the patient's finger or earlobe to measure the oxygen saturation level in the blood (ox/i means oxygen, and -meter means to measure). In a normal reading, 95%–100% of the blood is saturated by oxygen.
- Sputum (SPYOU-tum) is phlegm ejected through the mouth that can be examined for diagnostic purposes. Phlegm (FLEM) is thick mucus secreted by the tissues lining the respiratory passages.

Tuberculosis Testing

- Tuberculin skin testing is a screening test for tuberculosis in which the skin of the arm is injected with a harmless antigen extracted from TB bacteria. The tuberculin tine test is performed using an instrument with several small prongs called tines. A positive result indicates the possibility of exposure to the disease, and this response warrants further testing.
- The Mantoux PPD skin test is considered a more accurate skin test for diagnosing tuberculosis. A very small amount of PPD tuberculin (a purified protein derivative) is injected just under the top layer of the skin on the forearm. The site is checked for a reaction 48–72 hours later.

Treatment Procedures Of The Respiratory System

Medications and Their Administration

- An antitussive (an-tih-TUSS-iv), commonly known as cough medicine, is administered to prevent or relieve coughing (anti- means against, tuss means cough, and -ive means performs).
- A bronchodilator (brong-koh-dye-LAY-tor) is a medication that expands the opening of the passages into the lungs. At the first sign of an asthma attack, the patient uses a metered-dose inhaler to self-administer the bronchodilator.
- A metered-dose inhaler mixes a single dose of the medication with a puff of air and pushes it into the mouth via a chemical propellant.
- A nebulizer (NEB-you-lye-zer), also known as an atomizer, pumps air or oxygen through a liquid medicine to turn it into a vapor, which is then inhaled by the patient via a face mask or mouth piece.

The Nose, Throat, and Larynx
- Endotracheal intubation (en-doh-TRAY-kee-al in-too- BAY-shun) is the passage of a tube through the nose or mouth into the trachea to establish or maintain an open airway (endo- means within, trache means trachea, and -al means pertaining to). Intubation is the insertion of a tube, usually for the passage of air or fluids.
- Functional endoscopic sinus surgery (FESS) is a procedure performed using an endoscope in which chronic sinusitis is treated by enlarging the opening between the nose and sinus.
- A laryngectomy (lar-in-JECK-toh-mee) is the surgical removal of the larynx (laryng means larynx, and -ectomy means surgical removal).
- A laryngoplasty (lah-RING-goh-plas-tee) is the surgical repair of the larynx (laryng means larynx, and -plasty means surgical repair).
- Pharyngoplasty (fah-RING-goh-plas-tee) is the surgical repair of the pharynx (pharyng/o means pharynx, and -plasty means surgical repair).
- A pharyngotomy (far-ing-GOT-oh-mee) is a surgical incision of the pharynx (pharyng means pharynx and -otomy means a surgical incision).
- Septoplasty (SEP-toh-plas-tee) is the surgical repair or alteration of parts of the nasal septum (sept/o means septum, and -plasty means surgical repair).

The Trachea
- Tracheoplasty (TRAY-kee-oh-plas-tee) is the surgical repair of the trachea (trache/o means trachea, and -plasty means surgical repair).
- A tracheostomy(tray-kee-OS-toh-mee) is the creation of a stoma into the trachea and inserting a tube to facilitate the passage of air or the removal of secretions (trache means trachea, and -ostomymeans surgically creating an opening). Placement of this tube can be temporary or permanent. As used here, a stoma means a surgically created opening on a body surface.
- A tracheotomy (tray-kee-OT-oh-mee) is usually an emergency procedure in which an incision is made into the trachea to gain access to the airway below a blockage (trache means trachea, and -otomy means surgical incision).

The Lungs, Pleura, and Thorax
- A lobectomy(loh-BECK-toh-mee) is the surgical removal of a lobe of the lung (lob means lobe, and -ectomy means surgical removal). This term is also used to describe the removal of a lobe of the liver, brain, or thyroid gland.
- A pleurectomy (ploor-ECK-toh-mee) is the surgical removal of part of the pleura (pleur means pleura, and -ectomy means surgical removal).
- A pneumonectomy (new-moh-NECK-toh-mee) is the surgical removal of all or part of a lung (pneumon means lung, and -ectomy means surgical removal).

- Thoracentesis (thoh-rah-sen-TEE-sis) is the surgical puncture of the chest wall with a needle to obtain fluid from the pleural cavity (thor/a means chest, and -centesis means surgical puncture to remove fluid). This procedure is performed for diagnostic purposes or to drain excess fluid from severe pleural effusion.
- A thoracostomy (thoh-rah-KOS-toh-mee) is the surgical creation of an opening into the chest cavity (thorac means thorax or chest, and -ostomy means the surgical creation of an opening). This procedure is performed to establish drainage of empyema, which is pus in the pleural space.
- A thoracotomy (thoh-rah-KOT-toh-mee) is a surgical treatment of lung cancer by removing all or part of a lung (thorac means chest, and -otomy means surgical incision). This surgery involves cutting between the ribs on one side of the thorax and then removing the affected portion of the lung. A thoracotomy is also used for the visual examination of internal organs and the procurement of tissue specimens from the thorax.
- Video-assisted thoracic surgery (VATS) is the use of a video-assisted thoracoscope to view the inside of the chest cavity through very small incisions. A thoracoscope is a specialized endoscope used for treating the thorax. This procedure is used to obtain biopsy specimens to diagnose certain types of pneumonia, infections, or tumors of the chest wall. It is also used to treat repeatedly collapsing lungs.

Respiratory Therapy

- Diaphragmatic breathing, also known as abdominal breathing, is a relaxation technique used to relieve anxiety.
- A CPAP device (continuous positive airway pressure) is also known as a positive pressure ventilation device. This is treatment for sleep apnea that includes a mask, tubes, and a fan to create air pressure that pushes the tongue forward to maintain an open airway. Although this does not cure sleep apnea, it does reduce snoring and prevents dangerous apnea disturbances.
- A respirator is an apparatus for administering artificial respiration in cases of respiratory failure. For example, when a spinal cord injury destroys the natural breathing mechanism, the patient can continue to breathe through the use of a respirator. The term respirator also refers to any device that controls the quality of the air a person inhales. For example, it can also be a disposable dust mask or a piece of scuba diving equipment.
- A ventilator is a mechanical device for artificial ventilation of the lungs that is used to replace or supplement the patient's natural breathing function. The ventilator forces air into the lungs; exhalation takes place passively as the lungs contract.

Supplemental Oxygen

Supplemental oxygen is administered when the patient is unable to maintain an adequate oxygen saturation level in the blood. This oxygen is administered by the following methods.
- A nasal cannula is a small tube that divides into two nasal prongs.
- A rebreather mask allows the exhaled breath to be partially reused, delivering up to 60% oxygen.
- A non-rebreather mask allows higher levels of oxygen to be added to the air taken in by the patient.

Abbreviations Related To The Respiratory System
- bronchitis = BR, Br
- bronchoscopy = BRO, bronch
- Cheyne-Stokes breathing = CSB
- cystic fibrosis = CF
- diphtheria = diph
- Pneumocystis carinii pneumonia = PCP
- pneumothorax = Pno
- positive pressure ventilation = PPV
- sleep apnea syndromes = SAS
- upper respiratory infection = URI
-

Critical Thinking Exercise

The following story and questions are designed to stimulate critical thinking through class discussion or as a brief essay response. There are no right or wrong answers to these questions.

Sylvia Gaylord works as a legal aide on the twelfth floor of a tall glass-and-steel monument to modern architectural technology. On clear days, the views are spectacular. From her cubicle, Sylvia's eye catches the edge of the beautiful blue and white skyscape as she reaches for her inhaler. This is the third attack since she returned from lunch 4 hours ago—her asthma is really bad today. But if she leaves work early again, her boss will write her up for it. Sylvia concentrates on breathing normally.

Her roommate, Kelly, is a respiratory therapist at the county hospital. Kelly says Sylvia's asthma attacks are probably triggered by the city's high level of air pollution. That can't be true. They both run in the park every morning before work, and Sylvia rarely needs to use her inhaler. The problems start when she gets to work. The wheezing and coughing were so bad today that by the time she got up the elevator and into her cubicle, she could hardly breathe.

Last night, the cable news ran a story on the unhealthy air found in some buildings. They called it "sick building syndrome" and reported that certain employees developed allergic reactions just by breathing the air. "Hmmm," she thought, "It seems like more and more people are getting sick in our office. John has had the flu twice. Sid's bronchitis turned into bronchopneumonia, and Nging complains of sinusitis. Could this building have an air quality problem?"

Suggested Discussion Topics

1. Discuss which environmental factors might cause an asthma attack.
2. Discuss what Sylvia might do to find out if her building has an air quality problem.
3. What factors did Sylvia and Kelly consider as possible triggers for Sylvia's frequent attack?
4. If Sylvia's inhaler does not control her attack and her condition worsens, what steps should be taken promptly? Why?

Medical Terminology for Health Professions 4.0

CHAPTER 8

THE DIGESTIVE SYSTEM

This list contains essential word parts and medical terms for this chapter.

Word Parts

- an/o
- chol/e
- cholecyst/o
- col/o, colon/o
- -emesis
- enter/o
- esophag/o
- gastr/o
- hepat/o
- -lithiasis
- -pepsia
- -phagia
- proct/o
- rect/o
- sigmoid/o

Medical Terms

- aerophagia (ay-er-oh-FAY-jee-ah)
- amebic dysentery (ah-MEE-bik DIS-en-ter-ee)
- anastomosis (ah-nas-toh-MOH-sis)
- anorexia nervosa (an-oh-RECK-see-ah ner- VOH-sah)
- antiemetic (an-tih-ee-MET-ick)
- aphthous ulcers (AF-thus UL-serz)
- ascites (ah-SIGH-teez)
- bariatrics (bayr-ee-AT-ricks)
- borborygmus (bor-boh-RIG-mus)
- botulism (BOT-you-lizm)
- bulimia nervosa (byou-LIM-ee-ah ner-VOH-sah)
- cachexia (kah-KEKS-eeh-ah)

- cheilosis (kee-LOH-sis)
- cholangiography (koh-LAN-jee-og-rah-fee)
- cholangitis (koh-lan-JIGH tis)
- cholecystalgia (koh-lee-sis-TAL-jee-ah)
- cholecystectomy (koh-lee-sis-TECK-toh-mee)
- cholecystitis (koh-lee-sis-TYE-tis)
- choledocholithotomy (koh-led-oh-koh-lih-THOToh- mee)
- cholelithiasis (koh-lee-lih-THIGH-ah-sis)
- cholera (KOL-er-ah)
- cirrhosis (sih-ROH-sis)
- colonoscopy (koh-lun-OSS-koh-pee)
- Crohn's disease
- diverticulitis (dye-ver-tick-you-LYE-tis)
- diverticulosis (dye-ver-tick-you-LOH-sis)
- dyspepsia (dis-PEP-see-ah)
- dysphagia (dis-FAY-jee-ah)
- emesis (EM-eh-sis)
- enteritis (en-ter-EYE-tis)
- eructation (eh-ruk-TAY-shun)
- esophageal varices (eh-sof-ah-JEE-al VAYRih- seez)
- esophagogastroduodenoscopy (eh-sof-ah-goh-gastroh- dew-oh-deh-NOS-koh-pee)
- gastroduodenostomy (gas-troh-dew-oh-deh-NOStoh- mee)
- gastroesophageal reflux disease (gas-troh-eh-sofah- JEE-al REE flucks)
- gastrostomy tube (gas-TROS-toh-mee)
- hematemesis (hee-mah-TEM-eh-sis)
- Hemoccult test (HEE-moh-kult)
- hepatitis (hep-ah-TYE-tis)
- herpes labialis (HER-peez lay-bee-AL-iss)
- hiatal hernia (high-AY-tal HER-nee-ah)
- hyperemesis (high-per-EM-eh-sis)
- ileus (ILL-ee-us)
- inguinal hernia (ING-gwih-nal HERnee- ah)
- jaundice (JAWN-dis)
- melena (meh-LEE-nah)
- morbid obesity (MOR-bid oh-BEE-sih-tee) nasogastric intubation (nay-zoh-GAS-trick in-too- BAY-shun)
- obesity (oh-BEE-sih-tee)
- periodontium (pehr-ee-oh-DONshee- um)
- peristalsis (pehr-ih-STAL-sis)
- proctopexy (PROCK-toh-peck-see)
- regurgitation (ree-gur-jih-TAY-shun)
- salmonellosis (sal-moh-nel-LOH-sis)
- sigmoidoscopy (sig-moi-DOS-koh-pee)

- stomatorrhagia (stoh-mah-toh-RAY-jee-ah)
- trismus (TRIZ-mus)
- ulcerative colitis (UL-ser-ay-tiv koh-LYE-tis)
- volvulus (VOL-view-lus)
- xerostomia (zeer-oh-STOH-mee-ah)

Objectives

On completion of this chapter, you should be able to:
1. Identify and describe the major structures and functions of the digestive system.
2. Describe the processes of digestion, absorption, and metabolism.
3. Recognize, define, spell, and pronounce terms related to the pathology and the diagnostic and treatment procedures of the digestive system.

Structures Of The Digestive System

The major structures of the digestive system include the oral cavity (mouth), pharynx (throat), esophagus, stomach, small intestine, large intestine, rectum, and anus. The accessory organs of the digestive system aid with digestion, but are not part of the digestive system. These organs include the liver, gallbladder, and pancreas.

The Gastrointestinal Tract

The structures of the digestive system are also described as the gastrointestinal tract or GI tract (gastr/o means stomach, intestin means intestine, and -al means pertaining to).
- The upper GI tract consists of the mouth, esophagus, and stomach.
- The lower GI tract is made up of the small and large intestines (sometimes referred to as the bowels), plus the rectum, and anus.

The Oral Cavity

The major structures of the oral cavity, also known as the mouth, are the lips, hard and soft palates, salivary glands, tongue, teeth, and the periodontium.

The Lips

The lips, also known as labia, form the opening to the oral cavity (singular, labium). The term labia is also used to describe parts of the female genitalia. During eating, the lips hold food in the mouth and aid the tongue and cheeks in guiding food between the teeth for chewing. The lips also have important roles in breathing, speaking, and the expression of emotions.

The upper and lower labial frenum are narrow bands of tissue that attach the lips to the jaws.

The Palate

The palate (PAL-at) forms the roof of the mouth.

- The hard palate is the bony anterior portion of the palate that is covered with specialized mucous membrane. Rugae are irregular ridges or folds in this mucous membrane (singular, ruga).
- The soft palate is the flexible posterior portion of the palate. It has the important role of closing off the nasal passage during swallowing to prevent food and liquid from moving upward into the nasal cavity.
- The uvula (YOU-view-lah) hangs from the free edge of the soft palate. During swallowing, it moves upward with the soft palate. It also plays an important role in snoring and in the formation of some speech sounds.

The Tongue

The tongue is very strong, flexible, and muscular. It aids in speech and moves food during chewing and swallowing.
- The upper surface of the tongue is the dorsum. This surface has a tough protective covering and, in some areas, small bumps known as papillae (pah-PILL-ee) (singular, papilla). These papillae contain taste buds, which are the sensory receptors for the sense of taste.
- The sublingual surface of the tongue, and the tissues that lie under the tongue, are covered with delicate highly vascular tissues. Sublingual means under the tongue. Highly vascular means containing many blood vessels.
- It is the presence of this rich blood supply under the tongue that makes it suitable for administering certain medications by placing them sublingually where they are quickly absorbed into the bloodstream.
- The lingual frenum attaches the tongue to the floor of the mouth and limits its motion.

Soft Tissues of the Oral Cavity

- The periodontium (pehr-ee-oh-DON-shee-um) consists of the bone and soft tissues that surround and support the teeth (peri- means surrounding, odonti means the teeth, and -um is the noun ending).
- The gingiva (JIN-jih-vah), commonly known as the gums, is the specialized mucous membrane that surrounds the teeth, covers the bone of the dental arches, and lines the cheeks.

The Dental Arches

The boney structures of the oral cavity consist of the maxillary and mandibular arches. These structures, which are commonly referred to as the upper and lower jaws, firmly hold the teeth in position to facilitate chewing and speaking.
- The temporomandibular joint (tem-poh-roh-man- DIB-you-lar), commonly known as the TMJ, is formed at the back of themouth where the maxillary and mandibular arches come together. The maxillary arch, which is part of the skull, does not move. The mandibular arch, which is a separate bone, is the moveable component of this joint.

The Teeth

- The term dentition (den-TISH-un) refers to the natural teeth arranged in the upper and lower jaws.
- The human dentition includes four types of teeth: incisors and canines (also known as cuspids) that are used for biting and tearing, plus premolars (also known as bicuspids) and molars that are used for chewing and grinding.
- The primary dentition, also known as the deciduous dentition or baby teeth, consists of 20 teeth that are normally lost during childhood and are replaced by the permanent teeth. These teeth include: 8 incisors, 4 canines, 8 molars, and no premolars.
- The permanent dentition consists of 32 teeth that are designed to last a lifetime. These teeth include: 8 incisors, 4 canines, 8 premolars, and 12 molars.
- Edentulous (ee-DEN-too-lus) means without teeth. This term describes the situation after the natural permanent teeth have been lost.
- As used in dentistry, occlusion (ah-KLOO-zhun) describes any contact between the chewing surfaces of the upper and lower teeth.
- Malocclusion (mal-oh-KLOO-zhun) is any deviation from the normal positioning of the upper teeth against the lower teeth.

Structures and Tissues of the Teeth

The crown is the portion of a tooth that is visible in the mouth. It is covered with enamel, which is the hardest substance in the body.

- The roots of the tooth hold it securely in place within the dental arch. The roots are protected by cementum, which is strong, but not as hard as enamel.
- The cervix (neck) of the tooth is where the crown and root meet.
- Dentin makes up the bulk of the tooth structure and is protected on the outer surfaces by the enamel and cementum.
- The pulp consists of a rich supply of blood vessels and nerves that provide nutrients and innervation to the tooth. In the crown, the pulp is located in the pulp cavity. In the roots, the pulp continues through the root canals.

Saliva and Salivary Glands

Saliva is a colorless liquid that moistens the mouth, begins the digestive process, and lubricates food during chewing and swallowing. The three pairs of salivary glands (SALih- ver-ee) secrete saliva that is carried by ducts into the mouth.

- The parotid glands are located on the face in front of and slightly lower than each ear. The ducts for these glands are on the inside of the cheek near the upper molars.
- The sublingual glands and their ducts are located on the floor of the mouth under the tongue.

- The submandibular glands and their ducts are located on the floor of the mouth near the mandible.

The Pharynx

The pharynx (FAR-inks), which is the common passageway for both respiration and digestion.
- The epiglottis (ep-ih-GLOT-is) is a lid-like structure that closes off the entrance to the trachea (windpipe) to prevent food and liquids from moving from the pharynx during swallowing.

The Esophagus

- The esophagus (eh-SOF-ah-gus) is the muscular tube through which ingested food passes from the pharynx to the stomach.
- The lower esophageal sphincter, also known as the cardiac sphincter or the gastroesophageal sphincter, is a muscular ring controls the flow between the esophagus and stomach. This sphincter normally opens to allow the flow of food into the stomach and closes to prevent the stomach contents from regurgitating into the esophagus. Regurgitating means to flow backward.

The Stomach

- The stomach is a sac-like organ composed of the fundus (upper, rounded part), body (main portion), and antrum (lower part).
- Rugae (ROO-gay) are the folds in the mucosa lining the stomach. Glands located within these folds produce gastric juices that aid in digestion and mucus to create a protective coating on the lining of the stomach.
- The pylorus (pye-LOR-us) is the narrow passage that connects the stomach with the small intestine.
- The pyloric sphincter (pye-LOR-ick) is the ring-like muscle that controls the flow from the stomach to the duodenum of the small intestine.

The Small Intestine

The small intestine extends fromthe pyloric sphincter to the first part of the large intestine. The small intestine is a coiled organ up to 20 feet in length. The small intestine consists of three sections where food is digested and the nutrients are absorbed into the bloodstream.
- The duodenum (dew-oh-DEE-num) is the first portion of the small intestine. The duodenum extends from the pylorus to the jejunum.
- The jejunum (jeh-JOO-num) is the middle portion of the small intestine. The jejunum extends from the duodenum to the ileum.
- The ileum (ILL-ee-um), which is the last and longest portion of the small intestine, extends from the jejunum to the cecum of the large intestine.

The Large Intestine

The large intestine extends from the end of the small intestine to the anus. It is about twice as wide as the small intestine, but only one-fourth as long. It is here that the waste products of digestion are processed in preparation for excretion through the anus. The major parts of the large intestine are the cecum, colon, rectum, and anus.

The Cecum

The cecum (SEE-kum) is a pouch that lies on the right side of the abdomen. It extends from the end of the ileum to the beginning of the colon.

- The ileocecal sphincter (ill-ee-oh-SEE-kull) is the ringlike muscle that controls the flow from the ileum of the small intestine into the cecum of the large intestine.
- The vermiform appendix, commonly called the appendix, hangs from the lower portion of the cecum. The term vermiform refers to a worm-like shape. The appendix, which consists of lymphoid tissue.

The Colon

The colon, which is the longest portion of the large intestine, is subdivided into four parts:

- The ascending colon travels upward from the cecum to the undersurface of the liver. Ascending means upward.
- The transverse colon passes horizontally from right to left toward the spleen. Transverse means across.
- The descending colon travels down the left side of the abdominal cavity to the sigmoid colon. Descending means downward.
- The sigmoid colon (SIG-moid) is an S-shaped structure that continues from the descending colon above and joins with the rectum below. Sigmoid means curved like the letter S.

The Rectum and Anus

- The rectum, which is the widest division of the large intestine, makes up the last 4 inches of the large intestine and ends at the anus.
- The anus is the lower opening of the digestive tract. The flow of waste through the anus is controlled by the internal anal sphincter and the external anal sphincter.
- The term anorectal refers to the anus and rectum as a single unit (an/o means anus, rect means rectum, and -al means pertaining to).

Accessory Digestive Organs

The accessory organs of the digestive system are so named because they play a key role in the digestive process, but are not part of the gastrointestinal tract.

The Liver

The liver is a large organ located in the right upper quadrant of the abdomen (see Figures 8.7 and 8.8). It has several important functions related to removing toxins from the blood and turning food into the fuel and nutrients the body needs. The term hepatic means pertaining to the liver (hepat means liver, and -ic means pertaining to).

- The liver removes excess glucose, commonly known as blood sugar from the bloodstream and stores it as glycogen, which is a form of starch. When the blood sugar level is low, the liver converts glycogen back into glucose and releases it for use by the body.
- The liver also destroys old erythrocytes (red blood cells), removes toxins from the blood, and manufactures some blood proteins. Bilirubin (bill-ih-ROO-bin), which is the pigment produced from the destruction of hemoglobin, is released by the liver in bile.
- Bile, which aids in the digestion of fats, is a digestive juice secreted by the liver. Bile travels from the liver to the gallbladder, where it is concentrated and stored.

The Biliary Tree

- The biliary tree (BILL-ee-air-ee) provides the channels through which bile is transported from the liver to the small intestine. Biliary means pertaining to bile.
- Small ducts in the liver join together like branches to form the biliary tree. The trunk, which is just outside the liver, is known as the common hepatic duct.
- The bile travels from the liver through the common hepatic duct to the gallbladder where it enters and exits through the narrow cystic duct.
- The cystic duct leaving the gallbladder rejoins the common hepatic duct to form the common bile duct. The common bile duct joins the pancreatic duct, and together they enter the duodenum of the small intestine.

The Gallbladder

- The gallbladder is a pear-shaped organ about the size of an egg located under the liver. It stores and concentrates the bile for later use n The term cholecystic means pertaining to the gallbladder (cholecyst means gallbladder, and -ic means pertaining to).
- When bile is needed, the gallbladder contracts, forcing the bile out through the biliary tree.

The Pancreas

- The pancreas (PAN-kree-as) is a soft, 6 inch long oblong gland that is located behind the stomach. This gland has important roles in both the digestive and endocrine systems. The digestive functions are discussed here.

- The pancreas produces and secretes pancreatic juices that aid in digestion and contain sodium bicarbonate to help neutralize stomach acids and digestive enzymes. Pancreatic means pertaining to the pancreas (pancreat means pancreas, and -tic means pertaining to.)
- The pancreatic juices leave the pancreas through the pancreatic duct that joins the common bile duct just before the entrance into the duodenum.

Digestion

Digestion is the process by which complex foods are broken down into nutrients in a form the body can use. Digestive enzymes are responsible for the chemical changes that break foods down into simpler forms of nutrients for use by the body.

A nutrient is a substance, usually from food, that is necessary for normal functioning of the body. The primary nutrients are carbohydrates, fats, and proteins. Vitamins and minerals are essential nutrients, which are required only in small amounts.

Metabolism

- The term metabolism (meh-TAB-oh-lizm) includes all of the processes involved in the body's use of nutrients (metabol means change, and -ism means condition). It consists of two parts: anabolism and catabolism.
- Anabolism (an-NAB-oh-lizm) is the building up of body cells and substances from nutrients. Anabolism is the opposite of catabolism.
- Catabolism (kah-TAB-oh-lizm) is the breaking down of body cells or substances, releasing energy and carbon dioxide. Catabolism is the opposite of anabolism.

Absorption

- Absorption (ab-SORP-shun) is the process by which completely digested nutrients are transported to the cells throughout the body.
- The mucosa that lines the small intestine is covered with finger-like projections called villi (VILL-eye) (singular, villus). Each villus contains blood vessels and lacteals.
- The blood vessels absorb nutrients directly from the digestive system into the bloodstream for delivery to the cells of the body.
- Fats and fat-soluble vitamins cannot be transported directly by the bloodstream. Instead the lacteals, which are specialized structures of the lymphatic system, absorb these nutrients and transport them via lymphatic vessels. As these nutrients are being transported, they are filtered by the lymph nodes in preparation for their delivery to the bloodstream.

The Role of the Mouth, Salivary Glands, and Esophagus
- Mastication (mass-tih-KAY-shun), also known as chewing, breaks food down into smaller pieces, mixes it with saliva, and prepares it to be swallowed.
- A bolus (BOH-lus) is a mass of food that has been chewed and is ready to be swallowed
- During swallowing, food travels from the mouth into the pharynx and on into the esophagus.
- In the esophagus, food moves downward through the action of gravity and peristalsis. Peristalsis (pehr-ih- STAL-sis) is a series of wave-like contractions of the smooth muscles in a single direction.

The Role of the Stomach
- The gastric juices of the stomach contain hydrochloric acid and digestive enzymes to begin the digestive process. Few nutrients enter the bloodstream through the walls of the stomach.
- The churning action of the stomach works with the gastric juices by converting the food into chyme. Chyme (KYM) is the semifluid mass of partly digested food that passes out of the stomach, through the pyloric sphincter, and into the small intestine.

The Role of the Small Intestine
- The conversion of food into usable nutrients is completed as the chyme is moved through the small intestine by peristaltic action.
- In the duodenum, chyme is mixed with pancreatic juice and bile. The bile breaks apart large fat globules so enzymes in the pancreatic juices can digest the fats. This action is called emulsification and must be completed before the nutrients can be absorbed into the body.
- The jejunum secretes large amounts of digestive enzymes and continues the process of digestion.
- The primary function of the ileum is the absorption of nutrients from the digested food.

The Role of the Large Intestine
- The role of the entire large intestine is to receive the waste products of digestion and store them until they are eliminated from the body.
- Food waste enters the large intestine in liquid form. Excess water is reabsorbed into the body through the walls of the large intestine, helping to maintain the body's fluid balance, and the remaining waste forms into feces. Feces (FEE-seez), also known as stools, are solid body wastes expelled through the rectum and anus.
- Defecation (def-eh-KAY-shun), also known as a bowel movement, is the evacuation or emptying of the large intestine.
- The large intestine contains billions of bacteria, most of them harmless, which help break down organic waste material. This process produces

gas. Borborygmus (bor-boh-RIG-mus) is the rumbling noise caused by the movement of gas in the intestine.
- Flatulence (FLAT-you-lens), also known as flatus, is the passage of gas out of the body through the rectum.

Medical Specialties Related To The Digestive System

- Bariatrics (bayr-ee-AT-ricks) is the branch of medicine concerned with the prevention and control of obesity and associated diseases.
- A dentist holds a Doctor of Dental Surgery (DDS) or Doctor of Medical Dentistry (DMD) degree and specializes in diagnosing and treating diseases and disorders of teeth and tissues of the oral cavity.
- A gastroenterologist (gas-troh-en-ter-OL-oh-jist) is a physician who specializes in diagnosing and treating diseases and disorders of the stomach and intestines (gastr/o means stomach, enter means small intestine, and -ologist means specialist).
- An internist is a physician who specializes in diagnosing and treating diseases and disorders of the internal organs and related body systems.
- An orthodontist (or-thoh-DON-tist) is a dental specialist who prevents or corrects malocclusion of the teeth and related facial structures (orth means straight or normal, odont means the teeth, and -ist means specialist).
- A periodontist (pehr-ee-oh-DON-tist) is a dental specialist who prevents or treats disorders of the tissues surrounding the teeth (peri- means surrounding, odont means the teeth, and -ist means specialist).
- A proctologist (prock-TOL-oh-jist) is a physician who specializes in disorders of the colon, rectum, and anus (proct means anus and rectum, and -ologist means specialist).

Pathology Of The Digestive System

Tissues of the Oral Cavity

- Aphthous ulcers (AF-thus UL-serz), also known as canker sores or mouth ulcers, are grey-white pits with a red border in the soft tissues lining the mouth. Although the exact cause is unknown, the appearance of these very common sores is associated with stress, certain foods, or fever.
- Cheilosis (kee-LOH-sis), also known as cheilitis, is a disorder of the lips characterized by crack-like sores at the corners of the mouth (cheil means lips, and -osis means abnormal condition or disease).
- Herpes labialis (HER-peez lay-bee-AL-iss), also known as cold sores or fever blisters, are blister-like sores on the lips and adjacent facial tissue that are caused by the oral herpes simplex virus type 1 (HSV-1). Most adults have been infected by this extremely common virus, and in some, it becomes re-activated periodically, causing cold sores.
- Oral thrush develops when the fungus Candida albicans grows out of control. The symptoms are creamy white lesions on the tongue or inner cheeks, and this condition occurs most often in infants, older adults with

weakened immune systems, or individuals who have been taking antibiotics.
- Stomatomycosis (stoh-mah-toh-my-KOH-sis) is any disease of the mouth due to a fungus (stomat/o means mouth or oral cavity, myc means fungus, and -osis means abnormal condition or disease). See oral thrush.
- Stomatorrhagia (stoh-mah-toh-RAY-jee-ah) describes bleeding from any part of the mouth (stomat/o means mouth or oral cavity, and -rrhagia means bursting forth of blood).
- The term trismus (TRIZ-mus) describes any restriction to the opening of the mouth caused by trauma, surgery, or radiation associated with the treatment of oral cancer. This condition causes difficulty in speaking and affects the patient's nutrition due to impaired ability to chew and swallow.
- Xerostomia (zeer-oh-STOH-mee-ah), also known as dry mouth, is the lack of adequate saliva due to diminished secretions by the salivary glands (xer/o means dry, stom means mouth, and -ia means pertaining to). This condition can be due to medications or radiation of the salivary glands, and can cause discomfort, difficulty in swallowing, changes in the taste of food, and dental decay.

Cleft Lip and Cleft Palate
- A cleft lip, also known as a harelip, is a birth defect in which there is a deep groove of the lip running upward to the nose as a result of the failure of this portion of the lip to close during prenatal development.
- A cleft palate is the failure of the palate to close during the early development of the fetus. This opening can involve the upper lip, hard palate, and/or soft palate. If not corrected, this opening between the nose and mouth makes it difficult for the child to eat and speak. Cleft lip and cleft palate can occur singly or together and usually can be corrected surgically.

Dental Diseases
- Acute necrotizing ulcerative gingivitis (ANUG), also known as trench mouth, is caused by the abnormal growth of bacteria in the mouth. As this condition progresses, the inflammation, bleeding, deep ulceration, and the death of gum tissue become more severe. Necrotizing means causing ongoing tissue death.
- Bruxism (BRUCK-sizm) is the involuntary grinding or clenching of the teeth that usually occurs during sleep and is associated with tension or stress. Bruxism wears away tooth structure, damages periodontal tissues, and injures the temporomandibular joint.
- Dental calculus (KAL-kyou-luhs), also known as tartar, is dental plaque that has calcified (hardened) on the teeth. These deposits irritate the surrounding tissues and cause increasingly serious periodontal diseases.

- The term calculus is also used to describe hard deposits, such as gallstones or kidney stones, which form in other parts of the body.
- Dental caries (KAYR-eez), also known as tooth decay or a cavity, is an infectious disease caused by bacteria that destroy the enamel and dentin of the tooth. If the decay process is not arrested, the pulp can be exposed and become infected.
- Dental plaque (PLACK), which is a major cause of dental caries and periodontal disease, forms as soft deposits in sheltered areas near the gums and between the teeth. Dental plaque consists of bacteria and bacterial by-products. In contrast, the plaque associated with heart conditions consists of deposits of cholesterol that form within blood vessels.
- Gingivitis (jin-jih-VYE-tis) is the earliest stage of periodontal disease, and the inflammation affects only the gums (gingiv means gums, and -itis means inflammation).
- Halitosis (hal-ih-TOH-sis), also known as bad breath, is an unpleasant odor coming from the mouth that can be caused by dental diseases or respiratory or gastric disorders (halit means breath, and -osis means abnormal condition or disease).
- Periodontal disease, also known as periodontitis, is an inflammation of the tissues that surround and support the teeth (peri- means surrounding, odont means tooth or teeth, and -al means pertaining to). This progressive disease is classified according to the degree of tissue involvement. In severe cases, the gums and bone surrounding the teeth are involved.
- A temporomandibular disorder (tem-poh-roh-man- DIB-you-lar) part of the group of complex symptoms that include pain, headache, or difficulty in chewing that are related to the functioning of the temporomandibular joint.

The Esophagus
- Dysphagia (dis-FAY-jee-ah) is difficulty in swallowing (dys- means difficult, and -phagia means swallowing).
- Gastroesophageal reflux disease (gas-troh-eh-sof-ah- JEE-al REE-flucks), also known as GERD, is the upward flow of acid from the stomach into the esophagus (gastr/o means stomach, esophag means esophagus, and -eal means pertaining to). Reflux means a backward or return flow. When this occurs, the stomach acid irritates and damages the delicate lining of the esophagus.
- Pyrosis (pye-ROH-sis), also known as heartburn, is the burning sensation caused by the return of acidic stomach contents into the esophagus (pyr means fever or fire, and -osis means abnormal condition or disease).
- Esophageal varices (eh-sof-ah-JEE-al VAYR-ih-seez) are enlarged and swollen veins at the lower end of the esophagus (singular, varix). Severe bleeding occurs if one of these veins ruptures.

- A hiatal hernia (high-AY-tal HER-nee-ah) is a condition in which a portion of the stomach protrudes upward into the chest, through an opening in the diaphragm (hiat means opening, and -al means pertaining to). A hernia is the protrusion of a part or structure through the tissues that normally contain it. This condition can cause esophageal reflux and Pyrosis.

The Stomach

- Gastritis (gas-TRY-tis) is a common inflammation of the stomach lining that is often caused by the bacterium Helicobacter pylori (gastr means stomach, and -itis means inflammation).
- Gastroenteritis (gas-troh-en-ter-EYE-tis) is an inflammation of the mucous membrane lining the stomach and intestines (gastr/o means stomach, enter means small intestine, and -itis means inflammation).
- Gastrorrhea (gas-troh-REE-ah) is the excessive secretion of gastric juice or mucus in the stomach (gastr/o is stomach, and -rrhea means flow or discharge).

Peptic Ulcers

- Peptic ulcers (UL-serz) are sores that affect the mucous membranes of the digestive system (pept means digestion, and -ic means pertaining to). An ulcer is an erosion of the skin or mucous membrane. Peptic ulcers are caused by the bacterium Helicobacter pylori or by medications, such as aspirin, that irritate the mucous membranes.
- Gastric ulcers are peptic ulcers that occur in the stomach.
- Duodenal ulcers are peptic ulcers that occur in the upper part of the small intestine.
- A perforating ulcer is a complication of a peptic ulcer in which the ulcer erodes through the entire thickness of the organ wall.

Eating Disorders

- Anorexia (an-oh-RECK-see-ah) is the loss of appetite for food, especially when caused by disease.
- Anorexia nervosa (an-oh-RECK-see-ah ner-VOH-sah) is an eating disorder characterized by a false perception of body appearance. This leads to an intense fear of gaining weight and refusal to maintain a normal body weight. Voluntary starvation and excessive exercising often cause the patient to become emaciated. Emaciated means abnormally thin.
- Bulimia nervosa (byou-LIM-ee-ah ner-VOH-sah) is an eating disorder characterized by frequent episodes of binge eating followed by compensatory behaviors such as self-induced vomiting or the misuse of laxatives, diuretics, or other medications. The term bulimia means continuous, excessive hunger.
- Cachexia (kah-KEKS-eeh-ah) is a condition of physical wasting away due to the loss of weight and muscle mass that occurs in patients with

diseases such as advanced cancer or AIDS. Although these patients are eating enough, the wasting happens because their bodies are unable to absorb the nutrients.
- Pica (PYE-kah) is an abnormal craving or appetite for nonfood substances, such as dirt, paint, or clay that lasts for at least 1 month. Pica is not the same as the short-lasting abnormal food cravings that are sometimes associated with pregnancy.

Nutritional Conditions

- Dehydration is a condition in which fluid loss exceeds fluid intake and disrupts the body's normal electrolyte balance.
- Malnutrition is a lack of proper food or nutrients in the body due to a shortage of food, poor eating habits, or the inability of the body to digest, absorb, and distribute these nutrients.
- Malabsorption (mal-ab-SORP-shun) is a condition in which the small intestine cannot absorb nutrients from food that passes through it.

Obesity

- Obesity (oh-BEE-sih-tee) is an excessive accumulation of fat in the body. The term obese is usually used to refer to individuals who are more than 20%–30% over the established weight standards for their height, age, and gender. The term gender refers to the differences between men and women.
- Morbid obesity (MOR-bid oh-BEE-sih-tee) is the condition of weighing two to three times, or more, than the ideal weight or having a body mass index value greater than 39. As used here, the term morbid means a diseased state.
- The body mass index (BMI) is a number that shows body weight adjusted for height. The results fall into one of these categories: underweight, normal, overweight, or obese. A high BMI is one of many factors related to developing chronic diseases such as heart disease, cancer, or diabetes.
- Obesity is frequently present as a comorbidity with conditions such as hypertension and diabetes. Comorbidity means the presence of more than one disease or health condition in an individual at a given time.

Indigestion and Vomiting

- Aerophagia (ay-er-oh-FAY-jee-ah) is the excessive swallowing of air while eating or drinking, and is a common cause of gas in the stomach (aer/o means air, and -phagia means swallowing).
- Dyspepsia (dis-PEP-see-ah), also known as indigestion, is pain or discomfort in digestion (dys- means painful, and -pepsia means digestion).

- Emesis (EM-eh-sis), also known as vomiting, is the reflex ejection of the stomach contents through the mouth. Note that emesis is used both as a stand alone term and as a suffix.
- Eructation (eh-ruk-TAY-shun) is the act of belching or raising gas orally from the stomach.
- Hematemesis (hee-mah-TEM-eh-sis) is the vomiting of blood (hemat means blood, and -emesis means vomiting).
- Hyperemesis (high-per-EM-eh-sis) is extreme, persistent vomiting that can cause dehydration (hypermeans excessive, and -emesis means vomiting). During the early stages of pregnancy, this is known as morning sickness.
- Nausea (NAW-see-ah) is the urge to vomit.
- Regurgitation (ree-gur-jih-TAY-shun) is the return of swallowed food into the mouth.

Intestinal Disorders

- Colorectal carcinoma, also known as colon cancer, often first manifests itself in polyps in the colon.
- Diverticulosis (dye-ver-tick-you-LOH-sis) is the presence of a number of diverticula in the colon (diverticul means diverticulum, and -osis means abnormal condition or disease). A diverticulum (dye-ver-TICK-youlum) is a small pouch or sac occurring in the lining or wall of a tubular organ such as the colon (plural, diverticula).
- Diverticulitis (dye-ver-tick-you-LYE-tis) is the inflammation of one or more diverticula in the colon (diverticul means diverticulum, and -itis means inflammation).
- Enteritis (en-ter-EYE-tis) is an inflammation of the small intestine caused by eating or drinking substances contaminated with viral and bacterial pathogens (enter means small intestine, and -itis means inflammation).

Ileus

- Ileus (ILL-ee-us) is the partial or complete blockage of the small and/or large intestine. It is caused by the cessation (stopping) of intestinal peristalsis. Symptoms of ileus can include severe pain, cramping, abdominal distention, vomiting, and the failure to pass gas or stools. Postoperative ileus is a temporary impairment of bowel motility that is considered to be a normal response to abdominal surgery. It is often present for 24–72 hours depending on what part of the digestive system was treated.

Irritable Bowel Syndrome

- Irritable bowel syndrome (IBS), also known as spastic colon, is a common condition of unknown cause with symptoms that can include intermittent cramping, abdominal pain, bloating, constipation, and/or diarrhea. This condition, which is usually aggravated by stress, is not caused by pathogens (bacteria or viruses) or by structural changes.

Inflammatory Bowel Diseases

- Inflammatory bowel disease (IBD) is the general name for diseases that cause inflammation in the intestines. The two most common inflammatory bowel diseases are ulcerative colitis and Crohn's disease.
- These conditions are grouped together because both are chronic, incurable, and can affect the large and small intestines. They also have similar symptoms, which include abdominal pain, weight loss, fatigue, fever, rectal bleeding, and diarrhea.
- These conditions tend to occur at intervals of active disease known as flares alternating with periods of remission. These disorders are treated with medication and surgery to remove diseased portions of the intestine.

Ulcerative colitis

- Ulcerative colitis (UL-ser-ay-tiv koh-LYE-tis) is a chronic condition of unknown cause in which repeated episodes of inflammation in the rectum and large intestine cause ulcers and irritation (col means colon, and -itis means inflammation).
- Ulcerative colitis usually starts in the rectum and progresses upward to the lower part of the colon; however, it can affect the entire large intestine.
- Ulcerative colitis affects only the innermost lining and not the deep tissues of the colon.

Crohn's disease

- Crohn's disease (CD) is a chronic autoimmune disorder that can occur anywhere in the digestive tract; however, it is most often found in the ileum and in the colon.
- In contrast to ulcerative colitis, CD generally penetrates every layer of tissue in the affected area. This commonly results in scarring and thickening of the walls of the affected structures.
- The term regional ileitis is used to describe CD that affects the ileum. Ileitis is an inflammation of the ileum.
- The term Crohn's colitis is used to describe CD that affects the colon. Colitis is an inflammation of the colon.

Note: This term is not the same as the condition ulcerative colitis.

Intestinal Obstructions

- An intestinal obstruction is the partial or complete blockage of the small and/or large intestine caused by a physical obstruction. This blockage can result from many causes such as scar tissue or a tumor.

- Intestinal adhesions abnormally hold together parts of the intestine that normally should be separate. This condition, which is caused by inflammation or trauma, can lead to intestinal obstruction.
- In a strangulating obstruction, the blood flow to a segment of the intestine is cut off. This can lead to gangrene and perforation. Gangrene is tissue death that is usually associated with a loss of circulation. As used here, a perforation is a hole through the wall of a structure.
- Volvulus (VOL-view-lus) is the twisting of the intestine on itself that causes an obstruction. Volvulus is a condition that usually occurs in infancy.
- Intussusception (in-tus-sus-SEP-shun) is the telescoping of one part of the small intestine into the opening of an immediately adjacent part. This is a rare condition sometimes found in infants and young children.
- An inguinal hernia (ING-gwih-nal HER-nee-ah) is the protrusion of a small loop of bowel through a weak place in the lower abdominal wall or groin. This condition can be caused by obesity, pregnancy, heavy lifting, or straining to pass a stool.
- A strangulated hernia occurs when a portion of the intestine is constricted inside the hernia and its blood supply is cut off.

Anorectal Disorders
- An anal fissure is a small crack-like sore in the skin of the anus that can cause severe pain during a bowel movement. As used here, a fissure is a groove or cracklike sore of the skin.
- Bowel incontinence (in-KON-tih-nents) is the inability to control the excretion of feces.
- Constipation is defined as having a bowel movement fewer than three times per week. With constipation, stools are usually hard, dry, small in size, and difficult to eliminate.
- Diarrhea (dye-ah-REE-ah) is an abnormal frequent flow of loose or watery stools that can lead to dehydration (dia- means through, and -rrhea means flow or discharge).
- Hemorrhoids (HEM-oh-roids), also known as piles, occur when a cluster of veins, muscles, and tissues slip near or through the anal opening. The veins can become inflamed, resulting in pain, fecal leakage, and bleeding.
- Melena (meh-LEE-nah) is the passage of black, tarry, and foul-smelling stools (melan means black or dark, and -a is a noun ending). This appearance of the stools is caused by the presence of digested blood and often indicates an injury or disorder in the upper part of the gastrointestinal tract. In contrast, bright red blood in the stool usually indicates that the blood is coming from the lower part of the gastrointestinal tract.

The Liver

- Liver disorders are a major concern because the functioning of the liver is essential to the digestive process.
- Hepatitis (hep-ah-TYE-tis) is an inflammation of the liver (hepat means liver, and -itis means inflammation).
- Hepatomegaly (hep-ah-toh-MEG-ah-lee) is the abnormal enlargement of the liver (hepat/o means liver, and -megaly means enlargement).
- Jaundice (JAWN-dis) is a yellow discoloration of the skin, mucous membranes, and the eyes. This condition is caused by greater-than-normal amounts of bilirubin in the blood.

Cirrhosis

- Cirrhosis (sih-ROH-sis) is a progressive degenerative disease of the liver that is often caused by excessive alcohol use or by viral hepatitis B or C (cirrh means yellow or orange, and -osis means abnormal condition or disease). Degenerative means progressive deterioration resulting in the loss of tissue or organ function. The progress of cirrhosis is marked by the formation of areas of scarred liver tissue that are filled with fat. The liver damage causes abnormal conditions throughout the other body systems.
- Ascites (ah-SIGH-teez) is an abnormal accumulation of serous fluid in the peritoneal cavity. As used here, the term serous means a substance having a watery consistency.
- The term caput medusae describes the distended and engorged veins that are visible radiating from the umbilicus.
- The term hobnail liver describes the lumpy appearance of the liver surface due to cirrhosis.

Nonalcoholic Fatty Liver Disease

- The term nonalcoholic fatty liver disease (NAFLD) describes a range of conditions characterized by an accumulation of fat within the liver that affect people who drink little or no alcohol. Those with this condition most commonly are middle-aged individuals who are obese and may also have diabetes and elevated cholesterol.
- Steatosis (stee-ah-TOH-sis), which is the mildest type of this condition, is characterized by accumulations of fat within the liver that usually does not cause liver damage (steat/o means fat, and -osis means abnormal condition).
- Nonalcoholic steatohepatitis (NASH), which is a more serious form of this condition, consists of fatty accumulations plus liver-damaging inflammation (steat/o means fat, hepat means liver, and -itis mean inflammation).
- In some cases, this will progress to cirrhosis, irreversible liver scarring, or liver cancer.

The Gallbladder

- Cholangitis (koh-lan-JIGH-tis) is an acute infection of the bile duct characterized by pain in the upper-right quadrant of the abdomen, fever, and jaundice (choleang means bile duct, and -itis means inflammation).
- Cholecystalgia (koh-lee-sis-TAL-jee-ah) is pain in the gallbladder (cholecyst means gallbladder, and -algia means pain).
- Cholecystitis (koh-lee-sis-TYE-tis) is inflammation of the gallbladder, usually associated with gallstones blocking the flow of bile (cholecyst means gallbladder, and -itis means inflammation).
- A gallstone, also known as biliary calculus or a cholelith, is a hard deposit formed in the gallbladder and bile ducts due to the concretion of bile components (plural, calculi).
- Cholelithiasis (koh-lee-lih-THIGH-ah-sis) is the presence of gallstones in the gallbladder or bile ducts (chole means bile or gall, and -lithiasis means presence of stones).

DIAGNOSTIC PROCEDURES OF THE DIGESTIVE SYSTEM

- Abdominal computed tomography (CT) is a radiographic procedure that produces a detailed cross-section of the tissue structure within the abdomen, showing, for example, the presence of a tumor or obstruction.
- An abdominal ultrasound is a noninvasive test used to visualize internal organs by using very high frequency sound waves.
- An anoscopy (ah-NOS-koh-pee) is the visual examination of the anal canal and lower rectum (an/o means anus, and -scopy means visual examination). An anoscope, which is a short speculum, is used for this procedure. A speculum is an instrument used to enlarge the opening of any body cavity to facilitate inspection of its interior.
- A capsule endoscopy is a tiny video camera in a capsule that the patient swallows. For approximately 8 hours as it passes through the small intestine, this camera transmits images of the walls of the small intestine. The images are detected by sensor devices attached to the patient's abdomen and transmitted to a data recorder worn on the patient's belt.
- Cholangiography (koh-LAN-jee-og-rah-fee) is a radiographic examination of the bile ducts with the use of a contrast medium (cholangi/o means bile duct, and -graphy means the process of recording). This test is used to identify obstructions in the liver or bile ducts that slow or block the flow of bile from the liver. The resulting record is a cholangiogram.
- An esophagogastroduodenoscopy (eh-sof-ah-goh-gastroh- dew-oh-deh-NOS-koh-pee) is an endoscopic procedure that allows direct visualization of the upper GI tract which includes the esophagus, stomach, and upper duodenum (esophag/o means esophagus, gastr/o

means stomach, duoden/o means duodenum, and -scopy means visual examination).
- An upper GI series and a lower GI series are radiographic studies to examine the digestive system. A contrast medium is required to make these structures visible. A barium swallow is used for the upper GI series, and a barium enema is used for the lower GI series.
- Hemoccult test (HEE-moh-kult), also known as the fecal occult blood test, is a laboratory test for hidden blood in the stools (hem means blood, and -occult means hidden). A test kit is used to obtain the specimens at home, and these are then evaluated in a laboratory or physician's office.
- Stool samples are specimens of feces that are examined for content and characteristics. For example, fatty stools might indicate the presence of pancreatic problems. Cultures of the stool sample can be examined in the laboratory for the presence of bacteria or O & P. This abbreviation stands for ova (parasite eggs) and parasites.

Endoscopic Procedures

- An endoscope is an instrument used for visual examination of internal structures (endo- means within, and -scope means an instrument for visual examination). The following endoscopic examinations are used as preventive measure for the early detection of polyps that may be cancerous. Polyps are mushroom-like growths from the surface of mucous membrane. Not all polyps are malignant.
- Colonoscopy (koh-lun-OSS-koh-pee) is the direct visual examination of the inner surface of the entire colon from the rectum to the cecum (colon/o means colon, and -scopy means visual examination). A virtual colonoscopy uses x-rays and computers to produce two- and three-dimensional images of the colon.
- Sigmoidoscopy (sig-moi-DOS-koh-pee) is the endoscopic examination of the interior of the rectum, sigmoid colon, and possibly a portion of the descending colon (sigmoid/o means sigmoid colon, and -scopy is the visual examination).
- An enema is the placement of a solution into the rectum and colon to empty the lower intestine through bowel activity. An enema is part of the preparation for an endoscopic examination; however, enemas are also used to treat severe constipation.

Treatment Procedures Of The Digestive System

Medications

- Antacids, which neutralize the acids in the stomach, are taken to relieve the discomfort of conditions such as pyrosis or to help peptic ulcers heal.

- Acid reducers, which decrease the amount of acid produced by the stomach, are used to treat the symptoms of conditions such as gastroesophageal reflux disease.
- An antiemetic (an-tih-ee-MET-ick) is a medication that is administered to prevent or relieve nausea and vomiting (anti- means against, emet means vomit, and -ic means pertaining to).
- Laxatives are medications, or foods, given to stimulate bowel movements. Bulk-forming laxatives, such as bran, treat constipation by helping fecal matter retain water and remain soft as it moves through the intestines.
- Oral rehydration therapy (ORT) is a treatment in which a solution of electrolytes is administered in a liquid preparation to counteract the dehydration that can accompany severe diarrhea, especially in young children.

The Oral Cavity and Esophagus

- A dentalprophylaxis (proh-fih-LACK-sis) is the professional cleaning of the teeth to remove plaque and calculus. The term prophylaxis also refers to a treatment intended to prevent a disease or stop it from spreading. Examples include vaccination to provide immunity against a specific disease.
- A gingivectomy (jin-jih-VECK-toh-mee) is the surgical removal of diseased gingival tissue (gingiv means gingival tissue, and -ectomy means surgical removal).
- Maxillofacial surgery (mack-sill-oh-FAY-shul) is specialized surgery of the face and jaws to correct deformities, treat diseases, and repair injuries.
- Palatoplasty (PAL-ah-toh-plas-tee) is surgical repair of a cleft lip and/or palate (palat/o means palate, and -plasty means surgical repair).
- Stomatoplasty (STOH-mah-toh-plas-tee) is the surgical repair of the mouth (stomat/o means mouth or oral cavity, and -plasty means surgical repair).

The Stomach

- A gastrectomy (gas-TRECK-toh-mee) is the surgical removal of all or a part of the stomach (gastr means stomach, and -ectomy means surgical removal).
- Nasogastric intubation (nay-zoh-GAS-trick in-too- BAY-shun) is the placement of a feeding tube through the nose and into the stomach (nas/o means nose, gastr means stomach, and -ic means pertaining to). This tube, which is placed temporarily, provides nutrition for patients who cannot take sufficient nutrients by mouth.
- A gastrostomy tube (gas-TROS-toh-mee) is a surgically placed feeding tube from the exterior of the body into the stomach (gastr means stomach, and -ostomy means surgically creating an opening). This tube,

which is placed permanently, provides nutrition for patients who cannot swallow or take sufficient nutrients by mouth.
- Total parenteral nutrition (pah-REN-ter-al) is administered to patients who cannot, or should not, get their nutrition through eating. All of the patient's nutritional requirements are met through a nutritional liquid that is administered intravenously for 10–12 hours, once a day or five times a week. Parenteral means not in, or through, the digestive system.

Bariatric Surgery

- Bariatric surgery is performed to treat morbid obesity by restricting the amount of food that can enter the stomach and be digested. These procedures limit food intake and force dietary changes that enable weight reduction.
- Gastric bypass surgery surgically makes the stomach smaller and causes food to bypass the first part of the small intestine. This procedure is not reversible.
- A Gastric lap-band procedure involves placing a band around the exterior of the stomach to restrict the amount of food that can enter the stomach. This procedure has the advantage of being reversible through the removal of the band.

The Intestines

- A colectomy (koh-LECK-toh-mee) is the surgical removal of all, or part of, the colon (col means colon, and -ectomy means surgical removal).
- A diverticulectomy (dye-ver-tick-you-LECK-toh-mee) is the surgical removal of a diverticulum (diverticul means diverticulum, and -ectomy means surgical removal).
- A gastroduodenostomy (gas-troh-dew-oh-deh-NOStoh-mee) is the establishment of an anastomosis between the upper portion of the stomach, and the duodenum (gastr/o means stomach, duoden means first part of the small intestine, and -ostomy means surgically creating an opening). This procedure is performed to treat stomach cancer or to remove a malfunctioning pyloric valve.
- Anastomosis (ah-nas-toh-MOH-sis) is a surgical connection between two hollow or tubular structures (plural, anastomoses).
- An ileectomy (ill-ee-ECK-toh-mee) is the surgical removal of the ileum (ile means the ileum, and -ectomy means surgical removal. Note: This term is spelled with a double e.)

Ostomies

- An ostomy (OSS-toh-mee) is a surgical procedure to create an artificial opening between an organ and the body surface. This opening is called a stoma. Ostomy can be used alone as a noun to describe a procedure or as a suffix with the word part that describes the organ involved.

- An ileostomy (ill-ee-OS-toh-mee) is the surgical creation of an artificial excretory opening between the ileum, at the end of the small intestine, and the outside of the abdominal wall (ile means small intestine, and -ostomy means surgically creating an opening).
- A colostomy (koh-LAHS-toh-mee) is the surgical creation of an artificial excretory opening between the colon and the body surface (col means colon, and -ostomy means surgically creating an opening). The segment of the intestine below the ostomy is usually removed, and the fecal matter flows through the stoma into a disposable bag. A colostomy can be temporary, to divert feces from an area that needs to heal.

The Rectum and Anus

- A hemorrhoidectomy (hem-oh-roid-ECK-toh-mee) is the surgical removal of hemorrhoids (hemorrhoid means piles, and -ectomy means surgical removal). Rubber band ligation is often used instead of surgery. Rubber bands cut off the circulation at the base of the hemorrhoid, causing it to eventually fall off. Ligation means the tying off of blood vessels or ducts.
- A proctectomy (prock-TECK-toh-mee) is the surgical removal of the rectum (proct means rectum, and -ectomy means surgical removal).
- Proctopexy (PROCK-toh-peck-see) is the surgical fixation of a prolapsed rectum to an adjacent tissue or organ (proct/o means rectum, and -pexy means surgical fixation). Prolapse means the falling or dropping down of an organ or internal part. This can be performed as a laparoscopic procedure in which a laparoscope and instruments are inserted into the abdomen through small incisions. A laparoscope is a specialized endoscope used for the examination and treatment of abdominal conditions.
- Proctoplasty (PROCK-toh-plas-tee) is the surgical repair of the rectum (proct/o means rectum, and -plasty means surgical repair).

The Liver

- A hepatectomy (hep-ah-TECK-toh-mee) is the surgical removal of all or part of the liver (hepat means liver, and -ectomy means surgical removal).
- Hepatorrhaphy (hep-ah-TOR-ah-fee) means surgical suturing of the liver (hepat/o means liver, and -rrhaphy means surgical suturing).
- A liver transplant is an option for a patient whose liver has failed for a reason other than liver cancer. Because liver tissue regenerates, a partial liver transplant, in which only part of the organ is donated, can be adequate. A partial liver can be donated by a living donor whose blood and tissue types match.

The Gallbladder

- A choledocholithotomy (koh-led-oh-koh-lih-THOToh-mee) is an incision into the common bile duct for the removal of gallstones (choledoch/o means the common bile duct, lith means stone, and -otomy means surgical incision).
- A cholecystectomy (koh-lee-sis-TECK-toh-mee) is the surgical removal of the gallbladder. An open cholecystectomy is performed through an incision in the right side of the upper abdomen. A laparoscopic cholecystectomy, also known as a lap choley, is the surgical removal of the gallbladder using a laparoscope and other instruments inserted through three or four small incisions in the abdominal wall.

Abbreviations Related To The Digestive System

- bilirubin = BIL, Bil, bili
- cholecystectomy = CCE, chole
- cirrhosis = CIR, CIRR
- colonoscopy = COL
- colorectal carcinoma = CRC
- esophagogastroduodenoscopy = EGD
- esophageal varices = EV
- gastroenteritis = GE
- ileocecal sphincter = ICS
- inguinal hernia = IH
- intestinal obstruction = IO
- jaundice = j, jaund
- morbid obesity = MO
- peptic ulcers = PU
- temporomandibular disorders = TMD
- total parenteral nutrition = TPN
- ulcerative colitis = UC

Critical Thinking Exercise

The following story and questions are designed to stimulate critical thinking through class discussion or as a brief essay response. There are no right or wrong answers to these questions.

"Stick the landing and our team walks away with the gold!" Coach Schaefer meant to be supportive as she squeezed Claire's shoulder. "What you mean is beat Leia's score for the Riverview team and we'll win," Claire thought sarcastically. She watched as Leia's numbers were shown from her last vault. A 6.8 out of a possible 7. "Great, just great! She chooses a less difficult vault, but with that toothpick body she gets more height than I ever will!" She wondered if Leia was naturally that thin, or did she use the secret method—you can't gain weight if the food doesn't stay in your stomach.

All season it had been that way. Everyone seemed to be watching the rivalry between West High's Claire and Riverview's "tiny-mighty" Leia. Claire was pretty sure that her 10-pound weight loss had improved both her floor routine and her tricky dismount off the beam. "I'm less than a half point behind, so coach should be happy," she thought. But just last week, Coach Schaefer had a long talk with her when she got dizzy and fell off the balance beam. Coach had asked Claire the one question she hoped she'd never have to answer: "Just what have you been doing to lose the weight?"

Claire felt her hands sweat. "Just stick the landing," she told herself, but her body had a different

agenda. Starved for fuel, her muscles failed, she fell, and the gold slipped out of reach.

Suggested Discussion Topics

1. What do you think Claire is doing to lose weight?
2. What effects would anorexia or bulimia nervosa have on the long-term health of a young woman? Athletes sometimes abuse their bodies through dieting or drugs to achieve peak performances.
3. What should the groups that oversee competitive athletics do about this practice?
4. Imagine you have a daughter. How would you know if she had an eating disorder? How could you help her?

Medical Terminology for Health Professions 4.0

CHAPTER 9

THE URINARY SYSTEM

This list contains essential word parts and medical terms for this chapter.

Word Parts
- -cele
- cyst/o
- diah
- -ectasis
- glomerul/o
- lith/o
- -lysis
- nephr/o
- -pexy
- pyel/o
- -tripsy
- ur/o
- ureter/o
- urethr/o
- -uria

Medical Terms
- ablation (ab-LAY-shun)
- anuria (ah-NEW-ree-ah)
- benign prostatic hypertrophy (pros-TAT-ick high- PER-troh-fee)
- catheterization (kath-eh-ter-eye-ZAY-shun)
- cystitis (sis-TYE-tis)
- cystocele (SIS-toh-seel)
- cystolith (SIS-toh-lith)
- cystopexy (sis-toh-peck-see)
- cystoscopy (sis-TOS-koh-pee)
- dialysis (dye-AL-ih-sis)
- diuresis (dye-you-REE-sis)
- enuresis (en-you-REE-sis)

- epispadias (ep-ih-SPAY-dee-as)
- extracorporeal shockwave lithotripsy (LITH-ohtrip- see)
- glomerulonephritis (gloh-mer-you-loh-neh-FRY-tis)
- hemodialysis (hee-moh-dye-AL-ih-sis)
- hydronephrosis (high-droh-neh-FROH-sis)
- hydroureter (high-droh-you-REE-ter)
- hyperproteinuria (high-per-proh-tee-in-YOU-ree-ah)
- hypoproteinemia (high-poh-proh-tee-in-EE-mee-ah)
- hypospadias (high-poh-SPAY-dee-as)
- incontinence (in-KON-tih-nents)
- interstitial cystitis (in-ter-STISH-al sis-TYE-tis)
- intravenous pyelogram (in-trah-VEE-nus PYE-ehloh- gram)
- lithotomy (lih-THOT-oh-mee)
- nephrectasis (neh-FRECK-tah-sis)
- nephrolith (NEF-roh-lith)
- nephrolithiasis (nef-roh-lih-THIGH-ah-sis)
- nephrolysis (neh-FROL-ih-sis)
- nephropathy (neh-FROP-ah-thee)
- nephroptosis (nef-rop-TOH-sis)
- nephropyosis (nef-roh-pye-OH-sis)
- nephrostomy (neh-FROS-toh-me)
- nephrotic syndrome (neh-FROT-ick)
- neurogenic bladder (new-roh-JEN-ick)
- nocturia (nock-TOO-ree-ah)
- nocturnal enuresis (en-you-REE-sis)
- oliguria (ol-ih-GOO-ree-ah)
- percutaneous nephrolithotomy (per-kyou-TAYnee- us nef-roh-lih-THOT-oh-mee)
- peritoneal dialysis (pehr-ih-toh-NEE-al dye-AL-ih-sis)
- polycystic kidney disease (pol-ee-SIS-tick)
- polyuria (pol-ee-YOU-ree-ah)
- prostate-specific antigen
- prostatism (PROS tah-tizm)
- pyeloplasty (PYE-eh-loh-plas-tee)
- pyelotomy (pye-eh-LOT-oh-mee)
- suprapubic catheterization (soo-prah-PYOU-bick kath-eh-ter-eye-ZAY-shun)
- uremia (you-REE-mee-ah)
- ureterectasis (you-ree-ter-ECK-tah-sis)
- ureterolith (you-REE-ter-oh-lith)
- ureterorrhagia (you-ree-ter-oh-RAY-jee-ah)
- ureterorrhaphy (you-ree-ter-OR-ah-fee)
- urethritis (you-reh-THRIGH-tis)
- urethropexy (you-REE-throh-peck-see)

- urethrorrhagia (you-ree-throh-RAY-jee-ah)
- urethrostenosis (you-ree-throh-steh-NOH-sis)
- urethrostomy (you-reh-THROS-toh-mee)
- vesicovaginal fistula (ves-ih-koh-VAJ-ih-nahl FIStyou- lah)
- voiding cystourethrography (sis-toh-you-ree- THROG-rah-fee)
- Wilms tumor

Objectives

On completion of this chapter, you should be able to:
1. Describe the major functions of the urinary system.
2. Name and describe the structures of the urinary system.
3. Recognize, define, spell, and pronounce terms related to the pathology and the diagnostic and treatment procedures of the urinary system.

Functions Of The Urinary System

- The urinary system performs many functions that are important in maintaining homeostasis. Homeostasis is the process through which the body maintains a constant internal environment (home/o means constant, and -stasis means control). These functions include:
- Maintaining the proper balance of water, salts, and acids in the body by filtering the blood as it flows through the kidneys.
- Constantly filtering the blood to remove urea and other waste materials from the bloodstream. Urea (you-REEah) is the major waste product of protein metabolism.
- Converting these waste products and excess fluids into urine in the kidneys and excreting them from the body via the urinary bladder.

Structures Of The Urinary System

The urinary system, also referred to as the urinary tract, consists of two kidneys, two ureters, one bladder, and a urethra. The adrenal glands, which are part of the endocrine system, are located on the top of the kidneys.

The Kidneys

The kidneys constantly filter the blood to remove waste products and excess water. These are excreted as urine, which is 95% water and 5% other wastes.
- The term renal (REE-nal) means pertaining to the kidneys (ren means kidney or kidneys, and -al means pertaining to).
- The two kidneys are located retroperitoneally with one on each side of the vertebral column below the diaphragm. Retroperitoneal means pertaining to being located behind the peritoneum. The peritoneum is the membrane that lines the abdominal cavity.
- The renal cortex (REE-nal KOR-tecks) is the outer region of the kidney. It contains over one million microscopic units called nephrons. The cortex is the outer portion of an organ.

- The medulla (meh-DULL-ah) is the inner region of the kidney; it contains most of the urine-collecting tubules. A tubule is a small tube.

Nephrons

- A nephron (NEF-ron) is a functional unit of the kidney. These units form urine by the processes of filtration, reabsorption, and secretion. Reabsorption is the return to the blood of some of the substances that were removed during filtration.
- Each nephron contains a glomerulus (gloh-MER-youlus), which is a cluster of capillaries surrounded by a cup-shaped membrane called the Bowman's capsule (plural, glomeruli).
- Blood enters the kidney through the renal artery and flows into the nephrons. After being filtered in the capillaries of the glomerulus, the blood leaves the kidney through the renal vein.
- Waste products that were filtered out of the blood remain behind in the kidney where they pass through a series of urine-collecting tubules. When this process has been completed, the urine is transported to the renal pelvis where it is collected in preparation for entry into the ureters.
- Urochrome (YOU-roh-krome) is the pigment that gives urine its normal yellow-amber or straw color (ur/o means urine, and -chrome means color). The color of urine can be influenced by normal factors such as the amount of liquid consumed, and can also be changed by diseases and medications.

The Renal Pelvis

The renal pelvis is the funnel-shaped area within each kidney that is surrounded by renal cortex and medulla. This is where the newly formed urine collects before it flows into the ureters.

The Ureters

The ureters (you-REE-ters) are two narrow tubes, each about 10–12 inches long, which transport urine from the kidney to the bladder. Peristalsis, which is a series of wave-like contractions, moves urine down each ureter to the bladder. Urine drains from the ureters into the bladder through the ureteral orifices in the wall of the urinary bladder.

The Urinary Bladder

The urinary bladder is a hollow muscular organ that is a reservoir for urine before it is excreted from the body.

- The bladder is located in the anterior portion of the pelvic cavity behind the pubic symphysis. The bladder stores about one pint of urine.
- Like the stomach, the bladder is lined with rugae, which are folds that allow it to expand and contract.

- The trigone (TRY-gon) is the smooth triangular area on the inner surface of the bladder located between the openings of the ureters and urethra.

The Urethra
- The urethra (you-REE-thrah) is the tube extending from the bladder to the outside of the body. Caution: The spellings of ureter and urethra are very similar!
- Two urinary sphincters, one located at either end of the urethra, control the flow of urine from the bladder into the urethra and out of the urethra through the urethral meatus. A sphincter is a ring-like muscle that closes a passageway.
- The urethral meatus (you-REE-thrahl mee-AY-tus), also known as the urinary meatus, is the external opening of the urethra. Meatus means the external opening of a canal.
- The female urethra is approximately 1.5 inches long, and the urethral meatus is located between the clitoris and the opening of the vagina. In the female, the urethra conveys only urine.
- The male urethra is approximately 8 inches long, and the urethral meatus is located at the tip of the penis. This urethra transports both urine and semen.
- The prostate gland (PROS-tayt), which is part of the male reproductive system, surrounds the urethra. Most disorders of the prostate affect the male's ability to urinate.

The Excretion Of Urine
Urination, also known as voiding or micturition, is the normal process of excreting urine.
- As the bladder fills up with urine, pressure is placed on the base of the urethra, resulting in the urge to urinate or micturate. Urination requires the coordinated contraction of the bladder muscles and relaxation of the sphincters. This action forces the urine through the urethra and out through the urinary meatus.

Medical Specialties Related To The Urinary System
- A nephrologist (neh-FROL-oh-jist) is a physician who specializes in diagnosing and treating diseases and disorders of the kidneys (nephr means kidney, and -ologist means specialist).
- A urologist (you-ROL-oh-jist) is a physician who specializes in diagnosing and treating diseases and disorders of the urinary system of females and the genitourinary system of males (ur means urine, and -ologist means specialist). The term genitourinary refers to both the genital and urinary organs.

Pathology Of The Urinary System

Renal Failure

Renal failure, also known as kidney failure, is the inability of one or both of the kidneys to perform their functions. The body cannot replace damaged nephrons, and when too many nephrons have been destroyed, the result is kidney failure.

- Uremia (you-REE-mee-ah), also known as uremic poisoning, is a toxic condition resulting from renal failure in which kidney function is compromised and urea is retained in the blood (ur means urine, and -emia means blood condition).
- Acute renal failure (ARF) has sudden onset and is characterized by uremia. It can be fatal if not reversed promptly. This condition can be caused by many factors, including a sudden drop in blood volume or blood pressure due to injury or surgery.
- Chronic renal failure is the progressive loss of renal function, sometimes leading to uremia, which is caused by a variety of conditions such as kidney disease, diabetes mellitus, or hypertension.
- End-stage renal disease (ESRD) refers to the late stages of chronic renal failure in which there is irreversible loss of the function of both kidneys. Without dialysis or a kidney transplant, this condition is fatal.
- Hemolytic uremic syndrome (hee-moh-LIT-ick you- REE-mick) is a condition in which hemolytic anemia and thrombocytopenia cause acute renal failure and possibly death. This syndrome can be the result of an Escherichia coli (E. coli) infection in young children and the elderly.

Nephrotic Syndrome

- Nephrotic syndrome (neh-FROT-ick) is a condition in which very high levels of protein are lost in the urine and abnormally low levels of protein are present in the blood (nephr/o means kidney, and -tic means pertaining to). This is the result of damage to the kidney's glomeruli.
- Nephrosis (neh-FROH-sis) is any degenerative kidney disease causing nephrotic syndrome without inflammation (nephr means kidney, and -osis means abnormal condition or disease). The following are characteristics of diseases that are caused by the malfunctioning of the kidneys.
- Anuria (ah-NEW-ree-ah) is the absence of urine formation by the kidneys (an- means without, and -uria means urine).
- Edema (eh-DEE-mah) is excessive fluid in the body tissues.
- Hyperproteinuria (high-per-proh-tee-in-YOU-ree-ah) is the presence of abnormally high concentrations of protein in the urine (hyper- means excessive, protein means protein, and -uria means urine). This condition is often associated with hypoproteinemia.
- Hypoproteinemia (high-poh-proh-tee-in-EE-mee-ah) is the presence of abnormally low concentrations of protein in the blood (hypo- means

deficient or decreased, protein means protein, and -emia means blood condition). This condition is often associated with hyperproteinuria.

Nephropathy

- The term nephropathy (neh-FROP-ah-thee) means any disease of the kidney (nephr means kidney, and -pathy means disease). This definition includes both degenerative and inflammatory conditions.
- Diabetic nephropathy is a kidney disease characterized by hyperproteinuria, which is the result of thickening and hardening of the glomeruli caused by long-term diabetes mellitus.

The Kidneys

- Hydronephrosis (high-droh-neh-FROH-sis) is the dilation (swelling) of one or both kidneys (hydr/o means water, nephr means kidney, and -osis means abnormal condition or disease). This condition can be caused by problems associated with the backing up of urine due to an obstruction such as a stricture in the ureter or blockage in the opening from the bladder to the urethra, or in the urethra itself. A stricture is an abnormal band of tissue that narrows or completely blocks a body passage.
- Nephrectasis (neh-FRECK-tah-sis) is the distention of the pelvis of the kidney (nephr means kidney, and -ectasis means enlargement or stretching). Distention means enlarged or stretched.
- Nephritis (neh-FRY-tis) is an inflammation of the kidney or kidneys (nephr means kidney, and -itis means inflammation). The two most common causes of nephritis are infection or an autoimmune disease.
- Glomerulonephritis (gloh-mer-you-loh-neh-FRY-tis), also known as Bright's disease, is a type of kidney disease caused by inflammation of the glomeruli that causes red blood cells and proteins to leak into the urine (glomerul/o means glomeruli, nephr means kidney, and -itis means inflammation).
- Nephroptosis (nef-rop-TOH-sis), also known as a floating kidney, is the prolapse of a kidney (nephr/o means kidney, and -ptosis means droop or prolapse). Prolapse means slipping or falling out of place.
- Nephropyosis (nef-roh-pye-OH-sis), also known as pyonephrosis, is suppuration of the kidney (nephr/o means kidney, py means pus, and -osis means abnormal condition or disease). Suppuration means the formation or discharge of pus.
- Polycystic kidney disease (pol-ee-SIS-tick) is a genetic disorder characterized by the growth of numerous fluid-filled cysts in the kidneys (poly- means many, cyst means cyst, and -ic means pertaining to). These cysts, which slowly replace much of the mass of the kidney, reduce the kidney function, and this eventually leads to kidney failure.

- Renal colic (REE-nal KOLL-ick) is an acute pain in the kidney area that is caused by blockage during the passage of a kidney stone. Colic means spasmodic pains in the abdomen.
- A Wilms tumor is a malignant tumor of the kidney that occurs in young children. There is a high cure rate for this condition when this condition is treated promptly.

Stones

A stone, also known as calculus, is an abnormal mineral deposit that has formed within the body (plural, calculi). These stones vary in size from small sand-like granules to the size of marbles and are named for the organ or tissue where they are located. In the urinary system, stones are formed when waste products in the urine crystallize.
- The term nephrolithiasis (nef-roh-lih-THIGH-ah-sis) describes the presence of stones in the kidney (nephr/o means kidney, and -lithiasis means the presence of stones). As these stones travel with the urine, they are named for the location where they become lodged.
- A nephrolith (NEF-roh-lith), also known as renal calculus or a kidney stone, is found in the kidney (nephr/o means kidney, and -lith means stone).
- A ureterolith (you-REE-ter-oh-lith) is a stone located anywhere along the ureter (ureter/o means ureter, and -lith means stone).
- A cystolith (SIS-toh-lith) is a stone located within the urinary bladder (cyst/o means bladder, and -lith means stone).

The Ureters

- Hydroureter (high-droh-you-REE-ter) is the distention of the ureter with urine that cannot flow because the ureter is blocked (hydr/o means water, and -ureter means ureter).
- Ureterectasis (you-ree-ter-ECK-tah-sis) is the distention of a ureter (ureter means ureter, and -ectasis means enlargement).
- Ureterorrhagia (you-ree-ter-oh-RAY-jee-ah) is the discharge of blood from the ureter (ureter/o means ureter, and -rrhagia means bleeding).

Urinary Tract Infections

A urinary tract infection (UTI) usually begins in the bladder; however, these infections can affect all, or parts, of the urinary system. These infections occur more frequently in women because of the urethra is short and located near the openings to the vagina and rectum.
- Urethritis (you-reh-THRIGH-tis) is an inflammation of the urethra (urethr means urethra, and -itis means inflammation).
- Cystitis (sis-TYE-tis) is an inflammation of the bladder (cyst mean bladder, and -itis means inflammation).
- Pyelitis (pye-eh-LYE-tis) is an inflammation of the renal pelvis (pyel means renal pelvis, and -itis means inflammation).

- Pyelonephritis (pye-eh-loh-neh-FRY-tis) is an inflammation of both the renal pelvis and of the kidney (pyel/o means renal pelvis, nephr means kidney, and -itis means inflammation). This is usually caused by a bacterial infection that has spread upward from the bladder.

The Urinary Bladder
- Cystalgia (sis-TAL-jee-ah) and cystodynia both mean pain in the urinary bladder (cyst means bladder, and -algia means pain).
- A cystocele (SIS-toh-seel), also known as a fallen bladder, is a hernia of the bladder through the vaginal wall (cyst/o means bladder, and -cele means hernia).
- Interstitial cystitis (in-ter-STISH-al sis-TYE-tis) is a chronic inflammation within the walls of the bladder. The symptoms of this condition are similar to those of cystitis; however, they do not respond to traditional treatment. Interstitial means relating to spaces within a tissue or organ.
- Trigonitis (tryg-oh-NYE-tis) is an inflammation of the urinary bladder that is localized in the region of the trigone (trigon means trigone, and -itis means inflammation).
- A vesicovaginal fistula (ves-ih-koh-VAJ-ih-nahl FIStyou- lah) is an abnormal opening between the bladder and vagina that allows the constant flow of urine from the bladder into the vagina (vesic/o means bladder, vagin means vagina, and -al means pertaining to). A fistula is an abnormal passage between two internal organs.

Neurogenic Bladder
- Neurogenic bladder (new-roh-JEN-ick) is a urinary problem caused by interference with the normal nerve pathways associated with urination (neur/o means nervous system, and -genic means created by).
- Depending on the type of neurological disorder causing the problem, the bladder may empty spontaneously, resulting in incontinence. As used here, incontinence means the inability to control the voiding of urine. In contrast, the problem can prevent the bladder from emptying at all. This results in urinary retention with overflow leakage.
- Some of the causes of this condition are a tumor of the nervous system, trauma, neuropathy, or an inflammatory condition such as multiple sclerosis. Neuropathy is a peripheral nervous system disorder affecting nerves anywhere except the brain or the spinal cord.

The Urethra
- Urethrorrhagia (you-ree-throh-RAY-jee-ah) is bleeding from the urethra (urethr/o means urethra, and -rrhagia means bleeding).
- Urethrorrhea (you-ree-throh-REE-ah) is an abnormal discharge from the urethra (urethr/o means urethra, and -rrhea means flow or discharge). This condition is associated with some sexually transmitted diseases.
- Urethrostenosis (you-ree-throh-steh-NOH-sis) is narrowing of the urethra (urethr/o means urethra, and -stenosis means tightening or

narrowing). This condition occurs almost exclusively in men and is often associated with prostate enlargement. Abnormal Urethral Openings
- Epispadias (ep-ih-SPAY-dee-as) is a congenital abnormality of the urethral opening. In the male with epispadias, the urethral opening is located on the upper surface of the penis. In the female with epispadias, the urethral opening is in the region of the clitoris.
- Hypospadias (high-poh-SPAY-dee-as) is a congenital abnormality of the urethral opening. In the male with hypospadias, the urethral opening is on the under surface of the penis. In the female with hypospadias, the urethral opening is into the vagina.
- Paraspadias (par-ah-SPAY-dee-as) is a congenital abnormality in males in which the urethral opening is on the side of the penis.

The Prostate Gland
- Benign prostatic hypertrophy (pros-TAT-ick high- PER-troh-fee), also known as an benign prostatic hyperplasia, enlarged prostate, or prostatomegaly, is an abnormal enlargement of the prostate gland that occurs most often in men over age 50 (see Figure 9.9). This condition can make urination difficult. Hypertrophy is the general increase in bulk of a body part or organ that is not due to tumor formation.
- Prostatism (PROS-tah-tizm) is the condition of having symptoms resulting from compression or obstruction of the urethra due to benign prostatic hypertrophy (prostat means prostate gland, and -ism means condition of). This can produce difficulties with urination and with urinary retention.
- Prostate cancer is one of the most common cancers among men. The disease can grow slowly with no symptoms, or it can grow aggressively and spread throughout the body.
- Prostatitis (pros-tah-TYE-tis) is an inflammation of the prostate gland (prostat means prostate gland, and -itis means inflammation).

Urination
- Diuresis (dye-you-REE-sis) is the increased output of urine (diur means increasing the output of urine, and -esis means an abnormal condition).
- Dysuria (dis-YOU-ree-ah) is difficult or painful urination (dys- means painful, and -uria means urination). This condition is frequently associated with urinary tract infections.
- Enuresis (en-you-REE-sis) is the involuntary discharge of urine (en- means into, and -uresis means urination).
- Nocturnal enuresis (nock-TER-nal en-you-REE-sis) is urinary incontinence during sleep. It is also known as bed-wetting. Nocturnal means pertaining to night.
- Nocturia (nock-TOO-ree-ah) is excessive urination during the night (noct means night, and -uria means urination).

- Oliguria (ol-ih-GOO-ree-ah) means scanty urination (olig means scanty, and -uria means urination). Oliguria is the opposite of polyuria.
- Polyuria (pol-ee-YOU-ree-ah) means excessive urination (poly- means many, and -uria means urination). Polyuria is the opposite of oliguria.
- Urinary hesitancy is difficulty in starting a urinary stream. This condition is most common in older men with enlarged prostate glands. In younger people, the inability to urinate when another person is present is known as bashful bladder syndrome.
- Urinary retention is the inability to empty the bladder. This condition is also more common in men, and is frequently associated with an enlarged prostate gland.

Incontinence

- Incontinence (in-KON-tih-nents) means the inability to control the excretion of urine and feces.
- Urinary incontinence is the inability to control the voiding of urine.
- Stress incontinence is the inability to control the voiding of urine under physical stress such as running, sneezing, laughing, or coughing.
- Overactive bladder (OAB), also known as urge incontinence, occurs when the detrusor muscle in the wall of the bladder is too active. Symptoms can include urinary frequency, urgency, and accidental urination due to a sudden and unstoppable need to urinate.

Diagnostic Procedures Of The Urinary System

- Urinalysis (you-rih-NAL-ih-sis) is the examination of urine to determine the presence of abnormal elements (urin means urine, and -analysis means a study of the parts). These tests are discussed further in Chapter 15.
- A bladder ultrasound is the use of a handheld ultrasound transducer to measure the amount of urine remaining in the bladder after urination. A normal bladder holds between 300 and 400 ccs of urine. When more than this amount is still present after urination, the bladder is described as being distended (enlarged).
- Catheterization (kath-eh-ter-eye-ZAY-shun) is the insertion of a tube into the bladder in order to procure a sterile specimen for diagnostic purposes. It is also used to remove urine from the bladder when the patient is unable to urinate for other reasons. Another use is to place medication into the bladder.
- Cystography (sis-TOG-rah-fee) is a radiographic examination of the bladder after instillation of a contrast medium via a urethral catheter (cyst/o means bladder, and -graphy means the process of creating a picture or record). The resulting film is a cystogram.
- Cystoscopy (sis-TOS-koh-pee) is the visual examination of the urinary bladder using a cystoscope (cyst/o means bladder, and -scopy means visual examination). A specialized cystoscope is also for treatment

procedures such as the removal of tumors or the reduction of an enlarged prostate gland.
- An intravenous pyelogram (in-trah-VEE-nus PYE-ehloh- gram), also known as excretory urography, is a radiographic study of the kidneys and ureters (pyel/o means renal pelvis, and -gram means a picture or record). A contrast medium is administered intravenously to clearly define these structures in the resulting image. This examination is used to diagnose changes in the urinary tract resulting from kidney stones, infections, enlarged prostate, tumors, and internal injuries after an abdominal trauma.
- Computed tomography, also known as a CAT scan, is more commonly used as a primary tool for evaluation of the urinary system because it can be rapidly performed and provides additional imaging of the abdomen, which may reveal other potential sources for the patient's symptoms.
- A KUB (Kidneys, Ureters, Bladder) is a radiographic study of these structures without the use of a contrast medium. This study is also referred to as a flat-plate of the abdomen.
- Retrograde urography is a radiograph of the urinary system taken after dye has been placed in the urethra through a sterile catheter and caused to flow upward (backward) through the urinary tract.
- Voiding cystourethrography (sis-toh-you-ree-THROGrah- fee) is a diagnostic procedure in which a fluoroscope is used to examine the flow of urine fromthe bladder and through the urethra (cyst/o means bladder, urethr/o means urethra, and -graphy means the process of producing a picture or record). This procedure is often performed after cystography.

Diagnostic Procedures of the Prostate Gland

- A digital rectal examination is performed on men to screen for prostate enlargement, infection, and indications of prostate cancer. As used here, the term digital means performed with a gloved finger placed in the rectum to palpate the prostate gland. Palpate means the use of the hands to examine a body part.
- The prostate-specific antigen blood test is used to screen for prostate cancer. Commonly referred to as the PSA test, it measures the amount of prostatespecific antigen that is present in a blood specimen. The prostate-specific antigen is a protein produced by the cells of the prostate gland. The higher a man's PSA level, the more likely it is that cancer is present.

Treatment Procedures Of The Urinary System

Medications

Diuretics (dye-you-RET-icks) are medications administered to increase urine secretion in order to rid the body of excess water and salt.

Dialysis

Dialysis (dye-AL-ih-sis) is a procedure to remove waste products from the blood of a patient whose kidneys no longer function (dia- means complete or through, and -lysis means separation). The two types of dialysis in common use are hemodialysis and peritoneal dialysis.

Hemodialysis

- Hemodialysis (hee-moh-dye-AL-ih-sis) is the process by which waste products are filtered directly from the patient's blood (hem/o means blood, dia means complete or through, and -lysis means separation). Treatment is performed on a hemodialysis unit which is commonly referred to as an artificial kidney.
- A shunt implanted in the patient's arm is connected to the hemodialysis unit and arterial blood flows through the filters of the unit. A shunt is an artificial passage that allows the blood to flow between the body and the hemodialysis unit.
- The filters contain dialysate, which is a solution made up of water and electrolytes. This solution cleanses the blood by removing waste products and excess fluids. Electrolytes are the salts that conduct electricity and are found in the body fluid, tissue, and blood.
- The cleansed blood is returned to the body through a vein.
- These treatments each take several hours and must be repeated about three times a week.

Peritoneal Dialysis

- In peritoneal dialysis (pehr-ih-toh-NEE-al dye-AL-ih-sis) the lining of the peritoneal cavity acts as the filter to remove waste from the blood. The dialysate solution flows into the peritoneal cavity and the fluid is exchanged through a catheter implanted in the abdominal wall. This type of dialysis is used for renal failure and certain types of poisoning.
- Continuous ambulatory peritoneal dialysis provides ongoing dialysis as the patient goes about his or her daily activities. In this procedure, a dialysate solution is instilled from a plastic container worn under the patient's clothing. About every 4 hours, the used solution is drained back into this bag and the bag is discarded. A new bag is then attached, the solution is instilled, and the process continues.
- Continuous cycling peritoneal dialysis uses a machine to cycle the dialysate fluid during the night while the patient sleeps.

The Kidneys

- Nephrolysis (neh-FROL-ih-sis) is the freeing of a kidney from adhesions (nephr/o means kidney, and -lysis means setting free). An adhesion is a band of fibers that holds structures together abnormally.

Note: The suffix -lysis means setting free; however, it also means destruction. Therefore, the term nephrolysis can also describe a pathologic condition in which there is the destruction of renal cells.

- A nephropexy (NEF-roh-peck-see), also known as nephrorrhaphy, is the surgical fixation of a floating kidney (nephr/o means kidney, and -pexy means surgical fixation).
- A nephrostomy (neh-FROS-toh-mee) is the establishment of an opening from the pelvis of the kidney to the exterior of the body (nephr means kidney and -ostomy means creating an opening). In a kidney affected by hydronephrosis, this allows bypassing of the ureter because the urine from the kidney is drained directly through the back.
- Pyeloplasty (PYE-eh-loh-plas-tee) is the surgical repair of the renal pelvis (pyel/o means the renal pelvis, and -plasty means surgical repair).
- A pyelotomy (pye-eh-LOT-oh-mee) is a surgical incision into the renal pelvis (pyel means the renal pelvis, and -otomy means surgical incision). This procedure is performed to correct an obstruction of the junction between the renal pelvis and the ureter.
- Renal transplantation, commonly known as a kidney transplant, is the grafting of a donor kidney into the body to replace the recipient's failed kidneys. A single transplanted kidney, from either a living or nonliving donor, is capable of adequately performing all kidney functions.

Removal of Kidney Stones

- Extracorporeal shockwave lithotripsy (ESWL) is the destruction of stones with the use of high-energy ultrasonic waves traveling through water or gel. The fragments of these stones are then excreted in the urine. Extracorporeal means situated or occurring outside the body.
- Lithotripsy (LITH-ohtrip- see) means to crush a stone (lith/o means stone, and -tripsy means to crush).
- A nephrolithotomy (nef-roh-lih-THOT-oh-mee) is the surgical removal of a nephrolith (kidney stone) through an incision in the kidney (nephr/o means kidney, lith means stone, and -otomy means surgical incision).
- A percutaneous nephrolithotomy (per-kyou-TAY-nee-us nef-roh-lih-THOT-oh-mee) is performed by making a small incision in the back and inserting a nephroscope to crush and remove a kidney stone. Percutaneous means performed through the skin. A nephroscope is a specialized endoscope used in the treatment of the kidneys.

The Ureters

- A ureterectomy (you-ree-ter-ECK-toh-mee) is the surgical removal of a ureter (ureter means ureter, and -ectomy means surgical removal).
- Ureteroplasty (you-REE-ter-oh-plas-tee) is the surgical repair of a ureter (ureter/o means ureter, and -plasty means surgical repair).
- Ureterorrhaphy (you-ree-ter-OR-ah-fee) is the surgical suturing of a ureter (ureter/o means ureter, and -rrhaphy means surgical suturing).

The Urinary Bladder

- A cystectomy (sis-TECK-toh-mee) is the surgical removal of all or part of the urinary bladder (cyst means bladder, and -ectomy means surgical removal).
- Cystopexy (sis-toh-peck-see) is the surgical fixation of the bladder to the abdominal wall (cyst/o means bladder, and -pexy means surgical fixation).
- Cystorrhaphy (sis-TOR-ah-fee) is the surgical suturing of the bladder (cyst/o means bladder, and -rrhaphy means surgical suturing).
- A lithotomy (lih-THOT-oh-mee) is a surgical incision for the removal of a stone from the bladder (lith means stone, and -otomy means surgical incision). This term also is used to describe a physical examination position.

Catheterization

- Catheterization is performed to withdraw urine for diagnostic purposes, to control incontinence, or to place fluid, such as a chemotherapy solution, into the bladder.
- Urethral catheterization is performed by inserting a tube along the urethra and into the bladder.
- An indwelling catheter is one that remains inside the body for a prolonged time.
- Suprapubic catheterization (soo-prah-PYOU-bick kath-eh-ter-eye-ZAY-shun) is the placement of a catheter into the bladder through a small incision made through the abdominal wall just above the pubic bone.

The Urethra

- A meatotomy (mee-ah-TOT-oh-mee) is a surgical incision made in the urinary meatus to enlarge the opening (meat means meatus, and -otomy means surgical incision).
- Urethropexy (you-REE-throh-peck-see) is the surgical fixation of the urethra (urethr/o means urethra, and -pexy means surgical fixation). This procedure is usually performed to correct urinary stress incontinence.
- Urethrostomy (you-reh-THROS-toh-mee) is the surgical creation of a permanent opening between the urethra and the skin (urethr means urethra, and -ostomy means creating an opening).
- A urethrotomy (you-reh-THROT-oh-mee) is a surgical incision into the urethra for relief of a stricture (urethr means urethra, and -otomy means surgical incision).

Prostate Treatment

- Ablation (ab-LAY-shun), which is the term used to describe some types of treatment of prostate cancer, describes the removal of a body part or

the destruction of its function by surgery, hormones, drugs, heat, chemicals, electrocautery, or other methods.
- A prostatectomy (pros-tah-TECK-toh-mee) is the surgical removal of all or part of the prostate gland (prostat means prostate, and -ectomy means surgical removal). This procedure is performed to treat prostate cancer or to reduce an enlarged prostate gland.
- A radical prostatectomy, which is performed through the abdomen, is the surgical removal of the entire prostate gland, the seminal vesicles, and some surrounding tissues.
- A transurethral prostatectomy, also known as a TURP, is the removal of an overgrowth of tissue from the prostate gland through a resectoscope. A resectoscope is a specialized endoscopic instrument that resembles a cystoscope.
- Radiation therapy and hormone therapy are additional treatments used to control prostate cancer.

Urinary Incontinence Treatment

- Kegel exercises, which were named for Dr. Arnold Kegel, are a series of pelvic muscle exercises used to strengthen the muscles of the pelvic floor to control urinary stress incontinence in women.
- Bladder retraining is a program of urinating on a schedule with increasingly longer time intervals between scheduled urination. The goal is to reestablish voluntary bladder control and to break the cycle of frequency, urgency, and urge incontinence.

Abbreviations Related To The Urinary System

- benign prostatic hypertrophy = BPH
- catheterization = cath
- chronic renal failure = CRF
- cystoscopy = cysto
- intravenous pyelogram =
- polycystic kidney disease = PKD

Critical Thinking Exercise

The following story and questions are designed to stimulate critical thinking through class discussion or as a brief essay response. There are no right or wrong answers to these questions.

"Mom, they want me to play for the National Women's Hockey League!" Josie yelled as she ran into the living room. She had just finished practice, and the scouts had told her afterwards how impressed they were with her moves. Finally, her life long dream of winning an Olympic gold medal for Canada might actually come true! She'd had to make some sacrifices, like living at home after high school, but it looked like that would all pay off. As soon as she saw the looks on the faces of her parents, her smile disappeared.

"Honey, we just got back from the doctor. It turns out that your brother's recurrent bouts of pyelonephritis have led to irreversible renal damage. The nephrologist is recommending that Xavier have a kidney transplant," her mom explained with a pained look. "We know that he has a better chance if he has a related donor, but he could always go on hemodialysis and wait for a cadaver donor ..."

Josie saw her dreams of a hockey career fade away. After Xavier's third bout with nephrotic syndrome, the whole family had been tested for compatibility in case he needed a transplant. Josie was the only one with a positive cross-match. The doctors had explained to her then what it would mean if she decided to donate one of her kidneys, but Josie had brushed it off, assuming that her brother would get better. Now the voices of the doctors came back to her. "No contact sports after a nephrectomy," she heard them say, "There's too big a risk of rupturing the remaining kidney." Josie was faced with the toughest decision of all: she loved Xavier, but hockey was her life.

Suggested Discussion Topics

1. Discuss the long-term repercussions of being a living organ donor.
2. Imagine that you are Josie's mom or dad and one of your children has the opportunity to save the life of another one of your children. Would you encourage him or her to donate an organ?
3. If Josie decides to donate her kidney and then later chooses to continue playing hockey, what advice should her parents give her?
4. What options might be open to Josie's brother other than having his sister donate a kidney?

Medical Terminology for Health Professions 4.0

CHAPTER 10

THE NERVOUS SYSTEM

This list contains essential word parts and medical terms for this chapter.

Word Parts
- caus/o
- concuss/o
- contus/o
- encephal/o
- -esthesia
- esthet/o
- -graphy
- klept/o
- -mania
- mening/o
- myel/o
- neur/i, neur/o
- -phobia
- psych/o
- -tropic

Medical Terms
- acrophobia (ack-roh-FOH-bee-ah)
- Alzheimer's disease (ALTZ-high-merz)
- amyotrophic lateral sclerosis (ah-my-oh- TROH-fick)
- anesthetic (an-es-THET-ick)
- anesthetist (ah-NES-theh-tist)
- anxiety disorders
- autism (AW-tizm)
- Bell's palsy
- carotid ultrasonography (ul-trah-son-OG-rah-fee)
- causalgia (kaw-ZAL-jee-ah)
- cerebral contusion (SER-eh-bral kon-TOO-zhun)
- cerebral palsy (SER-eh-bral PAWL-zee)

- cerebrovascular accident (ser-eh-broh-VASkyou-lar)
- cervical radiculopathy (rah-dick-you-LOP-ah-thee)
- claustrophobia (klaws-troh-FOH-bee-ah)
- cognition (kog-NISH-un)
- coma (KOH-mah)
- concussion (kon-KUSH-un)
- cranial hematoma (hee-mah-TOH-mah)
- delirium (dee-LIR-ee-um)
- delirium tremens (dee-LIR-ee-um TREE-mens)
- delusion (dee-LOO-zhun)
- dementia (dee-MEN-shee-ah)
- dura mater (DOO-rah MAH-ter)
- dyslexia (dis-LECK-see-ah)
- echoencephalography (eck-oh-en-sef-ah-LOGrah-fee)
- electroencephalography (ee-leck-troh-en-sef-ah-LOG-rah-fee)
- encephalitis (en-sef-ah-LYE-tis)
- epidural anesthesia (ep-ih-DOO-ral an-es-THEEzee-ah)
- epilepsy (EP-ih-lep-see)
- factitious disorder (fack-TISH-us)
- Guillain-Barré syndrome (gee-YAHN-bah-RAY SIN-drohm)
- hallucination (hah-loo-sih-NAY-shun)
- hemorrhagic stroke (hem-oh-RAJ-ick)
- hydrocephalus (high-droh-SEF-ah-lus)
- hyperesthesia (high-per-es-THEE-zee-ah)
- hypochondriasis (high-poh-kon-DRY-ah-sis)
- ischemic stroke (iss-KEE-mick)
- lethargy (LETH-ar-jee)
- meningitis (men-in-JIGH-tis)
- meningocele (meh-NING-goh-seel)
- migraine headache (MY-grayn)
- multiple sclerosis (skleh-ROH-sis)
- myelitis (my-eh-LYE-tis)
- myelography (my-eh-LOG-rah-fee)
- narcolepsy (NAR-koh-lep-see)
- neurotransmitters (new-roh-trans-MIT-erz)
- obsessive-compulsive disorder
- panic attack
- paresthesia (pair-es-THEE-zee-ah)
- Parkinson's disease
- peripheral neuropathy (new-ROP-ah-thee)
- posttraumatic stress disorder
- Reye's syndrome
- schizophrenia (skit-soh-FREE-nee-ah)
- sciatica (sigh-AT-ih-kah)

- shaken baby syndrome
- syncope (SIN-koh-pee)
- trichotillomania (trick-oh-till-oh-MAY-nee-ah)
- trigeminal neuralgia (try-JEM-ih-nal new- RAL-jee-ah)

Objectives

On completion of this chapter, you should be able to:
1. Describe the functions and structures of the nervous system.
2. Identify the major divisions of the nervous system and describe the structures of each by location and function.
3. Identify the medical specialists who treat disorders of the nervous system.
4. Recognize, define, spell, and pronounce terms related to the pathology and the diagnostic and treatment procedures of the nervous system.
5. Recognize, define, spell, and pronounce terms related to the pathology and the diagnostic and treatment procedures of mental health disorders.

Structures Of The Nervous System

The major structures of the nervous system are the nerves, brain, spinal cord, and sensory organs. The sensory organs, which are the eyes, ears, nose, skin, and tongue, are discussed in other chapters.

Divisions of the Nervous System

For descriptive purposes, the nervous system is divided into two primary parts: the central and peripheral nervous systems.
- The central nervous system (CNS) includes the brain and spinal cord. The functions of the central nervous system are to receive and process information, and to regulate all bodily activity.
- The peripheral nervous system (PNS) includes the 12 pairs of cranial nerves extending from the brain and the 31 pairs of peripheral spinal nerves extending outward from the spinal cord. The function of the peripheral nervous system is to transmit nerve signals to, and from, the central nervous system.

The Nerves

- A nerve is one or more bundles of neurons that connect the brain and the spinal cord with other parts of the body.
- A tract is a bundle or group of nerve fibers located within the brain or spinal cord.
- Ascending nerve tracts carry nerve impulses toward the brain.
- Descending nerve tracts carry nerve impulses away from the brain.
- A ganglion (GANG-glee-on) is a nerve center made up of a cluster of nerve cell bodies outside the central nervous system (plural, ganglia or

ganglions). Note: The term ganglion also describes a benign, tumor-like cyst.
- The term innervation (in-err-VAY-shun) means the supply of nerves to a specific body part.
- A plexus (PLECK-sus) is a network of intersecting spinal nerves (plural, plexuses) (see Figure 10.9). This term also describes a network of intersecting blood or lymphatic vessels.
- Receptors are sites in the sensory organs (eyes, ears, skin, nose, and taste buds) that receive external stimulation. The receptors send the stimulus through the sensory neurons to the brain for interpretation.
- A stimulus is anything that excites (activates) a nerve and causes an impulse (plural, stimuli). An impulse is a wave of excitation transmitted through nerve fibers and neurons.

The Reflexes

- A reflex (REE-flecks) is an automatic, involuntary response to some change, either inside or outside the body. Examples of reflex actions include:
- Changes in the heart rate, breathing rate, and blood pressure.
- Coughing and sneezing.
- Responses to painful stimuli.

The Neurons

- Neurons (NEW-ronz) are the basic cells of the nervous system that allow different parts of the body to communicate with each other.
- The body has billions of neurons carrying nerve impulses throughout the body via an electrochemical process. This process creates patterns of neuron electrical activity known as brain waves. Different types of brain waves are produced during periods of intense activity, rest, and sleep.
- The three types of neurons are described according to their function. The memory aid A-C-E will help you remember their names, and S-A-M will help you remember their functions.

Neuron Parts

- Each neuron consists of a cell body, several dendrites, a single axon, and terminal end fibers.
- The dendrites (DEN-drytes) are the root-like processes that receive impulses and conduct them to the cell body. A process is a structure that extends out from the cell body.
- The axon (ACK-son) is a process that extends away from the cell body and conducts impulses away from the nerve cell. An axon can be more than three feet long. Many, but not all, axons are protected by a myelin sheath, which is a white fatty tissue covering.
- Terminal end fibers are the branching fibers at the end of the axon that lead the nervous impulse from the axon to the synapse.

- A synapse (SIN-apps) is the space between two neurons or between a neuron and a receptor organ. A single neuron can have a few, or several hundred, synapses.

Neurotransmitters

- Neurotransmitters (new-roh-trans-MIT-erz) are chemical substances that make it possible for messages to cross from the synapse of a neuron to the target receptor. There are between 200 and 300 known neurotransmitters, and each has a specialized function. Examples of neurotransmitters and their roles are shown below.
- Acetylcholine is released at some synapses in the spinal cord and at neuromuscular junctions; it influences muscle action.
- Dopamine is released within the brain. It is believed to be involved in mood and thought disorders and in abnormal movement disorders such as Parkinson's disease.
- Endorphins are naturally occurring substances that are produced by the brain to help relieve pain.
- Norepinephrine, which is released at synaptic nerve endings, responds to hypotension and physical stress.
- Serotonin, which is released in the brain, has roles in sleep, hunger, and pleasure recognition. It is also sometimes linked to mood disorders.

Glial Cells

Glial cells provide support and protection for neurons, and their four main functions are: (1) to surround neurons and hold them in place, (2) to supply nutrients and oxygen to neurons, (3) to insulate one neuron from another, and (4) to destroy and remove dead neurons.

The Myelin Sheath

- A myelin sheath (MY-eh-lin) is the protective covering made up of glial cells. This white sheath forms the white matter of the brain, and covers some parts of the spinal cord and the axon of most peripheral nerves.
- The portion of the nerve fibers that are myelinated are known as white matter. The term myelinated means having a myelin sheath. It is the color of this covering that makes these fibers white.
- The portion of the nerve fibers that are unmyelinated are known as gray matter. The termunmyelinated means lacking amyelin sheath. It is the lack of themyelin sheath that creates the gray color of the brain and spinal cord.

The Central Nervous System

The central nervous system is made up of the brain and spinal cord. These structures are protected externally by the bones of the craniumand the vertebrae of the spinal column. Within these bony structures, the brain and spinal cord are further protected by the meninges and the cerebrospinal fluid.

The Meninges
- The meninges (meh-NIN-jeez) are the system of membranes that enclose the brain and spinal cord of the central nervous (singular meninx). The meninges consist of three layers of connective tissue. These are the dura mater, arachnoid membrane, and the pia mater.

The Dura Mater
- The dura mater (DOO-rah MAH-ter) is the thick, tough, outermost membrane of the meninges. Dura means hard, and mater means mother.
- The inner surface of cranium (skull) is lined with dura mater.
- The inner surface of the vertebral column is known as the epidural space. This space, which is located between the walls of the vertebral column and the dura mater of the meninges, contains fat and supportive connective tissues to cushion the dura mater.
- In both the skull and vertebral column, the subdural space is located between the dura mater and the arachnoid membrane.

The Arachnoid Membrane
- The arachnoid membrane (ah-RACK-noid), which resembles a spider web, is the second layer of the meninges and is located between the dura mater and the pia mater. Arachnoid means having to do with spiders.
- The arachnoid membrane is loosely attached to the other meninges to allow space for fluid to flow between the layers.
- The subarachnoid space, which is located below the arachnoid membrane and above the pia mater, contains cerebrospinal fluid.

The Pia Mater
- The pia mater (PEE-ah MAH-ter), which is the third layer of the meninges, is located nearest to the brain and spinal cord. It consists of delicate connective tissue that contains a rich supply of blood vessels. Pia means tender or delicate, and mater means mother.

Cerebrospinal Fluid
Cerebrospinal fluid (ser-eh-broh-SPY-nal), also known as spinal fluid, is produced by special capillaries within the four ventricles located in the middle region of the cerebrum. Cerebrospinal fluid is a clear, colorless, and watery fluid that flows throughout the brain and around the spinal cord. The functions of this fluid are to:
- Cool and cushion these organs from shock or injury.
- Nourish the brain and spinal cord by transporting nutrients and chemical messengers to these tissues.

The Cerebrum
- The cerebrum (seh-REE-brum) is the largest and uppermost portion of the brain. It is responsible for all thought, judgment, memory, and emotion, as well as for controlling and integrating motor and sensory functions. Note that cerebrum and cerebellum are similar words, but refer to very different parts of the brain. Memory aid: The cerebellum is below the cerebrum.
- The term cerebral (SER-eh-bral) means pertaining to the cerebrum or to the brain (cerebr means brain, and -al means pertaining to).
- The cerebral cortex, which is made up of gray matter, is the outer layer of the cerebrum and is arranged in deep folds known as fissures. As used here, a fissure is a normally occurring deep groove. Skin fissures.

The Cerebral Hemispheres
The cerebrum is divided to create two cerebral hemispheres that are connected at the lower midpoint by the corpus callosum.
- The left cerebral hemisphere controls the majority of functions on the right side of the body. An injury to the left hemisphere produces sensory and motor deficits on the right side of the body.
- The right cerebral hemisphere controls most of functions on the left side of the body. An injury to the right hemisphere produces sensory and motor deficits on the left side of the body.
- The crossing of nerve fibers that makes this arrangement possible occurs in the brain stem.

The Cerebral Lobes
Each cerebral hemisphere is subdivided to create pairs of cerebral lobes. Each lobe is named for the bone of the cranium that covers it. The frontal lobe controls skilled motor functions,
memory, and behavior.
- The parietal lobe receives and interprets nerve impulses from sensory receptors in the tongue, skin, and muscles.
- The occipital lobe controls eyesight.
- The temporal lobe controls the senses of hearing and smell, and the ability to create, store, and access new information.

The Thalamus
- The thalamus (THAL-ah-mus), which is located below the cerebrum, produces sensations by relaying impulses to and from the cerebrum and the sense organs of the body.

The Hypothalamus
The hypothalamus (high-poh-THAL-ah-mus) is located below the thalamus.

The Cerebellum
- The cerebellum (ser-eh-BELL-um) is the second-largest part of the brain. It is located at the back of the head below the posterior portion of the cerebrum.
- The cerebellum receives incoming messages regarding movement within joints, muscle tone, and positions of the body. From here, messages are relayed to the different parts of the brain that control the motions of skeletal muscles.
- The general functions of the cerebellum are to produce smooth, coordinated movements, to maintain equilibrium, and to sustain normal postures.

The Brainstem
- The brainstem is the stalk-like portion of the brain that connects the cerebral hemispheres with the spinal cord. It is made up of three parts: the midbrain, pons, and medulla.
- The midbrain and pons (PONZ) provide conduction pathways to and from the higher and lower centers in the brain. They also control reflexes for movements of the eyes and head in response to visual and auditory stimuli. (Pons is the Latin word for bridge.)
- The medulla (meh-DULL-ah), which is located at the lowest part of the brainstem, is connected to the spinal cord. It controls basic survival functions, including the muscles that make possible respiration, heart rate, and blood pressure, as well as reflexes for coughing, sneezing, swallowing, and vomiting.

The Spinal Cord
- The spinal cord is a long, fragile tube-like structure that begins at the end of the brain stem and continues down almost to the bottom of the spinal column.
- The spinal cord contains all the nerves that affect the limbs and lower part of the body, and serves as the pathway for impulses traveling to and from the brain.
- The spinal cord is surrounded and protected by cerebrospinal fluid and the meninges.

The Peripheral Nervous System
- The peripheral nervous system consists of the 12 pairs of cranial nerves that extend from the brain, plus 31 pairs of spinal nerves that extending from the spinal cord. Peripheral means pertaining to body parts that are away from the center of the body. Three types of specialized peripheral nerves transmit signals to and from the central nervous system. These are autonomic, sensory, and somatic nerve fibers.
- Autonomic nerve fibers carry instructions to the organs and glands and from the autonomic nervous system.

- Sensory nerve fibers receive external stimuli, such as how something feels, and transmit this information to the brain where it is interpreted. Somatic nerve fibers, which are also known as motor nerve fibers, convey information that controls the body's voluntary muscular movements.

The Cranial Nerves
- The 12 pairs of cranial nerves originate from the undersurface of the brain. The two nerves of a pair are identical in function and structure, and each nerve of a pair serves half of the body.
- These cranial nerves are identified by Roman numerals and arenamedfor the area or function they serve.

The Peripheral Spinal Nerves
The 31 pairs of peripheralspinal nerves are grouped together, and named, based on the region of the body they innervate.

Medical Specialties Related To The Nervous System
- An anesthesiologist (an-es-thee-zee-OL-oh-jist) is a physician who specializes in administering anesthetic agents before and during surgery (an- means without, esthesi means feeling, and -ologist means specialist).
- An anesthetist (ah-NES-theh-tist) is amedical professional who specializes in administering anesthesia, but is not a physician, for example, a nurse anesthetist (an- means without, esthet means feeling, and -ist means specialist).
- A neurologist (new-ROL-oh-jist) is a physician who specializes in diagnosing and treating diseases and disorders of the nervous system (neur means nerve, and -ologist means specialist).
- A neurosurgeon is a physician who specializes in surgery of the nervous system.
- A psychiatrist (sigh-KYE-ah-trist) is a physician who specializes in diagnosing and treating chemical dependencies, emotional problems, and mental illness (psych means mind, and -iatrist means specialist).
- A psychologist (sigh-KOL-oh-jist) holds an advanced degree, but is not a medical doctor (MD). This specialist evaluates and treats emotional problems and mental illness (psych means mind, and -ologist means specialist).

Pathology Of The Nervous System

The Head and Meninges
- Cephalalgia (sef-ah-LAL-jee-ah), also known as a headache, is pain in the head (cephal means head, and -algia means pain).
- A migraine headache (MY-grayn), which can be preceded by a warning aura, is characterized by throbbing pain on one side of the head. As used

here, a warning aura is a sensation perceived by the patient that precedes a migraine. These headaches, which affect primarily women, are accompanied by nausea, vomiting, and sensitivity to light or sound.
- Cluster headaches are intensely painful headaches that affect one side of the head and may be associated with tearing of the eyes and nasal congestion. These headaches, which affect primarily men, are named for their repeated occurrence in groups or clusters.
- An encephalocele (en-SEF-ah-loh-seel), also known as a craniocele, is a congenital herniation of brain tissue through a gap in the skull (encephal/o means brain, and -cele means hernia). Congenital means present at birth, and herniation means protrusion of a structure from its normal position. Compare this with a meningocele.
- A meningocele (meh-NING-goh-seel) is the congenital herniation of the meninges through a defect in the skull or spinal column (mening/o means meninges, and -cele means hernia). Compare this with an encephalocele.
- Hydrocephalus (high-droh-SEF-ah-lus) is a condition in which excess cerebrospinal fluid accumulates in the ventricles of the brain (hydr/o means water, cephal means head, and -us is a singular noun ending). This condition can occur at birth or develop later on in life from obstructions related to meningitis, brain tumors, or other causes.
- Meningitis (men-in-JIGH-tis) is an inflammation of the meninges of the brain and spinal cord (mening means meninges, and -itis means inflammation). This condition, which can be fatal, is usually caused by a bacterial or viral infection and is characterized by fever, vomiting, intense headache, and a stiff neck. Compare with encephalitis.

Disorders of the Brain

- Alzheimer's disease (ALTZ-high-merz) is a group of disorders involving the parts of the brain that control thought, memory, and language. It is marked by progressive deterioration that affects both the memory and reasoning capabilities of an individual.
- The term cognition (kog-NISH-un) describes the mental activities associated with thinking, learning, and memory. Mild cognitive impairment is a memory disorder, usually associated with recently acquired information, that may be an early predictor of

Alzheimer's disease

- Dementia (dee-MEN-shee-ah) is a slowly progressive decline in mental abilities, including memory, thinking, and judgment, that is often accompanied by personality changes.
- Encephalitis (en-sef-ah-LYE-tis), which is an inflammation of the brain, can be caused by a viral infection such as rabies (encelphal means brain, and -itis means inflammation). Compare with meningitis.

- Parkinson's disease (PD) is a chronic, degenerative central nervous disorder characterized by fine muscle tremors, rigidity, and a slow or shuffling gait. Gait describes the manner of walking. This slow or shuffling gait is caused by the gradually progressive loss of control over movements due to inadequate levels of the neurotransmitter dopamine in the brain.
- Reye's syndrome (RS) is a potentially serious or deadly disorder in children that is characterized by vomiting and confusion. This syndrome usually follows a viral illness in which the child was treated with aspirin.
- Tetanus (TET-ah-nus), also known as lockjaw, is an acute and potentially fatal infection of the central nervous system caused by a toxin produced by the tetanus bacteria. Tetanus can be prevented through immunization. Without this protection, this condition is typically acquired through a deep puncture wound.

Brain Injuries

- Amnesia (am-NEE-zee-ah) is a memory disturbance characterized by a total or partial inability to recall past experiences. This condition can be caused by a brain injury, illness, or a psychological disturbance.
- A concussion (kon-KUSH-un) is a violent shaking up or jarring of the brain (concuss means shaken together, and -ion means condition or state of). A concussion may result in a temporary loss of awareness and function. Compare with a cerebral contusion.
- A cerebral contusion (SER-eh-bral kon-TOO-zhun) is the bruising of brain tissue as the result of a head injury that causes the brain to bounce against the rigid bone of the skull (contus means bruise, and -ion means condition). Compare with concussion.
- A cranial hematoma (hee-mah-TOH-mah) is a collection of blood trapped in the tissues of the brain (hemat means blood, and -oma means tumor).

Named for their location, the types of cranial hematomas include an epidural hematoma located above the dura mater or a subdural hematoma, which is located below the dura mater.

Traumatic Brain Injury

- A traumatic brain injury is a blow to the head or a penetrating head injury that damages the brain. Not all blows to the head result in damage to the brain. When an injury does occur, it can range from mild, with only a brief change in mental status, to severe, with longer lasting effects.
- The term coup describes an injury occurring within the skull near the point of impact, such as hitting the windshield in an auto accident. A contrecoup, also described as a counter blow, is an injury that occurs beneath the skull opposite to the area of impact.

- Shaken baby syndrome describes the results of a child being violently shaken by someone. This action can cause brain injury, blindness, fractures, seizures, paralysis, and death.

Levels of Consciousness
- Levels of consciousness (LOC) are terms used to describe alterations of consciousness caused by injury, disease, or substances such as medication, drugs, or alcohol.
- Being conscious is the state of being awake, alert, aware, and responding appropriately.
- Being unconscious is a state of being unaware and unable to respond to any stimuli including pain.
- Lethargy (LETH-ar-jee) is a lowered level of consciousness marked by listlessness, drowsiness, and apathy. As used here, apathy means indifference and a reduced level of activity. The term lethargic refers to a person who is at this level of consciousness.
- A stupor (STOO-per) is an unresponsive state from which a person can be aroused only briefly and with vigorous, repeated attempts.
- Syncope (SIN-koh-pee), also known as fainting, is the brief loss of consciousness caused by the decreased flow of blood to the brain.
- A coma (KOH-mah) is a profound (deep) state of unconsciousness marked by the absence of spontaneous eye movements, no response to painful stimuli, and the lack of speech. The term comatose refers to a person who is in a coma.
- A persistent vegetative state is a type of coma inwhich the patient exhibits alternating sleep and wake cycles; however, due to severe damage to certain areas of the brain, the person is unconscious even when appearing to be awake.

Delirium
- Delirium (dee-LIR-ee-um) is an acute condition of confusion, disorientation, disordered thinking and memory, agitation, and hallucinations. This condition is usually caused by a treatable physical condition, such as a high fever. An individual suffering from this condition is described as being delirious.

Strokes
- A stroke, or CVA, is properly known as a cerebrovascular accident (ser-eh-broh-VAS-kyou-lar). This condition is damage to the brain that occurs when the blood flow to the brain is disrupted because a blood vessel is either blocked or has ruptured. The location of the disruption determines the symptoms that will be present. Damage to the right side of the brain produces symptoms on the left side of the body. Damage to the left side of the brain produces symptoms on the right side of the body.

Ischemic Stroke

- An ischemic stroke (iss-KEE-mick), which is the most common type of stroke in older people, occurs when the flow of blood to the brain is blocked. This type of stroke may be caused by narrowing of the carotid artery or by a cerebral thrombosis. A cerebral thrombosis occurs when a blood clot blocks an artery that supplies blood to the cerebrum. This blockage damages the controls of movement, senses, and speech.
- A transient ischemic attack (TIA), pronounced as T-I-A, is the temporary interruption in the blood supply to the brain. Transient means passing quickly, and ischemic means pertaining to the disruption of the blood supply. Symptoms of a TIA include numbness, blurred vision, dizziness, or loss of balance. A TIA passes in less than an hour; however, this incident is often a warning sign that the individual is at risk for a more serious and debilitating stroke.
- Aphasia (ah-FAY-zee-ah), which is often caused by brain damage associated with a stroke, is the loss of the ability to speak, write, and/or comprehend the written or spoken word (a- means without, and -phasia means speech).

Hemorrhagic Stroke

- A hemorrhagic stroke (hem-oh-RAJ-ick), also known as a bleed, occurs when a blood vessel in the brain leaks. A bleed also occurs when an aneurysm within the brain ruptures. An aneurysm is a localized, weak, balloon-like enlargement of an artery wall. This type of stroke is less common than ischemic strokes and is often fatal. A hemorrhagic stroke affects the area of the brain damaged by the leaking blood.

Sleep Disorders

- Insomnia is the prolonged or abnormal inability to sleep. This condition is usually a symptom of another problem such as depression, pain, or excessive caffeine n Somnambulism (som-NAM-byou-lizm), also known as sleepwalking or noctambulism, is the condition of walking or performing some other activity without awakening (somn means sleep, ambul means to walk, and -ism means condition of).

The Spinal Cord

- Myelitis (my-eh-LYE-tis) is an inflammation of the spinal cord (myel means spinal cord and bone marrow, and -itis means inflammation). The term myelitis also means inflammation of bone marrow.
- A myelosis (my-eh-LOH-sis) is a tumor of the spinal cord (myel means spinal cord and bone marrow, and -osis means abnormal condition). Myelosis also means an abnormal proliferation of bone marrow tissue.
- Poliomyelitis (poh-lee-oh-my-eh-LYE-tis), also known as polio, is a highly contagious viral disease (poli/o means gray, myel means spinal cord and

bone marrow, and -itis means inflammation). There is no known cure for polio; however, it can be prevented through vaccination.
- Post-polio syndrome is the recurrence later in life of some polio symptoms in individuals who have had childhood poliomyelitis and have recovered from it.
- Spinal cord injuries are discussed in Chapter 4 under Paralysis.

Pinched Nerves

- Radiculitis (rah-dick-you-LYE-tis), also known as a pinched nerve, is an inflammation of the root of a spinal nerve that causes pain and numbness radiating down the affected limb (radicul means root or nerve root, and -itis means inflammation). This term usually applies to that portion of the root that lies between the spinal cord and the intervertebral canal of the spinal column.
- Cervical radiculopathy (rah-dick-you-LOP-ah-thee) is nerve pain caused by pressure on the spinal nerve roots in the neck region (radicul/o means nerve root, and -pathy means disease).
- Lumbar radiculopathy is nerve pain in the lower back caused by muscle spasms or by nerve root irritation from the compression of vertebral disks such as a herniated disk.

Multiple Sclerosis

- Multiple sclerosis (skleh-ROH-sis) is a progressive autoimmune disorder characterized by inflammation that causes demyelination of the myelin sheath. This scars the brain, spinal cord, and optic nerves and disrupts the transmission of nerve impulses. This damage leaves the patient with varying degrees of pain plus physical and cognitive problems.
- Demyelination is the loss of patches of the protective myelin sheath.
- The disease is characterized by periods of exacerbations, which are episodes of worsening symptoms that are also referred to as flares. Between these episodes, the patient may be in remission. Remission is a time during which the symptoms ease, but the disease has not been cured.

Nerves

- Amyotrophic lateral sclerosis (ah-my-oh-TROH-fick), also known as Lou Gehrig's disease, is a rapidly progressive neurological disease that attacks the nerve cells responsible for controlling voluntary muscles. Patients affected with this condition become progressively weaker until they are completely paralyzed and die.
- Bell's palsy is the temporary paralysis of the seventh cranial nerve that causes paralysis only of the affected side of the face. In addition, paralysis symptoms can include the inability to close the eye, pain, tearing, drooling, hypersensitivity to sound in the affected ear, and impairment of taste.

- Guillain-Barré syndrome (gee-YAHN-bah-RAY), also known as infectious polyneuritis, is an inflammation of the myelin sheath of peripheral nerves, characterized by rapidly worsening muscle weakness that can lead to temporary paralysis. This condition is an autoimmune reaction that can occur after certain viral infections or an immunization.
- Sciatica (sigh-AT-ih-kah) is inflammation of the sciatic nerve that results in pain, burning, and tingling along the course of the affected sciatic nerve through the thigh, leg, and foot.
- Trigeminal neuralgia (try-JEM-ih-nal new-RAL-jeeah) is characterized by severe lightning-like pain due to an inflammation of the fifth cranial nerve. These sudden, intense, brief attacks of sharp pain affect the cheek, lips, and gums only on the side of the face innervated by the affected nerve.

Cerebral Palsy

- Cerebral palsy (SER-eh-bral PAWL-zee) is a condition characterized by poor muscle control, spasticity, speech defects, and other neurologic deficiencies due to damage that affects the cerebrum. Spasticity is a condition in which certain muscles are continuously contracted. Palsy means paralysis of a body part that is often accompanied by loss of feeling and uncontrolled body movements, such as shaking.
- Cerebral palsy occurs most frequently in premature or low-birthweight infants.
- Cerebral palsy is usually caused by an injury that occurs during pregnancy, birth, or soon after birth.

Epilepsy and Seizures

- Epilepsy (EP-ih-lep-see) is a chronic neurological condition characterized by recurrent episodes of seizures of varying severity. Also known as a seizure disorder, epilepsy can usually be controlled with medication.
- A seizure (SEE-zhur) is a sudden surge of electrical activity in the brain that affects how a person feels or acts for a short time. Some seizures can hardly be noticed, whereas others cause a brief loss of consciousness. Seizures are symptoms of different disorders that can affect the brain and also can be caused by extreme high fever, brain injury, or brain lesions.

Abnormal Sensations

- Causalgia (kaw-ZAL-jee-ah) is persistent, severe burning pain that usually follows an injury to a sensory nerve (caus means burning, and -algia means pain).
- Complex regional pain syndrome, also known as reflex sympathetic dystrophy syndrome, is pain that occurs after an injury to an arm or a leg, a heart attack, stroke, or other medical problem. This condition is a

form of causalgia with burning pain that is much worse than would be expected due to the injury.
- Hyperesthesia (high-per-es-THEE-zee-ah) is a condition of abnormal and excessive sensitivity to touch, pain, or other sensory stimuli (hyper- means excessive, and -esthesia means sensation or feeling).
- Paresthesia (pair-es-THEE-zee-ah) refers to a burning or prickling sensation that is usually felt in the hands, arms, legs, or feet, but can also occur in other parts of the body (par- means abnormal, and -esthesia means sensation or feeling). These sensations may constitute the first symptoms of peripheral neuropathy or it may be a drug side effect.
- Peripheral neuropathy (new-ROP-ah-thee), also known as peripheral neuritis, is a disorder of the nerves that carry information to and from the brain and spinal cord. This produces pain, the loss of sensation, and the inability to control muscles, particularly in the arms or legs.
- Restless legs syndrome (RLS) is a neurological disorder characterized by uncomfortable feelings in the legs, producing a strong urge to move them. The sensation is usually most noticeable at night or when trying to rest.

Diagnostic Procedures Of The Nervous System
- Magnetic resonance imaging (MRI) and computed tomography (CT) are important neuroimaging tools because they facilitate the examination of the soft tissue structures of the brain and spinal cord.
- Carotid ultrasonography (ul-trah-son-OG-rah-fee) is an ultrasound study of the carotid artery (ultra- means beyond, son/o means sound, and -graphy means the process of producing a picture or record). This diagnostic test is performed to detect plaque buildup in the artery to predict or diagnose an ischemic stroke.
- Echoencephalography (eck-oh-en-sef-ah-LOG-rahfee) is the use of ultrasound imaging to diagnose a shift in the midline structures of the brain (ech/o means sound, encephal/o means brain, and -graphy means the process of producing a picture or record).
- Electroencephalography (ee-leck-troh-en-sef-ah- LOG-rah-fee) is the process of recording the electrical activity of the brain through the use of electrodes attached to the scalp (electr/o means electric, encephal/o means brain, and -graphymeans the process of producing a picture or record). The resulting record is an electroencephalogram. This electrical activity may also be displayed on a monitor as brain waves.
- Myelography (my-eh-LOG-rah-fee) is a radiographic study of the spinal cord after the injection of a contrast medium through a lumbar puncture (myel/o means spinal cord, and -graphy means the process of producing a picture or record). The resulting record is a myelogram.
- A lumbar puncture, also known as a spinal tap, is the process of obtaining a sample of cerebrospinal fluid by inserting a needle into the

subarachnoid space of the lumbar region to withdraw fluid. Changes in the composition of the cerebrospinal fluid can be an indication of injury, infection, or disease.

Treatment Procedures Of The Nervous System

Sedative and Hypnotic Medications
- Amobarbital (am-oh-BAR-bih-tal) is a barbiturate used as a sedative and hypnotic.
- A hypnotic depresses the central nervous system and usually produces sleep.
- An anticonvulsant (an-tih-kon-VUL-sant) is administered to prevent seizures such as those associated with epilepsy.
- Barbiturates (bar-BIT-you-raytz) are a class of drugs whose major action is a calming or depressed effect on the central nervous system.
- Phenobarbital (fee-noh-BAR-bih-tal) is a barbiturate used as a sedative and as an anticonvulsant.
- A sedative depresses the central nervous system to produce calm and diminished responsiveness without producing sleep. Sedation is the effect produced by a sedative.

Anesthesia

- Anesthesia (an-es-THEE-zee-ah) is the absence of normal sensation, especially sensitivity to pain, that is induced by the administration of an anesthetic (an- means without, and -esthesia means feeling).
- An anesthetic (an-es-THET-ick) is the medication used to induce anesthesia. The anesthetic may be topical, local, regional, or general (an- means without, esthet means feeling, and -ic means pertaining to).
- Topical anesthesia numbs only the tissue surface and is applied as a liquid, ointment, or spray.
- Local anesthesia causes the loss of sensation in a limited area by injecting an anesthetic solution near that area.
- Regional anesthesia, the temporary interruption of nerve conduction, is produced by injecting an anesthetic solution near the nerves to be blocked.
- Epidural anesthesia (ep-ih-DOO-ral an-es-THEEzee- ah) is regional anesthesia produced by injecting a local anesthetic into the epidural space of the lumbar or sacral region of the spine. When administered during childbirth, it numbs the nerves from the uterus and birth passage without stopping labor.
- Spinal anesthesia is produced by injecting an anesthetic into the subarachnoid space that is located below the arachnoid membrane and above the pia mater that surrounds the spinal cord.
- General anesthesia involves the total loss of body sensation and consciousness induced by anesthetic agents administered primarily by inhalation or intravenous injection.

The Brain
- A lobectomy (loh-BECK-toh-mee) is surgical removal of a portion of the brain to treat brain cancer or seizure disorders that cannot be controlled with medication.
- A thalamotomy (thal-ah-MOT-oh-mee) is a surgical incision into the thalamus (thalam means thalamus, and -otomy means surgical incision). This procedure, which destroys brain cells, is primarily performed to quiet the tremors of Parkinson's disease.

Nerves
- Neuroplasty (NEW-roh-plas-tee) is the surgical repair of a nerve or nerves (neur/o means nerve, and -plasty means surgical repair).
- Neurorrhaphy (new-ROR-ah-fee) is surgically suturing together the ends of a severed nerve (neur/o means nerve, and -rrhaphy means surgical suturing).
- A neurotomy (new-ROT-oh-mee) is a surgical incision or the dissection of a nerve (neur means nerve, and -otomy means a surgical incision).

Mental Health
Although described as being disorders of mental health, the causes of the following conditions also include congenital abnormalities, physical changes, substance abuse, medications, or any combination of these factors.

Anxiety Disorders
- Anxiety disorders are mental conditions characterized by excessive, irrational dread of everyday situations, or fear that is out of proportion to the real danger in a situation. Without treatment, an anxiety disorder can become chronic.
- A generalized anxiety disorder is characterized by chronic anxiety plus exaggerated worry and tension even when there is little or nothing to provoke these feelings. Physical symptoms associated with this condition include muscle tension, sleep disturbance, and restlessness.
- Obsessive-compulsive disorder is an anxiety disorder characterized by recurrent, unwanted obsessions (repetitive thoughts or impulses) and/or recurrent compulsions (unwanted impulses to act). Repetitive compulsive behaviors, such as hand washing, are often performed with the hope of preventing obsessive thoughts or making them go away. Performing these so-called "rituals" provides only temporary relief, and not performing them markedly increases anxiety.
- A panic disorder is an anxiety disorder characterized by unexpected and repeated episodes known as panic attacks. These attacks are caused by an unwarranted arousal of the sympathetic nervous system, which is the body's fight or flight response to danger.
- A panic attack is characterized by a group of intense emotional feelings that include apprehension, fearfulness, and terror. These emotions are

accompanied by physical symptoms that can include shortness of breath, feelings of unreality, sweating, heart palpitations, chest pain, and choking sensations.
- Posttraumatic stress disorder (PTSD) may develop after an event involving actual or threatened death or injury to the individual or someone else, during which the person felt intense fear, helplessness, or horror. Military service, a natural disaster, or a hostage situation can cause this disorder, with symptoms including diminished responsiveness to stimuli, anxiety, sleep disorders, persistent reliving of the event, and difficulty concentrating.

Phobias

- A phobia (FOH-bee-ah) is a persistent irrational fear of a specific thing or situation, strong enough to cause significant distress, to interfere with functioning, and to lead to the avoidance of the thing or situation that causes this reaction. There are countless types of phobias, and they are named by adding -phobia to the name of the object.
- Acrophobia (ack-roh-FOH-bee-ah) is an excessive fear of being in high places (acr/o means top, and -phobia means abnormal fear).
- Agoraphobia (ag-oh-rah-FOH-bee-ah) is an excessive fear of situations in which having a panic attack seems likely and/or dangerous or embarrassing. An example is a person who fears leaving the familiar setting of home and going out in public because social situations may provoke anxiety (agor/a means marketplace, and -phobia means abnormal fear).
- Arachnophobia (ah-rach-noh-FOH-bee-ah) is an excessive fear of spiders (arachn/o means spider, and -phobia means abnormal fear).
- Claustrophobia (klaws-troh-FOH-bee-ah) is an abnormal fear of being in narrow or enclosed spaces (claustr/o means barrier, and -phobia means abnormal fear).

Developmental Disorders

- Autism (AW-tizm), also known as autistic disorders, describes a group of conditions in which a young child cannot develop normal social relationships, compulsively follows repetitive routines, and frequently has poor communication skills.
- Asperger's syndrome is a less severely affected subgroup of the autism disorder spectrum. Individuals with Asperger's usually have normal or aboveaverage intelligence but are impaired in social interactions and nonverbal communication.
- An attention deficit disorder (ADD) is characterized by a short attention span and impulsive behavior that is inappropriate for the child's developmental age. The term attention deficit/hyperactivity disorder (ADHD) is sometimes used if there is a consistently high level of activity.

- Hyperactivity is restlessness or a continuing excess of movement. These conditions may persist into adulthood.
- Dyslexia (dis-LECK-see-ah), also known as a developmental reading disorder, is a learning disability characterized by substandard reading achievement due to the inability of the brain to process symbols.
- Learning disabilities are disorders found in children of normal intelligence who have difficulties in learning specific skills such as processing language or grasping mathematical concepts.
- A diagnosis of mental retardation is based on three criteria: (1) significant below-average intellectual functioning; (2) significant deficits in adaptive functioning; and (3) onset during the developmental period of life.

Dissociative Disorders

- Dissociative disorders occur when normal thought is separated from consciousness.
- Dissociative identity disorder, formerly known as multiple personality disorder, is a mental illness characterized by the presence of two or more distinct personalities, each with its own characteristics, which appear to exist within the same individual.

Factitious Disorders

- A factitious disorder (fack-TISH-us) is a condition in which an individual acts as if he or she has a physical or mental illness when he or she is not really sick. The term factitious means artificial, self-induced, or not naturally occurring. Visible symptoms are self-inflicted and the motivation is the patient's desire to receive attention and sympathy.
- A factitious disorder by proxy is a form of child abuse. Although seeming very concerned about the child's wellbeing, the mentally ill parent will falsify an illness in a child by making up, or inducing symptoms, and then seeking medical treatment, even surgery, for the child.

Impulse-Control Disorders

- Impulse-control disorders are a group of psychiatric disorders characterized by the inability to resist an impulse despite potential negative consequences. In additional to the examples listed below, this disorder includes compulsive shopping and gambling.
- Kleptomania (klep-toh-MAY-nee-ah) is a disorder characterized by repeatedly stealing objects neither for personal use nor for their monetary value (klept/o means to steal, and -mania means madness).
- Pyromania (pye-roh-MAY-nee-ah) is a disorder characterized by repeated, deliberate fire setting (pyr/o means fire, and -mania means madness).

- Trichotillomania (trick-oh-till-oh-MAY-nee-ah) is a disorder characterized by the repeated pulling out of one's own hair (trichotill/o means related to hair, and -mania means madness).

Mood Disorders
- A bipolar disorder is a condition characterized by cycles of severe mood changes shifting from highs (manic behavior) and severe lows (depression) that affect a person's attitude, energy, and ability to function.
- Manic behavior includes an abnormally elevated mood state, including inappropriate elation, increased irritability, severe insomnia, poor judgment, and inappropriate social behavior.
- Depression is a common mood disorder characterized by lethargy and sadness, as well as the loss of interest or pleasure in normal activities. Severe depression may lead to feelings of worthlessness and thoughts of death or suicide.
- Dysthymia (dis-THIGH-mee-ah), also known as a dysthymic disorder, is a low-grade chronic depression with symptoms that are milder than those of severe depression but are present on a majority of days for 2 or more years (dys- means bad, thym means mind, and -ia means condition).
- Seasonal affective disorder (SAD) is a seasonal bout of depression associated with the decrease in hours of daylight during winter months.

Personality Disorders
- A personality disorder is a chronic pattern of inner experience and behavior that causes serious problems with relationships and work. This pattern is pervasive and inflexible, has an onset in adolescence or early adulthood, is stable over time, and leads to distress or impairment.
- An antisocial personality disorder is a pattern of disregard for, and violation of, the rights of others. This pattern brings the individual into continuous conflict with society.
- A borderline personality disorder is characterized by impulsive actions, often with the potential for selfharm, as well as mood instability and chaotic relationships.
- A narcissistic personality disorder is a pattern of extreme preoccupation with the self and complete lack of empathy for others. Empathy is the ability to understand another person's mental and emotional state without becoming personally involved.

Psychotic Disorders
- A psychotic disorder (sigh-KOT-ick) is characterized by the loss of contact with reality and deterioration of normal social functioning.
- Catatonic behavior (kat-ah-TON-ick) is marked by a lack of responsiveness, stupor, and a tendency to remain in a fixed posture.

- A delusion (dee-LOO-zhun) is a false personal belief that is maintained despite obvious proof or evidence to the contrary. The belief is not one ordinarily accepted by other members of the individual's culture or religious faith.
- A hallucination (hah-loo-sih-NAY-shun) is a sensory perception (sight, touch, sound, smell, or taste) experienced in the absence of an external stimulation.
- Schizophrenia (skit-soh-FREE-nee-ah) is a psychotic disorder usually characterized by withdrawal from reality, illogical patterns of thinking, delusions, and hallucinations, and accompanied in varying degrees by other emotional, behavioral, or intellectual disturbances.

Somatoform Disorders

- A somatoform disorder (soh-MAT-oh-form) is characterized by physical complaints or concerns about one's body that are out of proportion to any physical findings or disease.
- A conversion disorder is characterized by serious temporary or ongoing changes in function, such as paralysis or blindness, that are triggered by psychological factors rather than by any physical cause.
- Hypochondriasis (high-poh-kon-DRY-ah-sis) is characterized by fearing that one has a serious illness despite appropriate medical evaluation and reassurance. A person exhibiting this syndrome is known as a hypochondriac.
- Malingering (mah-LING-ger-ing) is characterized by the intentional creation of false or grossly exaggerated physical or psychological symptoms. In contrast to a factitious disorder, this condition is motivated by incentives such as avoiding work.

Substance-Related Disorders

- Substance abuse is the addictive use of tobacco, alcohol, medications, or illegal drugs. This abuse leads to significant impairment in functioning, danger to one's self or others, and recurrent legal and/or interpersonal problems.
- Alcoholism (AL-koh-hol-izm) is chronic alcohol dependence with specific signs and symptoms upon withdrawal. Withdrawal is a psychological or physical syndrome (or both) caused by the abrupt cessation (stopping) of the use of alcohol or a drug in an addicted individual.
- Delirium tremens (dee-LIR-ee-um TREE-mens) is a disorder involving sudden and severe mental changes or seizures caused by abruptly stopping the use of alcohol.

Medications to Treat Mental Disorders

- An antidepressant is administered to prevent or relieve depression. Some of these medications are also used to treat obsessive-compulsive and generalized anxiety disorders and to help relieve chronic pain.

- An antipsychotic drug (an-tih-sigh-KOT-ick) is administered to treat symptoms of severe disorders of thinking and mood that are associated with neurological and psychiatric illnesses such as schizophrenia, mania, and delusional disorders (anti- means against, psych/o means mind, and -tropic means having an affinity for).
- An anxiolytic drug (ang-zee-oh-LIT-ick), also known as an antianxiety drug or tranquilizer, is administered to temporarily relieve anxiety and to reduce tension (anxi/o means anxiety, and -lytic means to destroy).
- Mood stabilizing drugs, such as lithium, are used to treat mood instability and bipolar disorders.
- A psychotropic drug (sigh-koh-TROP-pick) acts primarily on the central nervous system, where it produces temporary changes affecting the mind, emotions, and behavior (psych/o means mind, and -tropic means having an affinity for). These drugs are used as medications to control pain, and to treat narcolepsy and attention disorders.
- A stimulant works by increasing activity in certain areas of the brain to increase concentration and wakefulness. Drug therapies using stimulants have been effective in treating ADHD and narcolepsy. The overuse of stimulants, including caffeine, can cause sleeplessness and palpitations.

Psychological Therapies to Treat Mental Disorders

- In addition to drug treatments, mental disorders are often treated with individual or group therapy by a qualified psychotherapist.
- Psychoanalysis (sigh-koh-ah-NAL-ih-sis) is based on the idea that mental disorders have underlying causes stemming from childhood and can only be overcome by gaining insight into one's feelings and patterns of behavior.
- Behavioral therapy focuses on changing behavior by identifying problem behaviors, replacing them with appropriate behaviors, and using rewards or other consequences to make the changes.
- Cognitive therapy focuses on changing cognitions or thoughts that are affecting a person's emotions and actions. These are identified and then are challenged through logic, gathering evidence, and/or testing in action. The goal is to change problematic beliefs.
- Cognitive-behavioral therapy combines the techniques of cognitive and behavioral therapy.
- Hypnotherapy is the use of hypnosis to produce a relaxed state of focused attention in which the patient may be more willing to believe and act on suggestions.

Abbreviations Related To The Nervous System

- Alzheimer's disease = AD
- amyotrophic lateral sclerosis = ALS
- attention deficit hyperactivity disorder = ADHD

- cerebral palsy = CP
- cerebrospinal fluid = CSF
- electroencephalography = ECG
- epidural anesthesia = EPAN
- intracranial pressure = ICP
- levels of consciousness = LOC
- multiple sclerosis = MS
- obsessive-compulsive disorder = OCD

Critical Thinking Exercise

The following story and questions are designed to stimulate critical thinking through class discussion or as a brief essay response. There are no right or wrong answers to these questions.

Calle Washington read the information Dr. Thakker gave her with numb disbelief. "Multiple sclerosis is a neurological disorder characterized by demyelination of nerve fibers in the brain and spinal column. This disease may be progressively debilitating with symptoms that could include numbness, paralysis, ataxia, pain, and blindness. Some patients do experience life-threatening complications. This disease attacks young adults. It affects more women than men."

"Well, I sure fit the profile," thought Calle bitterly. She took a deep breath, trying to quiet the fluttering in her stomach. How could this happen now? Everything was so perfect. Her wedding gown was getting its last alterations, and the tickets for their honeymoon in Jamaica were in the desk drawer. Gabe was putting the final touches on the house where they planned on raising their family. She couldn't expect Gabe to waste his future caring for someone in a wheelchair, could she? Suddenly, her fairy tale life was turning into a nightmare.

Calle occasionally has the symptom of being off balance. If this happened suddenly, would this put the children she worked with at the day care center at risk? What would happen once her fellow teachers at the day care center noticed that? She would not risk hurting one of the children, but if she lost her job she'd lose her health insurance. Dr. Thakker had said there were new drugs for MS, but he'd mentioned that they were very expensive. And what about the children that she and Gabe both wanted? Could she still have a baby and take care of it?

"Maybe I should take out an ad that says '25-year-old female seeks cure for deadly disease before
marrying Prince Charming,'" she thought, trying to laugh through her tears ...

Suggested Discussion Topics

1. Which symptoms of Calle's condition might affect her job? She has been working with the youngest children. Should she consider resigning or could she ask for a different assignment?
2. Calle and Gabe decide to go ahead with the wedding. If they have children, is there a risk that Calle will transmit this condition? If Calle can not have children, what other options are open to have that would enable them to have the family they both want.

3. After their marriage, Calle will be covered by her husband's health insurance. Calle is ethical in completing her application for this coverage and mentions the MS diagnosis. But she has questions. Where could Calle get information as to whether or not the insurance company will ever cover her for this disease? Will her coverage begin immediately?
4. Calle is an excellent teacher and the children love her. In the past, her coworkers have commented, "I wish I could learn to be as good at this as you are." Even with multiple sclerosis, could Calle have a future in training other teachers? What other positive steps might she contemplate taking?

Scott J. Barnard

Medical Terminology for Health Professions 4.0

CHAPTER 11

SPECIAL SENSES: THE EYES AND EARS

This list contains essential word parts and medical terms for this chapter.

Word Parts
- blephar/o
- -cusis
- irid/o
- kerat/o
- myring/o
- ophthalm/o
- -opia
- opt/o
- ot/o
- phak/o
- presby/o
- retin/o
- scler/o
- trop/o
- tympan/o

Medical Terms
- adnexa (ad-NECK-sah)
- amblyopia (am-blee-OH-pee-ah)
- ametropia (am-eh-TROH-pee-ah)
- anisocoria (an-ih-so-KOH-ree-ah)
- astigmatism (ah-STIG-mah-tizm)
- barotrauma (bar-oh-TRAW-mah)
- blepharoptosis (blef-ah-roh-TOH-sis)
- cataract (KAT-ah-rakt)
- chalazion (kah-LAY-zee-on)
- cochlear implant (KOCK-lee-ar)

- conjunctivitis (kon-junk-tih-VYE-tis)
- dacryoadenitis (dack-ree-oh-ad-eh-NIGH-tis)
- diplopia (dih-PLOH-pee-ah)
- ectropion (eck-TROH-pee-on)
- emmetropia (em-eh-TROH-pee-ah)
- entropion (en-TROH-pee-on)
- esotropia (es-oh-TROH-pee-ah)
- eustachitis (you-stay-KYE-tis)
- exotropia (eck-soh-TROH-pee-ah)
- fluorescein angiography (flew-oh-RES-ee-in an-jee-OG-rah-fee)
- glaucoma (glaw-KOH-mah)
- hemianopia (hem-ee-ah-NOH-pee-ah)
- hordeolum (hor-DEE-oh-lum)
- hyperopia (high-per-OH-pee-ah)
- infectious myringitis (mir-in-JIGH-tis)
- iridectomy (ir-ih-DECK-toh-mee)
- iritis (eye-RYE-tis)
- keratitis (ker-ah-TYE-tis)
- labyrinthectomy (lab-ih-rin-THECK-toh-mee)
- laser trabeculoplasty (trah-BECK-you-lohplas-tee)
- mastoidectomy (mas-toy-DECK-toh-mee)
- myopia (my-OH-pee-ah)
- myringotomy (mir-in-GOT-oh-mee)
- nyctalopia (nick-tah-LOH-pee-ah)
- nystagmus (nis-TAG-mus)
- ophthalmoscopy (ahf-thal-MOS-koh-pee)
- optometrist (op-TOM-eh-trist)
- otitis media (oh-TYE-tis MEE-dee-ah)
- otomycosis (oh-toh-my-KOH-sis)
- otopyorrhea (oh-toh-pye-oh-REE-ah)
- otorrhagia (oh-toh-RAY-jee-ah)
- otosclerosis (oh-toh-skleh-ROH-sis)
- papilledema (pap-ill-eh-DEE-mah)
- periorbital edema
- presbycusis (pres-beh-KOO-sis)
- presbyopia (pres-bee-OH-pee-ah)
- pterygium (teh-RIJ-ee-um)
- radial keratotomy (ker-ah-TOT-oh-mee)
- retinopexy (RET-ih-noh-peck-see)
- scleritis (skleh-RYE-tis)
- stapedectomy (stay-peh-DECK-toh-mee)
- strabismus (strah-BIZ-mus)
- tarsorrhaphy (tahr-SOR-ah-fee)
- tinnitus (tih-NIGH-tus)

- tonometry (toh-NOM-eh-tree)
- tympanometry (tim-pah-NOM-eh-tree)
- tympanostomy tubes (tim-pan-OSS-toh-mee)
- vertigo (VER-tih-go)
- vitrectomy (vih-TRECK-toh-mee)
- xerophthalmia (zeer-ahf-THAL-mee-ah)

Objectives

On completion of this chapter, you should be able to:
1. Describe the functions and structures of the eyes and their accessory structures.
2. Recognize, define, spell, and pronounce terms related to the pathology and diagnostic and treatment procedures of the eyes and vision.
3. Describe the functions and structures of the ears.
4. Recognize, define, spell, and pronounce terms related to the pathology and diagnostic and treatment procedures of the ears and hearing.

Structures Of The Eyes

The structures of the eye include the eyeball and the adnexa that are attached to or surround the eyeball.

Adnexa of the Eyes

- The adnexa of the eyes, also known as adnexa oculi, are the structures outside the eyeball, and these include the orbit, eye muscles, eyelids, eyelashes, conjunctiva, and lacrimal apparatus.
- Adnexa (ad-NECK-sah) means appendages or accessory structures of an organ.

The Orbit

The orbit, also known as the eye socket, is the bony cavity of the skull that contains and protects the eyeball and its associated muscles, blood vessels, and nerves.

Muscles of the Eye

Six major eye muscles, which are arranged in three pairs, are attached to each eye. These are the superior and inferior oblique muscles, the superior and inferior rectus muscles, and the lateral and medial rectus muscles.

These muscles make a wide range of very precise eye movements possible.

The muscles of both eyes work together in coordinated movements that enable normal binocular vision (bin- means two, ocul means eye, and -ar means pertaining to). The term binocular refers the use of both eyes working together.

The Eyelids, Eyebrows, and Eye Lashes

- The upper and lower eyelids of each eye help protect the eyeball from foreign matter, excessive light, and injuries due to other causes.

- The canthus (KAN-thus) is the angle where the upper and lower eyelids meet (canth means corner of the eye, and -us is a singular noun ending) (plural, canthi).
- The inner canthus is where the eyelids meet nearest the nose.
- The epicanthus (ep-ih-KAN-thus) is a vertical fold of skin on either side of the nose.
- The outer canthus is where the eyelids meet farthest from the nose.
- The tarsus (TAHR-suhs), also known as the tarsal plate, is the framework within the upper and lower eyelids that provides the necessary stiffness and shape (tars means edge of the eyelid, and -us is a singular noun ending) (plural, tarsi). Note: Tarsus also refers to the seven tarsal bones of the instep.
- The eyebrows and eyelashes prevent foreign matter from reaching the eyes. The eyelashes consist of small hairs known as cilia (SIL-ee-ah). Cilia are also found in the nose.
- The edges of the eyelids contain oil-producing sebaceous glands.

The Conjunctiva

The conjunctiva (kon-junk-TYE-vah) is the transparent mucous membrane that lines the underside of each eyelid and continues to form a protective covering over the exposed surface of the eyeball (plural, conjunctivae).

The Lacrimal Apparatus

- The lacrimal apparatus (LACK-rih-mal), also known as the tear apparatus, consists of the structures that produce, store, and remove tears.
- The lacrimal glands, which secrete lacrimal fluid (tears), are located on the underside of the upper eyelid just above the outer corner of each eye. Lacrimation is the secretion of tears.
- The function of lacrimal fluid, also known as tears, is to maintain moisture on the anterior surface of the eyeball. Blinking distributes the lacrimal fluid across the eye.
- The lacrimal canal (LACK-rih-mal) consists of a duct at the inner corner of each eye. These ducts collect tears and empty them into the lacrimal sacs. Crying is the overflowing of tears from the lacrimal canals.
- The lacrimal sac, also known the tear sac, is an enlargement of the upper portion of the lacrimal duct.
- The lacrimal duct, also known as the nasolacrimal duct, is the passageway that drains excess tears into the nose.

The Eyeball

- The eyeball, also known as the globe, is a 1-inch sphere with only about one-sixth of its surface visible.
- The term optic means pertaining to the eye or sight (opt means sight, and -ic means pertaining to).

- Ocular (OCK-you-lar) means pertaining to the eye (ocul means eye, and -ar means pertaining to).
- Extraocular (eck-strah-OCK-you-lar) means outside the eyeball (extra- means on the outside, ocul means eye, and -ar means pertaining to).
- Intraocular (in-trah-OCK-you-lar) means within the eyeball (intra- means within, ocul means eye and -ar means pertaining to).

Walls of the Eyeball

- The walls of the eyeball are made up of three layers: the sclera, choroid, and retina.
- The sclera (SKLEHR-ah), also known as the white of the eye, maintains the shape of the eye and protects the delicate inner layers of tissue. This tough, fibrous tissue forms the outer layer of the eye, except for the part covered by the cornea. Note: The combining form scler/o means the white of the eye, and it also means hard.
- The choroid (KOH-roid), also known as the choroid coat, is the opaque middle layer of the eyeball that contains many blood vessels and provides the blood supply for the entire eye. Opaque means that light cannot pass through this substance.
- The retina (RET-ih-nah) is the sensitive innermost layer that lines the posterior segment of the eye. The retina receives nerve impulses and transmits them to the brain via the optic nerve. This is also known as the second cranial nerve.

Segments of the Eyeball

The interior of the eyeball is divided into the anterior and posterior segments.

Anterior Segment of the Eye

The anterior segment makes up the front one-third of the eyeball. This segment is divided into anterior and posterior chambers.

- The anterior chamber is located behind the cornea and in front of the iris. The posterior chamber is located behind the iris and in front of the ligaments holding the lens in place. Note: Don't confuse the posterior chamber with the posterior segment.
- These chambers are filled with aqueous fluid, also known as aqueous humor. Aqueous means watery or containing water. As used here, a humor is any clear body liquid or semifluid substance.
- Aqueous fluid helps the eye maintain its shape and nourishes the intraocular structures. This fluid is constantly filtered and drained through the trabecular meshwork and the canal of Schlemm.
- Intraocular pressure (IOP) is a measurement of the fluid pressure inside the eye. The rate at which aqueous fluid enters and leaves the eye regulates this pressure.

Posterior Segment of the Eye

- The posterior segment, which makes up the remaining two-thirds of the eyeball, is lined with the retina and filled with vitreous gel (VIT-ree-us). Also known as vitreous humor, this is a soft, clear, jelly-like mass that contains millions of fine fibers. These fibers, which are attached to the surface of the retina, help the eye maintain its shape.

Structures of the Retina

- The rods and cones of the retina receive images that have passed through the lens of the eye. These images are converted into nerve impulses and transmitted to the brain via the optic nerve. Rods are the black and white receptors, and cones are the color receptors.
- The macula (MACK-you-lah), also known as the macula lutea, is a clearly defined yellow area in the center of the retina. This is the area of sharpest central vision.
- The fovea centralis (FOH-vee-ah sen-TRAH-lis) is a pit in the middle of the macula. Color vision is best in this area because it contains a high concentration of cones and no rods.
- The optic disk, also known as the blind spot, is a small region in the eye where the nerve endings of the retina enter the optic nerve. This is called the blind spot because it does not contain any rods or cones to convert images into nerve impulses.
- The optic nerve transmits these nerve impulses from the retina to the brain.

The Uveal Tract

- The uveal tract (YOU-vee-ahl) is the pigmented layer of the eye. It has a rich blood supply and consists of the choroid, ciliary body, and iris.

The Ciliary Body

- The ciliary body (SIL-ee-ehr-ee), which is located within the choroid, is a set of muscles and suspensory ligaments that adjust the thickness of the lens to refine the focus of light rays on the retina.
- The ciliary body produces the aqueous fluid that fills the anterior segment of the eye.
- To focus on nearby objects, these muscles adjust the lens to make it thicker.
- To focus on distant objects, these muscles stretch the lens so it is thinner.

The Iris

- The iris is the colorful muscular layer of the eye that surrounds the pupil. The muscles within the iris control the amount of light that is allowed to enter the eye through the pupil.

- To decrease the amount of light, these circular muscles contract and make the pupil smaller.
- To increase the amount of light, the muscles dilate (relax) and make the pupil larger.

The Cornea, Pupil, and Lens

- The cornea (KOR-nee-ah) is the transparent outer surface of the eye covering the iris and pupil. It is the primary structure focusing light rays entering the eye.
- The pupil is the black circular opening in the center of the iris that permits light to enter the eye.
- The lens, also known as the crystalline lens, is the clear, flexible, curved structure that focuses images on the retina. The lens is contained within a clear capsule located behind the iris and pupil.

Normal Action of the Eyes

- Accommodation (ah-kom-oh-DAY-shun) is the process whereby the eyes make adjustments for seeing objects at various distances. These adjustments include contraction (narrowing) and dilation (widening) of the pupil, movement of the eyes, and changes in the shape of the lens.
- Convergence (kon-VER-jens) is the simultaneous inward movement of the eyes toward each other. This occurs in an effort to maintain single binocular vision as an object comes nearer.
- Emmetropia (em-eh-TROH-pee-ah) is the normal relationship between the refractive power of the eye and the shape of the eye that enables light rays to focus correctly on the retina (emmetr means in proper measure, and -opia means vision condition).
- Refraction, also refractive power, is the ability of the lens to bend light rays so they focus on the retina.
- Visual acuity (ah-KYOU-ih-tee) is the ability to distinguish object details and shape at a distance. Acuity means sharpness.

Medical Specialties Related To The Eyes

- An ophthalmologist (ahf-thal-MOL-oh-jist) is a physician who specializes in diagnosing and treating diseases and disorders of the eyes and vision (ophthalm means eye, and -ologist means specialist).
- An optometrist (op-TOM-eh-trist) holds a Doctor of Optometry degree and specializes in measuring the accuracy of vision to determine whether corrective lenses are needed (opt/o means vision, and -metrist means one who measures).

Vision

The Eyelids

- Blepharoptosis (blef-ah-roh-TOH-sis), also known simply as ptosis, is drooping of the upper eyelid that is usually due to paralysis (blephar/o means eyelid, and -ptosis means drooping or sagging).
- A chalazion (kah-LAY-zee-on), also known as an internal stye, is a localized swelling inside the eyelid resulting from obstruction a sebaceous gland. Compare with a hordeolum.
- Ectropion (eck-TROH-pee-on) is the eversion of the edge of an eyelid (ec- mean out, trop means turn, and -ion means condition). Eversion means turning outward. This usually affects the lower lid, thereby exposing the inner surface of the eyelid to irritation and preventing tears from draining properly. Ectropion is the opposite of entropion.
- Entropion (en-TROH-pee-on) is the inversion of the edge of an eyelid (en- means in, trop means turn, and -ion means condition). Inversion means turning inward. This usually affects the lower eyelid and causing the eyelashes to rub against the cornea. Entropion is the opposite of ectropion.
- A hordeolum (hor-DEE-oh-lum), also known as a stye, is a pus-filled lesion on the eyelid resulting from an infection in a sebaceous gland. Compare with a chalazion.
- Periorbital edema is swelling surrounding the eye or eyes (peri- means surrounding, orbit means eyeball, and -al means pertaining to). Edema means swelling of the tissues. This swelling can cause the eyes to be partially closed by the swollen eyelids. It can also give the face a bloated appearance. This swelling is associated with conditions including allergic reactions.

Additional Adnexa Pathology

- Conjunctivitis (kon-junk-tih-VYE-tis), also known as pinkeye, is an inflammation of the conjunctiva that is usually caused by an infection or allergy (conjunctiv means conjunctiva, and -itis means inflammation).
- Dacryoadenitis (dack-ree-oh-ad-eh-NIGH-tis) is an inflammation of the lacrimal gland that can be caused by a bacterial, viral, or fungal infection (dacry/o means tear, aden means gland, and -itis means inflammation). Signs and symptoms of this condition include sudden severe pain, redness, and pressure in the orbit of the eye.
- Subconjunctival hemorrhage is bleeding between the conjunctiva and the sclera. This common condition, which is usually caused by an injury, creates a red area over the white of the eye.
- Xerophthalmia (zeer-ahf-THAL-mee-ah), also known as dry eye, is drying of eye surfaces including the conjunctiva (xer means dry, ophthalm means eye, and -ia means abnormal condition). This condition is often

associated with aging. In addition, it can be due to systemic diseases such as rheumatoid arthritis or to a lack of vitamin A.

Uveal Tract, Cornea, Iris, and Sclera

- Iritis (eye-RYE-tis), also known as anterior uveitis, is an inflammation of the uveal tract affecting primarily structures in the front of the eye (ir means iris, and -itis means inflammation). This condition can be acute or chronic.
- A corneal abrasion is an injury, such as a scratch or irritation, to the outer layers of the cornea. Compare with corneal ulcer.
- A corneal ulcer is a pitting of the cornea caused by an infection or injury. Although these ulcers heal with treatment, they can leave a cloudy scar that impairs vision. Compare with corneal abrasion.
- Keratitis (ker-ah-TYE-tis) is an inflammation of the cornea (kerat means cornea, and -itis means inflammation).

Note: kerat/o also means hard. This condition can be due to many causes including bacterial, viral, or fungal infections.

- A pterygium (teh-RIJ-ee-um) is a benign growth on the cornea that can become large enough to distort vision.
- Scleritis (skleh-RYE-tis) is an inflammation of the sclera (scler means white of eye, and -itis means inflammation). This condition is usually associated with infections, chemical injuries, or autoimmune diseases.
- Synechia (sigh-NECK-ee-ah) is an adhesion that binds the iris to an adjacent structure such as the lens or cornea (plural, synechiae). An adhesion holds structures together abnormally.

The Eye

- Anisocoria (an-ih-so-KOH-ree-ah) is a condition in which the pupils are unequal in size (anis/o means unequal, cor means pupil, and -ia means abnormal condition). This condition can be congenital or caused by a head injury, aneurysm, or pathology of the central nervous system.
- A cataract (KAT-ah-rakt) is the loss of transparency of the lens that causes a progressive loss of visual clarity. The formation of most cataracts is associated with aging; however, this condition can be congenital or due to an injury or disease.
- PERRLA is an abbreviation meaning Pupils are Equal, Round, Responsive to Light and Accommodation. This is a diagnostic observation, and any abnormality here could indicate a head injury or damage to the brain.
- In a retinal detachment, also known as a detached retina, the retina is pulled away from its attachment to the choroid in the back of the eye.
- Floaters, also known as vitreous floaters, are particles of cellular debris that float in the vitreous fluid and cast shadows on the retina. Floaters occur normally with aging or in association with vitreous detachments, retinal tears, or intraocular inflammations.

- Nystagmus (nis-TAG-mus) is an involuntary, constant, rhythmic movement of the eyeball that can be congenital or caused by a neurological injury or drug use.
- Papilledema (pap-ill-eh-DEE-mah), also known as choked disk, is swelling and inflammation of the optic nerve at the point of entrance into the eye through the optic disk (papill means nipple-like, and -edema means swelling). This swelling is caused by increased intracranial pressure and can be due to a tumor pressing on the optic nerve.
- A retinal tear occurs when a hole develops in the retina as it is pulled away from its normal position. See vitreous detachment.
- Retinitis pigmentosa (ret-ih-NIGH-tis pig-men-TOHsah) is a progressive degeneration of the retina that affects night and peripheral vision. It can be detected by the presence of dark pigmented spots in the retina.
- Vitreous detachment occurs as aging causes the vitreous gel to slowly shrink. With this shrinkage, the fine fibers within the gel pull on the retinal surface. Usually the fibers break, allowing the vitreous to separate and shrink from the retina. In most cases, this condition is not sight-threatening and does not require treatment; however, if the fibers pull hard enough on the retina, they can cause a retinal tear.

Glaucoma

- Glaucoma (glaw-KOH-mah) is a group of diseases characterized by increased intraocular pressure that cause damage to the retinal nerve fibers and the optic nerve. This increase in pressure is caused by a blockage in the flow of fluid out of the eye. If left untreated, this pressure can cause the loss of peripheral vision and eventually blindness.
- Open-angle glaucoma, also known as chronic glaucoma, is the most common form of this condition. Here the trabecular meshwork gradually becomes blocked, and this causes a buildup of pressure. Symptoms of this condition are not noticed by the patient until the optic nerve has been damaged; however, it can be detected earlier through regular eye examinations including tonometry and visual field testing. See Diagnostic Procedures of the Eyes.
- In closed-angle glaucoma, also known as acute glaucoma, the opening between the cornea and iris narrows so that fluid cannot reach the trabecular meshwork. This narrowing can cause a sudden increase in the intraocular pressure that produces severe pain, nausea, redness of the eye, and blurred vision. Without immediate treatment, blindness can occur in as little as 2 days.

Macular Degeneration

- Macular degeneration (MACK-you-lar) is a gradually progressive condition in which the macula at the center of the retina is damaged,

resulting in the loss of central vision, but not in total blindness (macul means spot, and -ar mean pertaining to).
- Age-related macular degeneration occurs most frequently in older people and is the leading cause of legal blindness in those over age 60.
- Dry type macular degeneration, which accounts for 90% of cases, is caused by the deterioration of the cells of the macula.
- Wet type macular degeneration is caused by the formation of new blood vessels that produce small hemorrhages, damaging the macula.

Functional Defects
- Diplopia (dih-PLOH-pee-ah), also known as double vision, is the perception of two images of a single object (dipl means double, and -opia means vision condition). It is sometimes a symptom of a serious underlying disorder such as multiple sclerosis or a brain tumor.
- Hemianopia (hem-ee-ah-NOH-pee-ah) is blindness in one-half of the visual field (hemi- mean half, anmeans without, and -opia means vision).
- Monochromatism (mon-oh-KROH-mah-tizm), also known as color blindness, is the inability to distinguish colors (mon/o means one, chromat means color, and -ism means condition).
- Nyctalopia (nick-tah-LOH-pee-ah), also known as night blindness, is a condition in which an individual with normal daytime vision has difficulty seeing at night (nyctal means night, and -opia means vision condition).
- Presbyopia (pres-bee-OH-pee-ah) is the condition of common changes in the eyes that occur with aging (presby means old age, and -opia means vision condition). With age, near vision declines noticeably as the lens becomes less flexible and the muscles of the ciliary body become weaker. The result is that the eyes are no longer able to focus the image properly on the retina.

Strabismus
- Strabismus (strah-BIZ-mus) is a disorder in which the eyes point in different directions or are not aligned correctly because the eye muscles are unable to focus together.
- Esotropia (es-oh-TROH-pee-ah), also known as crosseyes, is strabismus characterized by an inward deviation of one or both eyes (eso- means inward, trop means turn, and -ia means abnormal condition). Esotropia is the opposite of exotropia.
- Exotropia (eck-soh-TROH-pee-ah), also known as walleye, is strabismus characterized by the outward deviation of one eye relative to the other (exo- means outward, trop means turn, and -ia means abnormal condition). Exotropia is the opposite of esotropia.

Refractive Disorders
- A refractive disorder is a focusing problem that occurs when the lens and cornea do not bend light so that it focuses properly on the retina.
- Ametropia (am-eh-TROH-pee-ah) is any error of refraction in which images do not focus properly on the retina (ametr means out of proportion, and -opia means vision condition). Astigmatism, hyperopia, and myopia are all forms of ametropia.
- Astigmatism (ah-STIG-mah-tizm) is a condition in which the eye does not focus properly because of uneven curvatures of the cornea.
- Hyperopia (high-per-OH-pee-ah), also known as farsightedness, is a defect in which light rays focus beyond the retina (hyper- means excessive and -opia means vision condition). This condition can occur in childhood, but usually causes difficulty after age 40. Hyperopia is the opposite of myopia.
- Myopia (my-OH-pee-ah), also known as nearsightedness, is a defect in which light rays focus in front of the retina. This condition occurs most commonly around puberty. Myopia is the opposite of hyperopia.

Blindness
Blindness is the inability to see. Although some sight remains, legal blindness is the point at which, under law, an individual is considered to be blind. A commonly used standard is that a person is legally blind when his or her best-corrected vision is reduced to 20/200 or less.
- Amblyopia (am-blee-OH-pee-ah) is a dimness of vision or the partial loss of sight, especially in one eye, without detectable disease of the eye (ambly means dim or dull, and -opia means vision condition).
- Scotoma (skoh-TOH-mah), also known as blind spot, is an abnormal area of absent or depressed vision surrounded by an area of normal vision.

Diagnostic Procedures Of The Eyes And Vision
- A Snellen chart (SC) is used to measure visual acuity. The results for each eye are recorded as a fraction with 20/20 being considered normal. The first number indicates the standard distance from the chart, which is 20 feet. The second number indicates the deviation from the norm based on the ability to read progressively smaller lines of letters on the chart.
- Refraction is an examination procedure to determine an eye's refractive error so that the best corrective lenses to be prescribed.
- A diopter (dye-AHP-tur) is the unit of measurement of a lens' refractive power.
- Ophthalmoscopy (ahf-thal-MOS-koh-pee), also known as funduscopy, is the visual examination of the fundus (back part) of the eye with an ophthalmoscope. This examination includes the retina, optic disk, choroid, and blood vessels.
- When ophthalmoscopy is performed as part of a complete eye examination, dilation is required. Dilation in preparation for an

examination of the interior of the eye is the artificial enlargement of the pupil through the use of mydriatic drops.
- Mydriatic drops (mid-ree-AT-ick) are medicated drops placed into the eyes that produce temporary paralysis. This paralysis forces the pupils to remain dilated (wide open) even in the presence of bright light.
- Slit-lamp ophthalmoscopy (ahf-thal-MOS-koh-pee) is a diagnostic procedure in which a narrow beam of light is focused onto parts of the eye to permit the ophthalmologist to examine the structures at the front of the eye including the cornea, iris, and lens.
- Tonometry (toh-NOM-eh-tree) is the measurement of intraocular pressure (ton/o means tension, and -metry means to measure). Abnormally high pressure can be an indication of glaucoma.

Specialized Diagnostic Procedures
- Fluorescein staining (flew-oh-RES-ee-in) is the application of fluorescent dye to the surface of the eye. This dye causes a corneal abrasion to appear bright green.
- Fluorescein angiography (flew-oh-RES-ee-in an-jee-OG-rah-fee) is a radiographic study of the blood vessels in the retina of the eye following the intravenous injection of a fluorescein dye as a contrast medium. The resulting angiograms are used to determine whether there is proper circulation in the retinal vessels.
- Visual field testing, also known as perimetry, is performed to determine losses in peripheral vision. Peripheral means occurring away from the center. Blank sections in the visual field can be symptomatic of glaucoma or an optic nerve disorder.

Treatment Procedures Of The Eyes And Vision
The Orbit and Eyelids
- An orbitotomy (or-bih-TOT-oh-mee) is a surgical incision into the orbit (orbit means bony socket, and -otomy means surgical incision). This procedure is performed for biopsy, abscess drainage, or to remove a tumor or foreign object.
- Tarsorrhaphy (tahr-SOR-ah-fee) is the partial, or complete, suturing together of the upper and lower eyelids (tars/o means eyelid, and -rrhaphy means surgical suturing). This procedure is sometimes performed to protect the eye when the lids are paralyzed and unable to close normally.

The Conjunctiva and Eyeball
- Conjunctivoplasty (kon-junk-TYE-voh-plas-tee) is the surgical repair of the conjunctiva (conjunctiv means conjunctiva, and -plasty means surgical repair).

- A corneal transplant, also known as keratoplasty, is the surgical replacement of a scarred or diseased cornea with clear corneal tissue from a donor.
- An iridectomy (ir-ih-DECK-toh-mee) is the surgical removal of a portion of the tissue of the iris (irid means iris, and -ectomy means surgical removal). This procedure is most frequently performed to treat closedangle glaucoma.
- An ocular prosthesis, also known as an artificial eye, may be fitted to wear over a malformed eye or to replace an eyeball that is either congenitally missing or has been surgically removed. A prosthesis is an artificial substitute for a diseased or missing body replacement part.
- A radial keratotomy (ker-ah-TOT-oh-mee) is a surgical procedure to treat myopia (kerat means cornea, and -otomy means surgical incision). During the surgery, incisions are made in the cornea to cause it to flatten. These incisions allow the sides of the cornea to bulge outward and thereby flatten the central portion of the cornea. This brings the focal point of the eye closer to the retina and improves distance vision. Compare with LASIK.
- Vitrectomy (vih-TRECK-toh-mee) is the removal of the vitreous fluid and its replacement with a clear solution (vitr means vitreous fluid, and -ectomy means removal). This procedure is sometimes performed to treat a retinal detachment or when diabetic retinopathy causes blood to leak and cloud the vitreous fluid.

Cataract Surgery

- Lensectomy (len-SECK-toh-mee) is the general term used to describe the surgical removal of a cataractclouded lens (lens means lens, and -ectomy means surgical removal).
- Phacoemulsification (fack-koh-ee-mul-sih-fih-KAYshun) is the use of ultrasonic vibration to shatter and remove the lens clouded by a cataract. This is performed through a very small opening, and the same opening is used to slide the intraocular lens into place (intra- means within, ocul means eye, and -ar mean pertaining to).
- An intraocular lens (IOL) is a surgically implanted replacement for a natural lens that has been removed.
- Pseudophakia (soo-doh-FAY-kee-ah) is an eye in which the natural lens has been replaced with an intraocular lens (pseudo/o means false, phak means lens, and -ia means abnormal condition).

Corrective Lenses

- Refractive errors in the eye can often be corrected with lenses that alter the angle of light rays before they reach the cornea. Concave lenses (curved inward) are used for myopia, or nearsightedness, and convex lenses (curved outward) for hyperopia (farsightedness).

- Corrective lenses can combine two or three different refractive powers, one above the other, to allow for better distance vision when looking up and near vision when looking down. Bifocals are lenses with two powers. Trifocals are lenses with three powers.
- Strabismus is sometimes treated with corrective lenses, or an eye patch, covering the stronger eye and thus strengthening the muscles in the weaker eye.
- Contact lenses are refractive lenses that float directly on the tear film in front of the eye. Rigid and gaspermeable lenses cover the central part of the cornea, and disposable soft lenses cover the entire cornea.

Laser Treatments of the Eyes

In the treatment of eye disorders, lasers are used for many reasons.
- A laser iridotomy (ir-ih-DOT-oh-mee) uses a focused beam of light to create a hole in the iris of the eye (irid means iris, and -otomy means surgical incision). This procedure is performed to treat closed-angle glaucoma by creating an opening that allows aqueous fluid to flow between the anterior and posterior chambers of the front part of the eye.
- Laser trabeculoplasty (trah-BECK-you-loh-plas-tee) is used to treat open-angle glaucoma by creating openings in the trabecular meshwork to allow fluid to drain properly.
- LASIK is the acronym for Laser-Assisted in Situ Keratomileusis (kerat/o means cornea, and -mileusis means carving). In situ means in its original place. LASIK is used to treat vision conditions, such as myopia, that are caused by the shape of the cornea. During this procedure, a flap is opened in the surface of the cornea and then a laser is used to change the shape of a deep corneal layer. Compare with radial keratotomy.
- Photocoagulation is the use of lasers to treat some forms of wet macular degeneration by sealing leaking or damaged blood vessels.
- Retinopexy (RET-ih-noh-peck-see) is used to reattach the detached area in a retinal detachment (retin/o means retina, and -pexy means surgical fixation).
- Lasers are used to treat retinal tears by sealing the torn portion.
- Lasers are used to remove clouded tissue that can have formed in the posterior portion of the lens capsule after cataract extraction.

Functions Of The Ears

The ears are the receptor organs of hearing, and their functions are to receive sound impulses and transmit them to the brain. The inner ear also helps to maintain balance.

The abbreviations relating to the ears, with the Latin words
from which they originated.

- The term auditory (AW-dih-tor-ee) means pertaining to the sense of hearing (audit means hearing or sense of hearing, and -ory means pertaining to).
- Acoustic (ah-KOOS-tick) means relating to sound or hearing (acous means hearing or sound, and -tic means pertaining to).

Structures Of The Ears

The ear is divided into three separate regions: the outer ear, the middle ear, and the inner ear.

The Outer Ear

- The pinna (PIN-nah), also known as the auricle, is the external portion of the ear. This structure catches sound waves and transmits them into the external auditory canal.
- The external auditory canal transmits sound waves from the pinna to the tympanic membrane (eardrum) of the middle ear.
- Cerumen (seh-ROO-men), also known as earwax, is secreted by ceruminous glands that line the auditory canal. This sticky yellow-brown substance has protective functions because it traps small insects, dust, debris,and certain bacteria to prevent them from entering the middle ear.

The Middle Ear

- The middle ear, which located between outer ear and the inner ear, transmits sound across this space.
- The tympanic membrane (tim-PAN-ick), also known as the eardrum, is located between the outer and middle ear. The word parts myring/o and tympan/o both mean tympanic membrane. When sound waves reach the eardrum, this membrane transmits the sound by vibrating.
- The middle ear is surrounded by the mastoid bone cells, which are hollow air spaces located in the mastoid process of the temporal bone.

The Auditory Ossicles

- The auditory ossicles (OSS-ih-kulz) are three small bones found in the middle ear. These bones transmit the sound waves from the eardrum to the inner ear by vibration. These bones, which are named for the Latin terms that describe their shapes, are the
- Malleus (MAL-ee-us), also known as the hammer.
- Incus (ING-kus), also known as the anvil.
- Stapes (STAY-peez), also known as the stirrup.

The Eustachian Tubes

- The eustachian tubes (you-STAY-shun), also known as the auditory tubes, are narrow tubes that lead from the middle ear to the nasal cavity and the throat. These tubes equalize the air pressure in the middle ear with that of the outside atmosphere.

The Inner Ear

- The inner ear, also known as the labyrinth, contains the sensory receptors for hearing and balance.
- The oval window, which is located under the base of the stapes, is the membrane that separates the middle ear from the inner ear. Vibrations enter the inner ear through this structure.
- The cochlea (KOCK-lee-ah) is the snail-shaped, fluidfilled structure that forms the inner ear. Located within the cochlea are the cochlear duct, the organ of Corti, the semicircular canals, and the acoustic nerves.
- The cochlear duct is a fluid filled cavity within the cochlea that vibrates when sound waves strike it.
- The organ of Corti receives the vibrations from the cochlear duct and relays them to the auditory nerve fibers. These fibers transmit them to the auditory center of the brain's cerebral cortex, where they are heard and interpreted.
- The three semicircular canals contain the liquid endolymph and sensitive hair-like cells. The bending of these hair-like cells in response to the movements of the head sets up impulses in nerve fibers to help maintain equilibrium. Equilibrium is the state of balance.
- The acoustic nerves (cranial nerve VIII) transmit this information to the brain, and the brain sends messages to muscles in all parts of the body to ensure that equilibrium is maintained.

Normal Action of the Ears

- Air conduction is the process by which sound waves enter the ear through the pinna. These waves then travel down the external auditory canal and strike the tympanic membrane between the outer and middle ear.
- Bone conduction occurs as the eardrum vibrates and moves the auditory ossicles. These bones conduct the sound waves through the middle ear to the oval window of the inner ear.
- Sensorineural conduction occurs when sound vibrations reach the inner ear. From here, the structures of the inner ear receive the sound waves and relay them to auditory nerve for transmission to the brain.

Medical Specialties Related To The Ears

- An audiologist (aw-dee-OL-oh-jist) specializes in the measurement of hearing function and in the rehabilitation of persons with hearing impairments (audi means hearing, and -ologist means specialist).

Pathology Of The Ears And Hearing

The Outer Ear

- Impacted cerumen is an accumulation of earwax that forms a solid mass by adhering to the walls of the external auditory canal. Impacted means lodged or wedged firmly in place.
- Otalgia (oh-TAL-gee-ah), also known as an earache, is pain in the ear (ot means ear, and -algia means pain).
- Otitis (oh-TYE-tis) means any inflammation of the ear (ot means ear, and -itis means inflammation). The second part of the term gives the location of the inflammation: otitis externa is an inflammation of external auditory canal; otitis media is an inflammation of the middle ear; and otitis interna is an inflammation of the inner ear.
- Otomycosis (oh-toh-my-KOH-sis), also known as swimmer's ear, is a fungal infection of the external auditory canal (ot/o means ear, myc means fungus, and -osis means abnormal condition).
- Otopyorrhea (oh-toh-pye-oh-REE-ah) is the flow of pus from the ear (ot/o means ear, py/o means pus, and -rrhea means flow or discharge).
- Otorrhagia (oh-toh-RAY-jee-ah) is bleeding from the ear (ot/o means ear, and -rrhagia means bleeding).

The Middle Ear

- Barotrauma (bar-oh-TRAW-mah) is pressure-related ear discomfort that can be caused by pressure changes when flying, driving in the mountains, scuba diving, or when the eustachian tube is blocked (bar/o means pressure, and -trauma means injury).
- Eustachitis (you-stay-KYE-tis), also known as salpingitis, is inflammation of the eustachian tube (eustach means eustachian tube, and -itismeans inflammation).
- Mastoiditis (mas-toy-DYE-tis) is an inflammation of any part of the mastoid bone cells (mastoid means mastoid process, and -itis means inflammation). This condition may develop when an infection in the middle ear that cannot be controlled with antibiotics spreads to the mastoid cells.
- Infectious myringitis (mir-in-JIGH-tis) is a contagious inflammation that causes painful blisters on the eardrum (myring means eardrum, and -itis means inflammation). This condition is associated with a middle ear infection.
- Otosclerosis (oh-toh-skleh-ROH-sis) is the ankylosis of the bones of the middle ear, resulting in a conductive hearing loss (ot/o means ear, and -sclerosis means abnormal hardening). Ankylosis means fused together. This condition is treated with a stapedectomy.
- Patulous eustachian tube (PAT-you-lus) is distention of the eustachian tube. Patulous means extended, spread wide open.

Otitis Media

- Otitis media (oh-TYE-tis MEE-dee-ah) is an inflammation of the middle ear.
- Acute otitis media is usually associated with an upper respiratory infection and is most commonly seen in young children. This condition can lead to a ruptured eardrum due to the buildup of pus or fluid in the middle ear.
- Serous otitis media is a fluid buildup in the middle ear that can follow acute otitis media or can be caused by obstruction of the eustachian tube.
- Acute purulent otitis media is a buildup of pus within the middle ear due to infection. Purulent means producing or containing pus.

The Inner Ear

- Labyrinthitis (lab-ih-rin-THIGH-tis) is an inflammation of the labyrinth that can result in vertigo and deafness (labyrinth means labyrinth, and -itis means inflammation).
- Vertigo (VER-tih-goh) is a sense of whirling, dizziness, and the loss of balance, that is often combined with nausea and vomiting. Although it is a symptom of many disorders, recurrent vertigo is sometimes associated with inner ear problems such as Ménière's syndrome.
- Ménière's syndrome is a rare chronic disease in which the amount of fluid in the inner ear increases intermittently, producing attacks of vertigo, a fluctuating hearing loss (usually in one ear), and tinnitus.
- Tinnitus (tih-NIGH-tus) is a ringing, buzzing, or roaring sound in one or both ears. It is often associated with hearing loss, and is more likely to occur when there has been prolonged exposure to loud noises.

Hearing Loss

- Deafness is the complete or partial loss of the ability to hear. It can range from the inability to hear sounds of a certain pitch or intensity, to a complete loss of hearing.
- Presbycusis (pres-beh-KOO-sis) is a gradual loss of sensorineural hearing that occurs as the body ages (presby means old age, and -cusis means hearing).
- A conductive hearing loss occurs when sound waves are prevented from passing from the air to the fluidfilled inner ear. Causes of this hearing loss include a buildup of earwax, infection, fluid in the middle ear, a punctured eardrum, otosclerosis, and scarring.
- A sensorineural hearing loss, also known as nerve deafness, develops when the auditory nerve or hair cells in the inner ear are damaged. The source of this hearing loss can be located in the inner ear, in the nerve from the inner ear to the brain, or in the brain.

Noise-Induced Hearing Loss

- A noise-induced hearing loss (NIHL) is a type of nerve deafness caused by repeated exposure to extremely loud noises such as a gunshot, or to moderately loud noise that continues for long periods of time.

Diagnostic Procedures Of The Ears And Hearing

- An audiological evaluation, also known as speech audiometry, is the measurement of the ability to hear and understand speech sounds based on their pitch and loudness. This testing is best achieved in a soundtreated room with earphones. The resulting graph is an audiogram that represents the ability to hear a variety of sounds at various loudness levels.
- Audiometry (aw-dee-OM-eh-tree) is the use of an audiometer to measure hearing acuity (audi/o means hearing, and -metry means to measure). An audiometer is an electronic device that produces acoustic stimuli of a set frequency and intensity.
- Sound is measured in two different ways. A hertz (Hz) is a measure of sound frequency that determines how high or low a pitch is. A decibel is commonly used as the measurement of the loudness of sound.
- An otoscope, which is used to examine the external ear canal.
- Monaural testing (mon-AW-rahl) involves one ear (mon- means one, aur means hearing, and -al means pertaining to). Compare with binaural testing.
- Binauraltesting (bye-NAW-rul or bin-AW-rahl) involves both ears (bi- means two, aur means hearing, and -al means pertaining to). Compare with monaural testing.
- Tympanometry (tim-pah-NOM-eh-tree) is the use of air pressure in the ear canal to test for disorders of the middle ear (tympan/o means eardrum, and -metry means to measure). The resulting record is a tympanogram.

This is used to test for middle ear fluid buildup or eustachian tube obstruction, or to evaluate a conductive hearing loss.

Treatment Procedures Of The Ears And Hearing

The Outer Ear

Otoplasty (OH-toh-plas-tee) is the surgical repair of the pinna of the ear (ot/o means ear, and -plasty means surgical repair).

The Middle Ear

- A mastoidectomy (mas-toy-DECK-toh-mee) is the surgical removal of mastoid cells (mastoid means mastoid process, and -ectomy means surgical removal). This procedure is used to treat a mastoiditis that cannot be controlled with antibiotics or in preparation for the placement of a cochlear implant.

- A myringotomy (mir-in-GOT-oh-mee) is the surgical incision in the eardrum to create an opening for the placement of tympanostomy tubes (myring means eardrum, and -otomy means surgical incision).
- Tympanostomy tubes (tim-pan-OSS-toh-mee), also known as pediatric ear tubes, are tiny ventilating tubes placed through the eardrum to provide ongoing drainage for fluids and to relieve pressure that can build up after childhood ear infections.
- Tympanoplasty (tim-pah-noh-PLAS-tee) is the surgical correction of a damaged middle ear, either to cure chronic inflammation or to restore function (tympan/o means eardrum, and -plasty means a surgical repair).
- A stapedectomy (stay-peh-DECK-toh-mee) is the surgical removal of the top portion of the stapes bone and the insertion of a small prosthetic device known as a piston that conducts sound vibrations to the inner ear.

The Inner Ear

- Fenestration (fen-es-TRAY-shun) is a surgical procedure in which a new opening is created in the labyrinth to restore hearing (fenestra means window, and -tion means process).
- A hearing aid is an external electronic device that uses a microphone to detect sounds. The sounds may be coded into a digital representation and are filtered to best compensate for the hearing loss before being amplified into the ear canal. Sensorineural hearing loss can sometimes be corrected with a hearing aid.
- A labyrinthectomy (lab-ih-rin-THECK-toh-mee) is the surgical removal of all or a portion of the labyrinth (labyrinth means labyrinth, and -ectomy means surgical removal). This procedure is performed to relieve uncontrolled vertigo; however, this procedure causes a complete hearing loss in the affected ear.
- A labyrinthotomy (lab-ih-rin-THOT-oh-mee) is a surgical incision between two of the fluid chambers of the labyrinth to allow the pressure to equalize (labyrinth means labyrinth, and -otomy means a surgical incision). This procedure is performed to relieve severe vertigo; however, about half of patients suffer some loss of high tone hearing in the affected ear.

Cochlear Implant

- A cochlear implant (KOCK-lee-ar) is an implanted electronic device that can give a deaf person a useful auditory understanding of the environment and/or hearing and help them to understand speech. The external speech processor captures sounds and converts them into digital signals. Electrodes implanted in the cochlea receive the signals and stimulate the auditory nerve. The brain receives these signals and perceives them as sound.

Abbreviations Related To The Special Senses
- astigmatism = AS
- cataract = CAT
- conjunctivitis = CI
- diopter = D, Dptr
- emmetropia = EM, em
- fluorescein angiography = FA, FAG
- glaucoma = G, glc
- macular degeneration = MD
- radial keratotomy = RK
- retinal detachment = RD
- visual acuity = V, VA

Critical Thinking Exercise

The following story and questions are designed to stimulate critical thinking through class discussion or as a brief essay response. There are no right or wrong answers to these questions.

William Davis is 62 years old. He was employed as a postal worker until his declining eyesight forced him into early retirement a few months ago. His wife, Mildred, died last year of complications from diabetes after a prolonged and expensive hospitalization. Mr. Davis does not trust the medical community and because of this distrust, he has not been to a doctor since his wife's death.

Mr. Davis is not considered legally blind, but his presbyopia and the advancing cataract in his right eye are starting to interfere with his ability to take care of himself. He still drives to the market once a week, but other drivers get angry and honk at him. He pays for his groceries with a credit card because he is afraid the cashier will cheat him if he accidentally gives her the wrong bills. He complains that the cleaning lady hides things from him and deliberately leaves the furniture out of place. When she leaves, he can't find his slippers or an ashtray. Yesterday, he put his lit pipe down in a wooden bowl by accident.

His son insists on taking him to see the ophthalmologist who treated his wife's diabetic retinopathy. Dr. Hsing believes Mr. Davis's sight can be improved in the right eye by performing cataract surgery. Mr. Davis listens in fear as the doctor explains. "Without this procedure, your sight will only get worse."

Mr. Davis thinks about all the medical procedures that were tried on Mildred, and she died anyway. He doesn't want to go into the hospital, and he doesn't want any operations. But his son is talking about taking away his car if he doesn't do something about his failing sight. "What more can be taken away from me?" he thinks bitterly. "First my wife, then my job, and now my independence."

Suggested Discussion Topics

1. Discuss how Mr. Davis's loss of sight is affecting the way he treats others and is treated by them.
2. Mr. Davis is a patient at the clinic where you work. Discuss the ways you would adjust your usual routine to accommodate his needs.

3. Discuss why cataract surgery would be scary to Mr. Davis and what Dr. Hsing and his staff could do to ease his apprehension.
4. If Mr. Davis does not go ahead with the surgery, what help might he receive from an agency for the visually impaired? What groups might be available to help him deal with his grief and depression?

Scott J. Barnard

CHAPTER 12

SKIN: THE INTEGUMENTARY SYSTEM

This list contains essential word parts and medical terms for this chapter.

Word Parts

- bi/o
- derm/o, dermat/o
- erythr/o
- hidr/o
- hirsut/o
- kerat/o
- lip/o
- melan/o
- myc/o
- onych/o
- pedicul/o
- rhytid/o
- seb/o
- urtic/o
- xer/o

Medical Terms

- actinic keratosis (ack-TIN-ick kerr-ah-TOH-sis)
- albinism (AL-bih-niz-um)
- alopecia (al-oh-PEE-shee-ah)
- blepharoplasty (BLEF-ah-roh-plas-tee)
- bulla (BULL-ah)
- carbuncle (KAR-bung-kul)
- cellulitis (sell-you-LYE-tis)
- chloasma (kloh-AZ-mah)
- cicatrix (sick-AY-tricks)
- comedo (KOM-eh-doh)
- debridement (day-breed-MON)
- dermatitis (der-mah-TYE-tis)

- diaphoresis (dye-ah-foh-REE-sis)
- dysplastic nevi (dis-PLAS-tick NEE-vye)
- ecchymosis (eck-ih-MOH-sis)
- eczema (ECK-zeh-mah)
- erythema (er-ih-THEE-mah)
- erythroderma (eh-rith-roh-DER-mah)
- exfoliative dermatitis (ecks-FOH-lee-ay-tiv eh-rith-roh-DER-mah)
- folliculitis (foh-lick-you-LYE-tis)
- furuncles (FYOU-rung-kulz)
- granuloma (gran-you-LOH-mah)
- hematoma (hee-mah-TOH-mah)
- hirsutism (HER-soot-izm)
- ichthyosis (ick-thee-OH-sis)
- impetigo (im-peh-TYE-go)
- keloid (KEE-loid)
- keratosis (kerr-ah-TOH-sis)
- koilonychia (koy-loh-NICK-ee-ah)
- lipedema (lip-eh-DEE-mah)
- lipoma (lih-POH-mah)
- lupus erythematosus (LOO-pus er-ih-theemah- TOH-sus)
- macule (MACK-youl)
- malignant melanoma (mel-ah-NOH-mah)
- miliaria (mill-ee-AYR-ee-ah)
- necrotizing fasciitis (fas-ee-EYE-tis)
- onychocryptosis (on-ih-koh-krip-TOH-sis)
- onychomycosis (on-ih-koh-my-KOH-sis)
- papilloma (pap-ih-LOH-mah)
- papule (PAP-youl)
- paronychia (par-oh-NICK-ee-ah)
- pediculosis (pee-dick-you-LOH-sis)
- petechiae (pee-TEE-kee-ee)
- pruritus (proo-RYE-tus)
- psoriasis (soh-RYE-uh-sis)
- purpura (PUR-pew-rah)
- purulent (PYOU-roo-lent)
- rhytidectomy (rit-ih-DECK-toh-mee)
- rosacea (roh-ZAY-shee-ah)
- scabies (SKAY-beez)
- scleroderma (sklehr-oh-DER-mah)
- seborrhea (seb-oh-REE-ah)
- squamous cell carcinoma (SKWAY-mus)
- strawberry hemangioma (hee-man-jee-OH-mah)
- tinea (TIN-ee-ah)
- urticaria (ur-tih-KARE-ree-ah)

- verrucae (veh-ROO-kee)
- vitiligo (vit-ih-LYE-goh)
- wheal (WHEEL)
- xeroderma (zee-roh-DER-mah)

Objectives

On completion of this chapter, you should be able to:
1. Identify and describe the functions and structures of the integumentary system.
2. Identify the medical specialists associated with the integumentary system.
3. Recognize, define, spell, and pronounce the terms used to describe the pathology and the diagnostic and treatment procedures related to the skin.
4. Recognize, define, spell, and pronounce terms used to describe the pathology and the diagnostic and treatment procedures related to hair, nails, and sebaceous glands.

Functions Of The Integumentary System

The integumentary system (in-teg-you-MEN-tah-ree), which is made up of the skin and its related structures, performs important functions in maintaining the health of the body.

Functions of the Skin

The skin forms the protective outer covering of the entire body.
- The skin waterproofs the body and prevents fluid loss.
- Intact (unbroken) skin plays an important role in the immune system by blocking the entrance of pathogens into the body.
- Skin is the major receptor for the sense of touch.
- Skin helps the body manufacture vitamin D, an essential nutrient, from the sun's ultraviolet light, while screening out some harmful ultraviolet radiation.

Functions of Related Structures

- The related structures of the integumentary system are the sebaceous glands, sweat glands, hair, and nails.
- The sebaceous glands (seh-BAY-shus) secrete sebum (oil) that lubricates the skin and discourages the growth of bacteria on the skin.
-
- The sweat glands help regulate body temperature and water content by secreting sweat. A small amount of metabolic waste is also excreted through the sweat glands.
- Hair helps control the loss of body heat.
- Nails protect the dorsal surface of the last bone of each toe and finger.

The Structures Of The Skin And Its Related Structures

The Skin
- Skin covers the external surfaces of the body. The average adult has two square yards of skin, making it the largest bodily organ.
- The terms cutaneous (kyou-TAY-nee-us) means relating to the skin (cutane means skin, and -ous means pertaining to). The skin is a complex system of specialized tissues and is made up of three basic layers: the epidermis, dermis, and the subcutaneous layer.

The Epidermis
- The epidermis (ep-ih-DER-mis), which is the outermost layer of the skin, is made up of several specialized epithelial tissues.
- Epithelial tissues (ep-ih-THEE-lee-al) form a protective covering for all of the internal and external surfaces of the body.
- Squamous epithelial tissue (SKWAY-mus) forms the upper layer of the epidermis. Squamous means scalelike. This layer consists of flat, scaly cells that are continuously shed.
- The epidermis, which does not contain any blood vessels or connective tissue, is dependent on lower layers for nourishment.
- The basal layer is the lowest layer of the epidermis. It is here that cells are produced and then pushed upward. When these cells reach the surface, they die and become filled with keratin.
- Keratin (KER-ah-tin) is a fibrous, water-repellent protein. Soft keratin is a primary component of the epidermis. Hard keratin is found in the hair and nails.
- The basal cell layer also contains special cells called melanocytes (MEL-ah-noh-sights). These cells produce and contain a dark brown to black pigment called melanin. The type and amount of melanin pigment determines the color of the skin. It also produces spots of color such as freckles.
- Melanin has the important function of protecting the skin against some of the harmful ultraviolet rays of the sun. Ultraviolet (UV) refers to light that is beyond the visible spectrum at the violet end. Some UV rays help the skin produce vitamin D; however, other rays damage the skin.

The Dermis
- The dermis (DER-mis), also known as the corium, is the thick layer of living tissue directly below the epidermis. It contains connective tissue, blood and lymph vessels, and nerve fibers. It also contains the associated structures of the skin, which are the hair follicles plus the sebaceous and sweat glands. Sensory nerve endings in the dermis are the sensory receptors stimuli such as touch, temperature, pain, and pressure.

Tissues Within the Dermis
- Collagen (KOL-ah-jen), which means glue, is a tough, yet flexible, fibrous protein material found in the skin and in the bones, cartilage, tendons, and ligaments.
- Mast cells, which are found in the connective tissue of the dermis, respond to injury, infection, or allergy by producing and releasing substances, including heparin and histamine.
- Heparin (HEP-ah-rin), which is released in response to an injury, is an anticoagulant. An anticoagulant prevents blood clotting.
- Histamine (HISS-tah-meen), which is released in response to allergens, causes the signs of an allergic response, including itching and increased mucus secretion.

The Subcutaneous Layer
- The subcutaneous layer, which is located just below the skin, connects the skin to the surface muscles.
- This layer is made up of loose connective tissue and adipose tissue (AD-ih-pohs). Adipose means fat.
- Cellulite is a term sometimes used to describe deposits of dimpled fat. This is not a medical term, and medical authorities agree that cellulite is simply ordinary fatty tissue. Note: Do not confuse cellulite with cellulitis, which is discussed later in this chapter.
- Lipocytes (LIP-oh-sights), also known as fat cells, are predominant in the subcutaneous layer where they manufacture and store large quantities of fat (lip/o means fat, and -cytes means cells).

The Sebaceous Glands
- Sebaceous glands (seh-BAY-shus) are located in the dermis layer of the skin and are closely associated with hair follicles.
- These glands secrete sebum (SEE-bum), which is released through ducts opening into the hair follicles. From here, the sebum moves onto the surface and lubricates the skin.
- Because sebum is slightly acidic, it discourages the growth of bacteria on the skin.
- The milk-producing mammary glands, which are modified sebaceous glands, are sometimes classified with the integumentary system.

The Sweat Glands
Sweat glands, also known as sudoriferous glands, are tiny, coiled glands found on almost all body surfaces. They are most numerous in the palms of the hands, the soles of the feet, the forehead, and the armpits.
- Pores are the openings on the surface of the skin for the ducts of the sweat glands.

- Perspiration, also known as sweat, is secreted by sweat glands and is made up of 99% water plus some salt and metabolic waste products.
- Perspiring, also known as sweating, is one way in which the body excretes excess water. As the sweat evaporates into the air it also cools the body. Body odor associated with sweat comes from the interaction of the perspiration with bacteria on the skin's surface.
- Hidrosis (high-DROH-sis) is the production and excretion of sweat.

The Hair

Hair fibers are rod-like structures composed of tightly fused, dead protein cells filled with hard keratin. The darkness and color of the hair is determined by the amount and type of melanin produced by the melanocytes that surround the core of the hair shaft.

- Hair follicles are the sacs that hold the root of the hair fibers. The shape of the follicle determines whether the hair is straight or curly.
- Although hair is dead tissue, it appears to grow because the cells at the base of the follicle divide rapidly and push the old cells upward. As these cells are pushed upward, they harden and undergo pigmentation.
- The arrector pili (ah-RECK-tor PYE-lye) are tiny muscle fibers attached to the hair follicles that cause the hair to stand erect. In response to cold or fright, these muscles contract, causing raised areas of skin known as goose bumps. This action reduces heat loss through the skin.

The Nails

- An unguis (UNG-gwis), commonly known as a fingernail or toenail, is the keratin plate protecting the dorsal surface of the last bone of each finger and toe (plural, ungues). Each nail consists of these parts.
- The nail body, which is translucent, is closely molded the surface of the underlying tissues. It is made up of hard, keratinized plates of epidermal cells.
- The nail bed, which joins the nail body to the underlying connective tissue, nourishes the nail. The blood vessels here give the nail its characteristic pink color.
- The free edge, which is the portion of the nail not attached to the nail bed, extends beyond the tip of the finger or toe.
- The lunula (LOO-new-lah) is a pale half-moon-shaped region at every nail root that is generally most easily seen in the thumbnail (plural, lunulae). This is the active area of the nail, where new keratin cells form. Lunula means little moon.
- The cuticle is a narrow band of epidermis attached to the surface of the nail just in front of the root, protecting the new keratin cells as they form. Cuticle means little skin.
- The nail root fastens the nail to the finger or toe by fitting into a groove in the skin.

- A dermatologist (der-mah-TOL-oh-jist) is a physician who specializes in diagnosing and treating disorders of the skin (dermat means skin, and -ologist means specialist).
- A cosmetic surgeon, also known as a plastic surgeon, is a physician who specializes in the surgical restoration and reconstruction of body structures. As used here, plastic refers to the suffix -plasty, meaning surgical repair.

Pathology of the integumentary System

The Sebaceous Glands

- Acne vulgaris (ACK-nee vul-GAY-ris), commonly known as acne, is a chronic inflammatory disease characterized by pustular eruptions of the skin caused by an overproduction of sebum. Although often triggered by hormones in puberty and adolescence, it also occurs in adults. Vulgaris is a Latin term meaning common.
- A comedo (KOM-eh-doh) is a noninfected lesion formed by the buildup of sebum and keratin in a hair follicle (plural, comedones). Comedones are often associated with acne vulgaris. When a sebum plug is exposed to air, it oxidizes and becomes a blackhead.
- A sebaceous cyst (seh-BAY-shus SIST) is a closed sac associated with a sebaceous gland that is found just under the skin. These cysts contain yellow, fatty material and are usually found on the face, neck, or trunk.
- Seborrhea (seb-oh-REE-ah) is overactivity of the sebaceous glands that results in the production of an excessive amount of sebum (seb/o means sebum, and -rrhea means flow or discharge).
- Seborrheic dermatitis (seb-oh-REE-ick der-mah-TYE-tis) is an inflammation that causes scaling and itching of the upper layers of the skin or scalp. Extensive dandruff is a form of seborrheic dermatitis, as is the scalp rash in infants known as cradle cap. In contrast, mild dandruff is usually caused by a yeast-like fungus on the scalp.
- A seborrheic keratosis (seb-oh-REE-ick kerr-ah-TOH-sis) is a benign skin growth that has a waxy or "pasted-on" look. These growths, which can vary in color from light tan to black, occur most commonly in the elderly.

The Sweat Glands

- Anhidrosis (an-high-DROH-sis) is the abnormal condition of lacking sweat in response to heat (an- means without, hidr means sweat, and -osis means abnormal condition).
- Diaphoresis (dye-ah-foh-REE-sis) is profuse sweating dia- means through or complete, phor means movement, and -esis means abnormal condition). This is a normal condition when brought on by heat or exertion, but can also be the body's response to emotional or physical distress.

- Hyperhidrosis (high-per-high-DROH-sis) is a condition of sweating in one area or over the whole body (hyper- means excessive, hidr means sweat, and -osis means abnormal condition).
- Miliaria (mill-ee-AYR-ee-ah), also known as heat rash and prickly heat, is an intensely itchy rash caused by blockage of the sweat glands by bacteria and dead cells. Caution: Do not confuse this condition with the infectious disease malaria.
- Sleep hyperhidrosis, commonly known as night sweats, is the occurrence of excessive hyperhidrosis during sleep. There are many potential causes of this condition, including menopause, certain medications, and some infectious diseases.

The Hair

- Folliculitis (foh-lick-you-LYE-tis) is an inflammation of the hair follicles (follicul means the hair follicle, and -itis means inflammation). This condition is especially common on the limbs and in the beard area of men.

Excessive Hairiness

- Hirsutism (HER-soot-izm) is the presence of excessive body and facial hair in women, usually occurring in a male pattern (hirsut means hairy, and -ism means condition). This condition can be hereditary or caused by a hormonal imbalance.

Abnormal Hair Loss

- Alopecia (al-oh-PEE-shee-ah), also known as baldness, is the partial or complete loss of hair, most commonly on the scalp (alopec means baldness, and -ia means condition).
- Alopecia areata is an autoimmune disorder that attacks the hair follicles, causing well-defined bald areas on the scalp or elsewhere on the body. This condition often begins in childhood. Areata means occurring in patches.
- Alopecia capitis totalis is an uncommon condition characterized by the loss of all the hair on the scalp. Capitis means head.
- Alopecia universalis is the total loss of hair on all parts of the body. Universalis means total.
- Female pattern baldness is a condition in which the hair thins in the front and on the sides of the scalp and sometimes on the crown. This condition rarely leads to total hair loss.
- Male pattern baldness is a common hair-loss pattern in men, with the hairline receding from the front to the back until only a horseshoe-shaped area of hair remains in the back and at the temples.

Medical Terminology for Health Professions 4.0

The Nails

- Clubbing is abnormal curving of the nails that is often accompanied by enlargement of the fingertips. This condition can be hereditary, but usually is caused by changes associated with oxygen deficiencies related to coronary or pulmonary disease.
- Koilonychia (koy-loh-NICK-ee-ah), also known as spoon nail, is a malformation of the nails in which the outer surface is concave or scooped out like the bowl of a spoon (koil means hollow or concave, onych means fingernail or toenail, and -ia means condition). Koilonychia is often an indication of iron-deficiency anemia.
- Onychia (oh-NICK-ee-ah), also known as onychitis, is an inflammation of the matrix of the nail that usually results in the loss of the nail (onych means fingernail or toenail, and -ia means condition).
- Onychocryptosis (on-ih-koh-krip-TOH-sis) is commonly known an ingrown toenail (onych/o means fingernail or toenail, crypt means hidden, and -osis means abnormal condition). The edges of a toenail, usually on the big toe, curve inward and cut into the skin. The affected area is prone to inflammation or infection.
- Onychomycosis (on-ih-koh-my-KOH-sis) is a fungal infection of the nail (onych/o means fingernail or toenail, myc means fungus, and -osis means abnormal condition). Depending on the type of fungus involved, this condition can cause the nails to turn white, yellow, green, or black and to become thick or brittle.
- Onychophagia (on-ih-koh-FAY-jee-ah) means nail biting or nail eating (onych/o means fingernail or toenail, and -phagia means eating or swallowing).
- Paronychia (par-oh-NICK-ee-ah) is an acute or chronic infection of the skin fold around a nail (parmeans near, onych means fingernail or toenail, and -ia means condition).
- Albinism (AL-bih-niz-um) is a genetic condition characterized by a deficiency or the absence of pigment in the skin, hair, and irises of the eyes (albin means white, and -ism means condition). This condition is the result of a missing enzyme that is necessary for the production of melanin. A person with this condition is known as an albino.
- Chloasma (kloh-AZ-mah), also known as melasma or the mask of pregnancy, is a pigmentation disorder characterized by brownish spots on the face. This can occur during pregnancy, especially among women with dark hair and fair skin, and usually disappears after delivery.
- Melanosis (mel-ah-NOH-sis) is any condition of unusual deposits of black pigment in different parts of the body (melan means black, and -osis means abnormal condition).
- Vitiligo (vit-ih-LYE-goh) is a skin condition resulting from the destruction of the melanocytes due to unknown causes. Vitiligo is characterized by irregular patches of white skin. Hair growing in an affected area is also white.

Bleeding into the Skin

- A contusion (kon-TOO-zhun) is an injury to underlying tissues without breaking the skin and is characterized by discoloration and pain (contus means bruise, and -ion means condition). The discoloration is caused by an accumulation of blood within the skin.
- An ecchymosis (eck-ih-MOH-sis), also known as a bruise, is a large, irregular area of purplish discoloration due to bleeding under the skin (ecchym means pouring out of juice, and -osis means abnormal condition) (plural, ecchymoses).
- Purpura (PUR-pew-rah) is the appearance of multiple purple discolorations on the skin caused by bleeding underneath the skin (purpur means purple, and -a is a noun ending). These areas of discoloration are smaller than ecchymosis and larger than petechiae.
- Petechiae (pee-TEE-kee-ee) are very small, pinpoint hemorrhages that are less than 2 mm in diameter (singular, petechia). These hemorrhages sometimes result from high fevers.
- A hematoma (hee-mah-TOH-mah), which is usually caused by an injury, is a swelling of clotted blood trapped in the tissues (hemat means blood, and -oma means tumor). The body eventually resorbs this blood. A hematoma is often named for the area where it occurs. For example, a subungual hematoma is blood trapped under a finger or toenail.

Surface Lesions

- A lesion (LEE-zhun) is a pathologic change of the tissues due to disease or injury. Skin lesions are described by their appearance, location, color, and size as measured in centimeters (cm).
- A crust, also known as scab, is a collection of dried serum and cellular debris.
- A macule (MACK-youl), also known as a macula, is a discolored, flat spot that is less than 1 cm in diameter. Freckles, or flat moles, are examples of macules.
- A nodule is a solid, raised skin lesion that is larger than 0.5 cm in diameter and deeper than a papule. In acne vulgaris, nodules can cause scarring.
- A papule (PAP-youl) is a small, raised red lesion that is less than 0.5 cm in diameter and does not contain pus. Small pimples and insect bites are types of papules.
- A plaque (PLACK) is a scaly, solid raised area of closely spaced papules. For example, the lesions of psoriasis are plaques.

Note: The term plaque also means a fatty buildup in the arteries and a soft substance that forms on the teeth.

- Scales are flakes or dry patches made up of excess dead epidermal cells. Some shedding of scales is normal; however, excessive shedding is associated with skin disorders such as psoriasis.

- Verrucae (veh-ROO-kee), also known as warts, are small, hard skin lesions caused by the human papilloma virus (singular, verruca). Plantar warts develop on the sole of the foot.
- A wheal (WHEEL), also known as a welt, is a small bump that itches. Wheals can appear as a symptom of an allergic reaction.

Fluid-Filled Lesions

- An abscess (AB-sess) is a closed pocket containing pus that is caused by a bacterial infection. An abscess can appear on the skin or within other structures of the body. Purulent (PYOU-roo-lent) means producing or containing pus.
- A cyst (SIST) is an abnormal sac containing gas, fluid, or a semisolid material. The term cyst can also refer to a sac or vesicle elsewhere in the body. The most common type of skin cyst is a sebaceous cyst.
- A pustule (PUS-tyoul), also known as a pimple, is a small, circumscribed lesion containing pus. Circumscribed means contained within a limited area. Pustules can be cause by acne vulgaris, impetigo, or other infections.
- A vesicle (VES-ih-kul) is a small blister, less than 0.5 cm in diameter, containing watery fluid. For example, the rash of poison oak consists of vesicles.
- A bulla (BULL-ah) is a large blister that is usually more than 0.5 cm in diameter (plural, bullae).

Lesions Through the Skin

- An abrasion (ah-BRAY-zhun) is an injury in which superficial layers of skin are scraped or rubbed away. The term abrasion also describes a treatment that involves scraping or rubbing away skin.
- A pressure sore, previously known as a decubitus ulcer or bedsore, is an ulcerated area in which prolonged pressure has caused tissue death. Without proper care, open sores quickly become infected.
- A fissure is a groove or crack-like break in the skin. In tinea pedis (athlete's foot), fissures are commonly present between the toes. The term fissure also describes normal folds in the contours of the brain.
- A laceration (lass-er-AY-shun) is a torn or jagged wound, or an accidental cut wound.
- A puncture wound is a deep hole made by a sharp object such as a nail. The risk for infection, especially tetanus, is greater with this type of wound. A needlestick injury, which can transmit infection, is an accidental puncture caused by a used hypodermic needle.
- An ulcer (UL-ser) is an open lesion of the skin or mucous membrane resulting in tissue loss around the edges. Note: Ulcers also occur inside the body.

Birthmarks

- A port-wine stain is a large, reddish-purple discoloration of the face or neck. This discoloration will not resolve without treatment. See Laser Treatment of Skin Conditions later in this chapter.
- A strawberry hemangioma (hee-man-jee-OH-mah) is a soft, raised, dark-reddish-purple birthmark (hem means blood, angi/o means blood or lymph vessels, and -oma means tumor). A hemangioma is a benign tumor made up of newly formed blood vessels. These birthmarks often, but not always, resolve by the age 5 without treatment.

Dermatitis

- The term dermatitis (der-mah-TYE-tis) means an inflammation of the skin (dermat means skin, and -itis means inflammation). This condition, which takes many forms, usually includes redness, swelling, and itching.
- Contact dermatitis (CD) is a localized allergic response caused by contact with an irritant, for example, as seen with diaper rash. It is also caused by exposure to an allergen, such as an allergic reaction to latex gloves.
- Eczema (ECK-zeh-mah) is a form of persistent or recurring dermatitis that is usually characterized by redness, itching, and dryness, with possible blistering, cracking, oozing, or bleeding. This chronic condition appears to be an abnormal response of the body's immune system.
- Pruritus (proo-RYE-tus), also known as itching, is associated with most forms of dermatitis (prurit means itching, and -us is a singular noun ending).

Erythema

- Erythema (er-ih-THEE-mah) is redness of the skin due to capillary dilation (erythem means flushed, and -a is a noun ending).
- Erythema multiforme is a skin disorder resulting from a generalized allergic reaction to an illness, infection, or medication. This reaction, which affects the skin and/or mucous membranes, is characterized by a rash that may appear as nodules or papules (raised red bumps), macules (flat discolored areas), or vesicles or bullae (blisters).
- Erythema infectiosum, also known as fifth disease, is a mildly contagious viral infection that is common in childhood. This infection produces a red, lace-like rash on the child's face that looks as if the child has been slapped.
- Erythema pernio, also known as chilblains, is a purple-red inflammation that occurs when the small blood vessels below the skin are damaged, usually due to exposure to cold and damp weather. When restores full circulation, the affected areas begin to itch; however, they usually heal without treatment.
- Erythroderma (eh-rith-roh-DER-mah) is abnormal redness of the entire skin surface (erythr/o means red, and -derma means skin).

- Sunburn is a form of erythema in which skin cells are damaged by exposure to the ultraviolet rays in sunlight. This damage increases the chances of later developing skin cancer.
- Exfoliative dermatitis (ecks-FOH-lee-ay-tiv eh-rithroh- DER-mah) is a condition in which there is widespread scaling of the skin, often with pruritus, erythroderma, and hair loss. It may occur in severe cases of many common skin conditions, include eczema, psoriasis, and allergic reactions.

General Skin Conditions

- Dermatosis (der-mah-TOH-sis) is a general term used to denote skin lesions or eruptions of any type that are not associated with inflammation (dermat means skin, and -osis means abnormal condition).
- Ichthyosis (ick-thee-OH-sis) is a group of hereditary disorders characterized by dry, thickened, and scaly skin (ichthy means dry or scaly, and -osis means abnormal condition). These conditions are caused either by the slowing of the skin's natural shedding process or by a rapid increase in the production of the skin's cells.
- Lipedema (lip-eh-DEE-mah), also known as painful fat syndrome, is a chronic abnormal condition that is characterized by the accumulation of fat and fluid in the tissues just under the skin of the hips and legs (lip means fat, and -edema means swelling). This condition usually affects women and, even when weight is lost, this localized excess fat does not go away.
- Lupus erythematosus (LOO-pus er-ih-thee-mah-TOHsus), also known as lupus, is an autoimmune disorder characterized by a red, scaly rash on the face and upper trunk. In addition to the skin, this condition also attacks the connective tissue in other body systems, especially in the joints.
- Psoriasis (soh-RYE-uh-sis) is a common skin disorder characterized by flare-ups in which red papules covered with silvery scales occur on the elbows, knees, scalp, back, or buttocks
- Rosacea (roh-ZAY-shee-ah), which is also known as adult acne, is characterized by tiny red pimples and broken blood vessels. This chronic condition of unknown cause usually develops individuals with fair skin, between 30 and 60 years of ages.
- Rhinophyma (rye-noh-FIGH-muh), also known as bulbous nose, usually occurs in older men (rhin/o means nose, and -phyma means growth). This condition is characterized by hyperplasia (overgrowth) of the tissues of the nose and is associated with advanced rosacea.
- Scleroderma (sklehr-oh-DER-mah) is an autoimmune disorder in which the connective tissues become thickened and hardened, causing the skin to become hard and swollen (scler/o means hard, and -derma means skin). This condition can also affect the joints and internal organs.

- Urticaria (ur-tih-KARE-ree-ah), also known as hives, are itchy wheals caused by an allergic reaction (urtic means rash, and -aria means connected with).
- Xeroderma (zee-roh-DER-mah), also known as xerosis, is excessively dry skin (xer/o means dry, and -derma means skin).

Bacterial Skin Infections

- A carbuncle (KAR-bung-kul) is a cluster of connected furuncles (boils).
- Cellulitis (sell-you-LYE-tis) is an acute, rapidly spreading infection within the connective tissues that is characterized by malaise, swelling, warmth, and red streaks. Malaise is a feeling of general discomfort or uneasiness that is often the first indication of an infection or other disease.
- Furuncles (FYOU-rung-kulz), also known as boils, are large, tender, swollen areas caused by a staphylococcal infection around hair follicles or sebaceous glands.
- Gangrene (GANG-green), which is tissue necrosis (death), is most commonly caused by a loss of circulation to the affected tissues. The tissue death is followed by bacterial invasion that causes putrefaction, and if this infection enters the bloodstream, it can be fatal. Putrefaction is decay that produces foulsmelling odors.
- Impetigo (im-peh-TYE-goh) is a highly contagious bacterial skin infection that commonly occurs in children. This condition is characterized by isolated pustules that become crusted and rupture.
- Necrotizing fasciitis (fas-ee-EYE-tis) is a severe infection caused by Group A strep bacteria (also known as flesh-eating bacteria). Necrotizing means causing tissue death, and fasciitis is inflammation of fascia. These bacteria normally live harmlessly on the skin; however, if they enter the body through a skin wound, this serious infection can result. If untreated, the infected body tissue is destroyed, and the illness can be fatal.
- Pyoderma (pye-oh-DER-mah) is any acute, inflammatory, pus-forming bacterial skin infection such as impetigo (py/o means pus, and -derma means skin).

Fungal Skin Infections

- Tinea (TIN-ee-ah) is a fungal infection that can grow on the skin, hair, or nails. This condition is also known as ringworm, not because a worm is involved, but because as the fungus grows, it spreads out in a worm-like circle leaving normal-looking skin in the middle.
- Tinea capitis is found on the scalps of children. Capitis means head.
- Tinea corporis is a fungal infection of the skin on the body. Corporis means body.
- Tinea cruris, also known as jock itch, is found in the genital area.

- Tinea pedis, also known as athlete's foot, is found between the toes and on the feet. Pedis means feet.
- Tinea versicolor, also known as pityriasis versicolor, is a fungal infection that causes painless, discolored areas on the skin. Versicolor means a variety of color.

Parasitic Skin Infestations

- An infestation is the dwelling of microscopic parasites on external surface tissue. Some parasites live temporarily on the skin. Others lay eggs and reproduce there.
- Pediculosis (pee-dick-you-LOH-sis) is an infestation with lice (pedicul means lice, and -osis means abnormal condition). The lice eggs, known as nits, must be destroyed in order to get rid of the infestation. There are three types of lice, each attracted to a specific part of the body:
- Pediculosis capitis is an infestation with head lice.
- Pediculosis corporis is an infestation with body lice.
- Pediculosis pubis is an infestation with lice in the pubic hair and pubic region.
- Scabies (SKAY-beez) is a skin infection caused by an infestation with the itch mite, which causes small, itchy bumps and blisters due to tiny mites that burrow into the top layer of human skin to lay their eggs. Medications applied to the skin kill the mites; however, itching may persist for several weeks.

Skin Growths

- A callus (KAL-us) is a thickening of part of the skin on the hands or feet caused by repeated rubbing. A clavus, or corn, is a callus in the keratin layer of the skin covering the joints of the toes, usually caused by ill-fitting shoes.
- A cicatrix (sick-AY-tricks) is a normal scar resulting from the healing of a wound (plural, cicatrices).
- Granulation tissue is the tissue that normally forms during the healing of a wound. This tissue eventually forms the scar.
- Granuloma (gran-you-LOH-mah) is a general term used to describe small, knot-like swellings of granulation tissue in the epidermis (granul meaning granular, and -oma means tumor). Granulomas can result from inflammation, injury, or infection.
- A keloid (KEE-loid) is an abnormally raised or thickened scar that expands beyond the boundaries of the incision (kel means growth or tumor, and -oid means resembling). A tendency to form keloids is often inherited, and is more common among people with dark-pigmented skin.
- A keratosis (kerr-ah-TOH-sis) is any skin growth, such as a wart or a callus, in which there is overgrowth and thickening of the skin (kerat means hard or horny, and -osis means abnormal condition).

- Note: kerat/o also refers to the cornea of the eye (plural, keratoses).
- A lipoma (lih-POH-mah) is a benign, slow-growing fatty tumor located between the skin and the muscle layer (lip means fatty, and -oma means tumor). This fatty tumor is usually harmless, and treatment is rarely necessary unless the tumor is in a bothersome location, is painful, or is growing rapidly.
- Nevi (NEE-vye), also known as moles, are small, dark, skin growths that develop from melanocytes in the skin (singular, nevus). Normally, these growths are benign. In contrast, dysplastic nevi (dis-PLAS-tick NEE-vye) are atypical moles that can develop into skin cancer.
- A papilloma (pap-ih-LOH-mah) is a benign, superficial wart-like growth on the epithelial tissue or elsewhere in the body, such as in the bladder (papill means resembling a nipple, and -oma means tumor.)
- Polyp (POL-ip) is a general term used most commonly to describe a mushroom-like growth from the surface of a mucous membrane, such as a polyp in the nose. These growths have many causes and are not necessarily malignant.
- Skin tags are small, flesh-colored or light-brown polyps that hang from the body by fine stalks. Skin tags are benign and tend to enlarge with age.

Skin Cancer

Skin cancer is a harmful, malignant growth on the skin, which can have many causes, including repeated severe sunburns or long-term exposure to the sun. There are three main types of skin cancer: basal cell carcinoma, squamous cell carcinoma, and melanoma.

- An actinic keratosis (ack-TIN-ick kerr-ah-TOH-sis) is a precancerous skin growth that occurs on sun-damaged skin. It often looks like a red scaly patch and feels like sandpaper. Precancerous describes a growth that is not yet malignant; however, if not treated, it is likely to become malignant.
- A basal cell carcinoma is a malignant tumor of the basal cell layer of the epidermis. This is the most common, and least harmful, type of skin cancer because it is slow growing and rarely spreads to other parts of the body. The lesions, which occur mainly on the face or neck and tend to bleed easily, are usually pink, smooth, and are raised with a depression in the center.
- Squamous cell carcinoma (SKWAY-mus) originates as a malignant tumor of the scaly squamous cells of the epithelium; however, it can quickly spread to other body systems. These cancers begin as skin lesions that appear to be sores that will not heal or that have a crusted look.
- Malignant melanoma (mel-ah-NOH-mah), also known as melanoma, is a type of skin cancer that occurs in the melanocytes (melan means black, and -oma means tumor). This is the most serious type of skin cancer and often the first signs are changes in the size, shape, or color of a mole.

Burns

A burn is an injury to body tissues caused by heat, flame, electricity, sun, chemicals, or radiation. The severity of a burn is described according to the percentage of the total body skin surface affected (more than 15% is considered serious).

Diagnostic Procedures Of The Integumentary System

- A biopsy (BYE-op-see) is the removal of a small piece of living tissue for examination to confirm or establish a diagnosis (bi means pertaining to life, and -opsy means view of).
- In an incisional biopsy, a piece, but not all, of the tumor or lesion is removed. The term incision means to cut into.
- In an excisional biopsy, the entire tumor or lesion and a margin of surrounding tissue are removed. Excision means the complete removal of a lesion or organ.
- In a needle biopsy, a hollow needle is used to remove a core of tissue for examination.
- Exfoliative cytology is a technique in which cells are scraped from the tissue and examined under a microscope. To exfoliate means to remove a specimen in flakes or scales.

Treatment Procedures Of The Integumentary System

Preventive Measures

Sunscreen that blocks out the harmful ultraviolet B (UVB) rays is sometimes measured in terms of the strength of the sun protection factor. Some sunscreens also give protection against ultraviolet A (UVA rays).

Tissue Removal

- Cauterization (kaw-ter-eye-ZAY-zhun) is the destruction of tissue by burning.
- Chemabrasion, also known as chemical peel, is the use of chemicals to remove the outer layers of skin to treat acne scaring, fine wrinkling, and keratoses.
- Cryosurgery (krye-oh-SIR-jur-ee) is the destruction or elimination of abnormal tissue cells, such as warts or tumors, through the application of extreme cold by using liquid nitrogen (cry/o means cold, and -surgery means operative procedure).
- Curettage (kyou-reh-TAHZH) is the removal of material from the surface by scraping. One use of this technique is to remove basal cell tumors.
- Debridement (day-breed-MON) is the removal of dirt, foreign objects, damaged tissue, and cellular debris from a wound to prevent infection and to promote healing.

- Dermabrasion (der-mah-BRAY-zhun) is a form of abrasion involving the use of a revolving wire brush or sandpaper. It is used to remove acne and chickenpox scars as well as for facial skin rejuvenation.
- Incision and drainage (I & D) involves incision (cutting open) of a lesion, such as an abscess, and draining the contents.
- Mohs surgery is a technique used to treat skin cancer. Individual layers of cancerous tissue are removed and examined under a microscope one at a time until all cancerous tissue has been removed.

Cosmetic Procedures

- Blepharoplasty (BLEF-ah-roh-plas-tee), also known as a lid lift, is the surgical reduction of the upper and lower eyelids by removing excess fat, skin, and muscle (blephar/o means eyelid, and -plasty means surgical repair).
- Botox is a formulation of botulinum toxin type A. This is the neurotoxin that is responsible for the form of food poisoning known as botulism. Botox injections, which temporarily block the nerve signals to the injected muscle, reduce moderate to severe frown lines for up to 3–4 months. Frown lines are located between the eyebrows.
- Collagen replacement therapy is a form of soft-tissue augmentation used to soften facial lines or scars or to make lips appear fuller. Tiny quantities of collagen are injected under a line or scar to boost the skin's natural supply of collagen. The effect usually lasts for 3–12 months.
- Dermatoplasty (DER-mah-toh-plas-tee), also known as a skin graft, is the replacement of damaged skin with healthy tissue taken from a donor site on the patient's body (dermat/o means skin, and -plasty means surgical repair).
- Electrolysis is the use of electric current to destroy hair follicles in order to produce the relatively permanent removal of undesired hair (electr/o means electric, and -lysis means destruction).
- Lipectomy (lih-PECK-toh-mee) is the surgical removal of fat beneath the skin (lip means fat, and -ectomy means surgical removal).
- Liposuction (LIP-oh-suck-shun), also known as suction-assisted lipectomy, is the surgical removal of fat beneath the skin with the aid of suction.
- Rhytidectomy (rit-ih-DECK-toh-mee), also known as a facelift, is the surgical removal of excess skin and fat around the face to eliminate wrinkles (rhytid means wrinkle, and -ectomy means surgical removal).
- Sclerotherapy (sklehr-oh-THER-ah-pee) is used in the treatment of spider veins. Spider veins are small, nonessential veins that can be seen through the skin. This treatment involves injecting a sclerosing solution (saline solution) into the vein being treated. This solution irritates the tissue, causing the veins to collapse and disappear.

Abbreviations Related To The Integumentary System

- alopecia areata = AA
- basal cell carcinoma = BCC, BCCA
- cauterization = caut
- cryosurgery = CRYO
- debridement = debm
- eczema = Ecz, Ez
- lupus erythematosus = LE
- malignant melanoma = MM, mm
- necrotizing fasciitis = NF
- psoriasis = PS, Ps
- sclerotherapy = ST
- squamous cell carcinoma = SCC

Critical Thinking Exercise

The following story and questions are designed to stimulate critical thinking through class discussion or as a brief essay response. There are no right or wrong answers to these questions.

"OK, guys, we're late again." Shaylene Boulay calls out to her two oldest sons, Nathan Jr., 10, and Carl, 12. Grabbing the lunches Nate Sr. packed, she walks out the back door. "Come on, Michel, school time!" Shaylene peers under the porch for her 5-year-old. Their house is only a mile from the waterfront, and he loves to race cars between their dog Bubba's big paws in the cool sand underneath the porch. "Look at you!" As Shaylene dusts him off and heads to the truck, she notices that the rash of blisters on his leg is still bright red. "Must be ant bites, she thinks."

"Have a good day!" Shaylene hands Nathan and Carl their lunches as they hop out of the truck at the middle school. Next stop, Oak Creek Elementary. As Michel starts to get out, clutching his brown lunch bag tightly, his kindergarten teacher comes rushing over. "Michel, what are you doing here today? Didn't you give your mother the note from the nurse?"

"What note? Michel, honey, did you forget to give Mama something from school?" Michel smiles sheepishly and reaches into his shorts pocket for a wadded up piece of paper. The note says: "We believe Michel has impetigo. Since this condition is very contagiou, please consult your doctor as soon as possible. We will need a note from him before we can allow Michel to reenter class."

"Oh, no," Shaylene thinks. "I'm due for my shift at the diner in 15 minutes. Nobody's home to watch Miche and we don't have the money to see Dr. Gaines again. And what if this rash on my arm is that thing Michel has?" She sits clutching the wheel of the old pickup, asking herself over and over, "What am I gonna do?"

Suggested Discussion Topics

1. Discuss why the school wants Michael to have completed treatment before he returns to class.
2. You work in Dr. Gaines's office and you know that the Boulay's appointment today is about a potential contagious rash. What precautions should you take when the family arrives?
3. Discuss how you might explain to Shaylene what impetigo is, how it spreads, and what she can do to prevent her other children from getting it.
4. Shaylene is in a very difficult, and all too common, situation. Discuss possible answers to her question "What am I gonna do?"

CHAPTER 13

THE ENDOCRINE SYSTEM

This list contains essential word parts and medical terms for this chapter.

Word Parts
- acr/o
- adren/o
- crin/o
- -dipsia
- glyc/o
- gonad/o
- -ism
- pancreat/o
- parathyroid/o
- pineal/o
- pituitar/o
- polyh somat/o thym/o
- thyr/o, thyroid/o

Medical Terms
- acromegaly (ack-roh-MEG-ah-lee)
- Addison's disease (AD-ih-sonz)
- adrenalitis (ah-dree-nal-EYE-tis)
- aldosteronism (al-DOSS-teh-roh-niz-em)
- antidiuretic hormone (an-tih-dye-you-RET-ick)
- calcitonin (kal-sih-TOH-nin)
- chemical thyroidectomy (thigh-roi-DECKtoh- mee)
- Conn's syndrome
- cortisol (KOR-tih-sol)
- cretinism (CREE-tin-izm)
- Cushing's syndrome (KUSH-ingz)
- diabetes insipidus (dye-ah-BEE-teez in-SIP-ih-dus)
- diabetes mellitus (dye-ah-BEE-teez mel-EYE-tus)
- diabetic retinopathy (ret-ih-NOP-ah-thee)

263

- electrolytes (ee-LECK-troh-lytes)
- epinephrine (ep-ih-NEF-rin)
- estrogen (ES-troh-jen)
- exophthalmos (eck-sof-THAL-mos)
- follicle-stimulating hormone follicle (FOL-lick-kul)
- fructosamine test (fruck-TOHS-ah-meen)
- gestational diabetes (jes-TAY-shun-al dyeah- BEE-teez)
- gigantism (jigh-GAN-tiz-em)
- glucagon (GLOO-kah-gon)
- glucose (GLOO-kohs)
- glycogen (GLYE-koh-jen)
- Graves' disease (GRAYVZ dih-ZEEZ)
- gynecomastia (guy-neh-koh-MAS-tee-ah)
- Hashimoto's thyroiditis (hah-shee-MOH-tohz thigh-roi-DYE-tis)
- hypercalcemia (high-per-kal-SEE-mee-ah)
- hypercrinism (high-per-KRY-nism)
- hyperglycemia (high-per-glye-SEE-mee-ah)
- hyperinsulinism (high-per-IN-suh-lin-izm)
- hyperpituitarism (high-per-pih-TOO-ih-tah-rizm)
- hyperthyroidism (high-per-THIGH-roid-izm)
- hypoglycemia (high-poh-gly-SEE-mee-ah)
- hypothyroidism (high-poh-THIGH-roid-izm)
- insulinoma (in-suh-lin-OH-mah)
- interstitial cell-stimulating hormone
- laparoscopic adrenalectomy (ah-dree-nal- ECK-toh-mee)
- leptin (LEP-tin)
- luteinizing hormone (LOO-tee-in-eye-zing)
- myxedema (mick-seh-DEE-mah)
- norepinephrine (nor-ep-ih-NEF-rin)
- oxytocin (ock-sih-TOH-sin)
- pancreatalgia (pan-kree-ah-TAL-jee-ah)
- pancreatitis (pan-kree-ah-TYE-tis)
- pheochromocytoma (fee-oh-kroh-moh-sigh- TOH-mah)
- pinealoma (pin-ee-ah-LOH-mah)
- pituitarism (pih-TOO-ih-tar-izm)
- pituitary adenoma (pih-TOO-ih-tair-ee adeh- NOH-mah)
- polydipsia (pol-ee-DIP-see-ah)
- polyphagia (pol-ee-FAY-jee-ah)
- polyuria (pol-ee-YOU-ree-ah)
- progesterone (proh-JES-ter-ohn)
- prolactinoma (proh-lack-tih-NOH-mah)
- testosterone (tes-TOS-teh-rohn)
- thymectomy (thigh-MECK-toh-mee)
- thymitis (thigh-MY-tis)

- thymosin (THIGH-moh-sin)
- thyroxine (thigh-ROCK-sin)

Objectives

On completion of this chapter, you should be able to:
1. Describe the role of the endocrine glands in maintaining homeostasis.
2. Name and describe the functions of the primary hormones secreted by each of the endocrine glands.
3. Recognize, define, spell, and pronounce terms relating to the pathology and the diagnostic and treatment procedures of the endocrine glands.

Structures Of The Endocrine System

There are 13 major glands of the endocrine system:
- One pituitary gland (divided into two lobes)
- One pineal gland
- One thyroid gland
- Four parathyroid glands
- One thymus
- One pancreas (pancreatic islets)
- Two adrenal glands
- Two gonads (ovaries in females, testes in males)

Specialized Types of Hormones

There are several specialized types of hormones that do not fit the tradition hormone definition.

Steroids

- A steroid (STEHR-oid) is any one of a large number of hormone-like substances secreted by endocrine glands or artificially produced as medications to relieve swelling and inflammation in conditions such as asthma.
- Anabolic steroids (an-ah-BOL-ick STEHR-oidz) are chemically related to the male sex hormone testosterone. These have been used illegally by athletes to increase strength and muscle mass. Serious side effects of anabolic steroid use include liver damage, altered body chemistry, testicular shrinkage, and breast development in males, plus unpredictable mood swings and violence.

Hormones Secreted by Fat Cells

- Fat is not commonly thought of as an endocrine gland; however, research has revealed that fat cells do secrete at least one, and possibly more, hormones that play an important role in the balance and health of the body.
- Leptin (LEP-tin) is a hormone secreted by adipocytes (fat cells).

- Leptin leaves the fat cells and travels in the bloodstream to brain centers. Here, it acts to control the balance of food intake and energy expenditure.
- Leptin also affects female reproduction, immune function, and the function of many other hormones, including insulin.

Neurohormones

- Unlike the hormones, which are secreted by endocrine glands, neurohormones (new-roh-HOR-mohnz) are secreted by specialized cells of the brain. Although produced in the brain, they are able to affect cells throughout distant parts of the body.

Medical Specialties Related To The Endocrine System

- An endocrinologist (en-doh-krih-NOL-oh-jist) is a physician who specializes in diagnosing and treating diseases and malfunctions of the endocrine glands (endocrin means to secrete within, and -ologist means specialist).

Pathology Of The Endocrine System

- Endocrinopathy (en-doh-krih-NOP-ah-thee) is any disease caused by a disorder of the endocrine system (endo- means within, crin/o means to secrete, and -pathy means disease).
- Hypercrinism (high-per-KRY-nism) is a condition due to excessive secretion of any gland, especially an endocrine gland (hyper- means excessive, crin means to secrete, and -ism means condition). Hypercrinism is the opposite of hypocrinism.
- Hypocrinism (high-poh-KRY-nism) is a condition caused by deficient secretion of any gland, especially an endocrine gland (hypo- means deficient, crin means to secrete, and -ism means condition). Hypocrinism is the opposite of hypercrinism.

The Pituitary Gland

The pea-sized pituitary gland (pih-TOO-ih-tair-ee), which is composed of anterior and posterior lobes, hangs from the infundibulum below the hypothalamus, which is part of the brain. An infundibulum is a stalk-like structure.

Secretions of the Pituitary Gland: Anterior Lobe

- The adrenocorticotropic hormone (ACTH) stimulates the adrenal cortex to secrete cortisol.
- The follicle-stimulating hormone (FSH) stimulates the secretion of estrogen and the growth of ova (eggs) in the ovaries of the female. In the male, it stimulates the production of sperm in the testicles.
- The growth hormone (GH), also known as a somatotropic hormone, regulates the growth of bone, muscle, and other body tissues (somat/o means body and -tropic means having an affinity for).

- The interstitial cell-stimulating hormone (ICSH) stimulates ovulation in the female. In the male, it stimulates the secretion of testosterone.
- The lactogenic hormone (LTH), also known as prolactin, stimulates and maintains the secretion of breast milk in the mother after childbirth.
- The luteinizing hormone (LOO-tee-in-eye-zing) stimulates ovulation in the female and production of the female sex hormone progesterone. In the male, LH it stimulates the secretion of testosterone.
- The melanocyte-stimulating hormone (MSH) increases the production of melanin in melanocytes, thereby causing darkening the pigmentation of the skin.
- The thyroid-stimulating hormone (TSH) stimulates the growth and secretions of the thyroid gland.

Secretions of the Pituitary Gland: Posterior Lobe
- The antidiuretic hormone (an-tih-dye-you-RET-ick) maintains the water balance within the body by promoting the reabsorption of water through the kidneys. When more antidiuretic hormone is secreted, less urine is produced. In contrast, a diuretic is a medication that is administered to increase urine secretion.
- Oxytocin (ock-sih-TOH-sin) (OXT) stimulates uterine contractions during childbirth (oxy- means swift, and -tocin means labor). After childbirth, oxytocin stimulates the flow of milk from the mammary glands. Pitocin is a synthetic form of oxytocin that is administered to induce or speed up labor.

Pathology of the Pituitary Gland
- Acromegaly (ack-roh-MEG-ah-lee) is abnormal enlargement of the extremities (hands and feet) that is caused by excessive secretion of growth hormone after puberty (acr/o means extremities, and -megaly means abnormal enlargement). Contrast with gigantism.
- Gigantism (jigh-GAN-tiz-em), also known as giantism, is abnormal overgrowth of the entire body that is caused by excessive secretion of the growth hormone before puberty. Contrast with acromegaly.
- Hyperpituitarism (high-per-pih-TOO-ih-tah-rizm) is pathology resulting in the excessive secretion by the anterior lobe of the pituitary gland (hyper- means excessive, pituitar means pituitary, and -ism means condition). Hyperpituitarism is the opposite of hypopituitarism.
- Hypopituitarism (high-poh-pih-TOO-ih-tah-rizm) is a condition of reduced secretion due to the partial, or complete, loss of the function of the anterior lobe of the pituitary gland (hypo- means deficient, pituitar means pituitary, and -ism means condition). Hypopituitarism is the opposite of hyperpituitarism.
- Pituitarism (pih-TOO-ih-tar-izm) is any disorder of pituitary function (pituitar means pituitary, and -ism means condition).

- A pituitary adenoma (pih-TOO-ih-tair-ee ad-eh-NOHmah), also known as a pituitary tumor, is a slowgrowing, benign tumor of the pituitary gland. The two types of these tumors are functioning and nonfunctioning pituitary tumors. Functioning pituitary tumors often produce hormones in large and unregulated amounts. Nonfunctioning pituitary tumors do not produce significant amounts of hormones.
- A prolactinoma (proh-lack-tih-NOH-mah), also known as a prolactin-producing adenoma, is a benign tumor of the pituitary gland that causes it to produce too much prolactin. In females, this overproduction causes infertility and changes in menstruation. In males, it causes impotence.

Diabetes Insipidus
- Diabetes insipidus (dye-ah-BEE-teez in-SIP-ih-dus) is caused by insufficient production of the antidiuretic hormone or by the inability of the kidneys to respond appropriately to this hormone.
- When there is an insufficient quantity of ADH, too much fluid to be excreted by the kidneys. This causes extreme polydipsia (excessive thirst) and polyuria (excessive urination). If this problem is not controlled, it can become a very serious condition due to dehydration.

Treatment Procedures of the Pituitary Gland
The human growth hormone, also known as recombinant GH, is a synthetic version of the growth hormone that is administered to stimulate growth when the natural supply of growth hormone is insufficient for normal development.

The Pineal Gland
The pineal gland (PIN-ee-al) is very small endocrine gland that is located in the central portion of the brain.

Functions of the Pineal Gland
The pineal gland, also known as the pineal body, influences the sleep-wakefulness cycle.

Secretion of the Pineal Gland
- The pineal gland secretes the hormone melatonin (melah- TOH-nin), which influences the sleep and wakefulness portions of the circadian cycle. The term circadian cycle refers to the biological functions that occur within a 24-hour period.

Pathology and Treatment of the Pineal Gland
- A pinealoma (pin-ee-ah-LOH-mah) is a tumor of the pineal gland that can disrupt the production of melatonin (pineal means pineal gland, and -oma means tumor). This tumor can also cause insomnia by disrupting the circadian cycle.

- A pinealectomy (pin-ee-al-ECK-toh-mee) is the surgical removal of the pineal gland (pineal means pineal gland, and -ectomy means surgical removal).

The Thyroid Gland

The butterfly-shaped thyroid gland lies on either side of the larynx, just below the thyroid cartilage.

Functions of the Thyroid Gland

- One of the primary functions of the thyroid gland is to regulate the body's metabolism. The term metabolism describes all of the processes involved in the body's use of nutrients, including the rate at which they are utilized.
- Thyroid secretions also influence growth and the functioning of the nervous system.

Secretions of the Thyroid Gland

- The two primary thyroid hormones are thyroxine (thigh-ROCK-sin) and triiodothyronine (try-eye-ohdoh- THIGH-roh-neen). The rate of metabolism is influenced by these hormones. The rate of secretion of these hormones is controlled by the thyroid-stimulating hormone produced by the anterior lobe of the pituitary gland.
- Calcitonin (kal-sih-TOH-nin), which is secreted by cells of the thyroid gland, works with the parathyroid hormone to regulate the calcium levels in the blood and tissues. Calcitonin decreases blood levels by moving calcium into storage in the bones and teeth. Compare with the function of the parathyroid hormone.

Pathology of the Thyroid Gland Insufficient Thyroid Secretion

- Hashimoto's thyroiditis (hah-shee-MOH-tohz thighroi- DYE-tis), also known as chronic lymphocytic thyroiditis, is an autoimmune disease in which the body's own antibodies attack and destroy the cells of the thyroid gland.
- Hypothyroidism (high-poh-THIGH-roid-izm), also known as an underactive thyroid, is caused by a deficiency of thyroid secretion (hypo- means deficient, thyroid means thyroid, and -ism means condition). Symptoms include fatigue, depression, sensitivity to cold, and a decreased metabolic rate.
- Cretinism (CREE-tin-izm) is a congenital form of hypothyroidism. If treatment is not started soon after birth, cretinism causes arrested physical and mental development.
- Myxedema (mick-seh-DEE-mah), which is also known as adult hypothyroidism, is caused by extreme deficiency of thyroid secretion. Symptoms include swelling, particularly around the eyes and cheeks, fatigue, and a subnormal temperature.

Excessive Thyroid Secretion

- Hyperthyroidism (high-per-THIGH-roid-izm), also known as thyrotoxicosis, is an imbalance of metabolism caused by the overproduction of thyroid hormones (hyper- means excessive, thyroid means thyroid, and -ism means condition). Symptoms include an increased metabolic rate, sweating, nervousness, and weight loss.
- A thyroid storm, also known as a thyrotoxic crisis, is a relatively rare, life-threatening condition caused by exaggerated hyperthyroidism. Patients experiencing a thyroid storm may complain of fever, chest pain, palpitations, shortness of breath, tremors, increased sweating, disorientation, and fatigue.

Graves' Disease

- Graves' disease (GRAYVZ dih-ZEEZ), which is an autoimmune disorder that is caused by hyperthyroidism, is characterized by goiter and/or exophthalmos.
- Goiter (GOI-ter), also known as thyromegaly, is an abnormal nonmalignant enlargement of the thyroid gland (thyr/o means thyroid, and -megaly means abnormal enlargement). This enlargement produces a swelling in the front of the neck. A simple goiter usually occurs when the thyroid gland is not able to produce enough thyroid hormone to meet the body's needs.
- Exophthalmos (eck-sof-THAL-mos) is an abnormal protrusion of the eyeball out of the orbit.

Diagnostic and Treatment Procedures Related to the Thyroid Gland

- A thyroid-stimulating hormone assay is a diagnostic test to measure the circulating blood level of thyroid-stimulating hormone. This test is used to detect abnormal thyroid activity resulting from excessive pituitary stimulation.
- A thyroid scan, which measures thyroid function, is a form of nuclear medicine.
- An antithyroid drug is a medication administered to slow the ability of the thyroid gland to produce thyroid hormones.
- A chemical thyroidectomy (thigh-roi-DECK-tohmee), also known as radioactive iodine therapy, is the administration of radioactive iodine to destroy thyroid cells. This procedure, which disables at least part of the thyroid gland, is used to treat chronic hyperthyroid disorders such as Graves' disease.
- A lobectomy (loh-BECK-toh-mee) is the surgical removal of one lobe of the thyroid gland. This term is also used to describe the removal of a lobe of the liver, brain, or lung.
- Synthetic thyroid hormones are administered to replace lost thyroid function.

The Parathyroid Glands

The four parathyroid glands, each of which is about the size of a grain of rice, are embedded in the posterior surface of the thyroid gland.

Functions of the Parathyroid Glands

The primary function of the parathyroid glands is to regulate calcium levels throughout the body. These calcium levels are important to the smooth functioning of the muscular and nervous systems.

Secretions of the Parathyroid Glands

The parathyroid hormone works with the hormone calcitonin that is secreted by the thyroid gland. Together, they regulate the calcium levels in the blood and tissues. The parathyroid hormone increases calcium levels in the blood by mobilizing the release of calcium from storage in the bones and teeth. Compare with the function of the calcitonin.

Pathology and Treatment of the Parathyroid Glands

- Hyperparathyroidism (high-per-par-ah-THIGH-roidizm), which is the overproduction of the parathyroid hormone, causes the condition known as hypercalcemia (hyper-means excessive, parathyroid means parathyroid, and -ism means condition). Primary hyperparathyroidism is due to a disorder of the parathyroid gland. Secondary hyperparathyroidism is due to a disorder elsewhere in the body, such as kidney failure. Hyperparathyroidism is the opposite of hypoparathyroidism.
- Hypercalcemia (high-per-kal-SEE-mee-ah) is characterized by abnormally high concentrations of calcium circulating in the blood instead of being stored in the bones (hyper- means excessive, calc means calcium, and -emia means blood condition). This can lead to weakened bones and the formation of kidney stones. Hypercalcemia is the opposite of hypocalcemia.
- Hypocalcemia (high-poh-kal-SEE-mee-ah) is characterized by abnormally low levels of calcium in the blood (hypo- means deficient, calc means calcium, and -emia means blood condition). Hypocalcemia is the opposite of hypercalcemia.
- Hyperparathyroidism (high-per-par-ah-THIGH-roidizm) is the overproduction of the parathyroid hormone (hyper- means excessive, parathyroid means parathyroid, and -ism means condition). This condition causes hypercalcemia that can lead to weakened bones and the formation of kidney stones. Hyperparathyroidism is the opposite of hypoparathyroidism.
- Osteitis fibrosa is a complication of hyperparathyroidism in which bone becomes softened and deformed, and may develop cysts. This condition can be caused by overproduction of parathyroid hormone or by parathyroid cancer.

- Hypoparathyroidism (high-poh-par-ah-THIGH-roidizm) is caused by an insufficient or absent secretion of the parathyroid hormone (hypo- means deficient, parathyroid means parathyroid, and -ism means condition). This condition causes hypocalcemia, and in severe cases, it leads to tetany. Tetany is the condition of periodic, painful muscle spasms and tremors. Hypoparathyroidism is the opposite of hyperparathyroidism.
- A parathyroidectomy (par-ah-thigh-roi-DECK-tohmee), which is the surgical removal of one or more of the parathyroid glands, is performed to control hyperparathyroidism.

The Thymus

The thymus (THIGH-mus) is located near the midline in the anterior portion of the thoracic cavity. It is posterior to (behind) the sternum and slightly superior to (above) the heart.

Functions of the Thymus

The thymus functions as part of the endocrine system by secreting a hormone that functions as part of the immune system.

Secretions of the Thymus

Thymosin (THIGH-moh-sin) stimulates the maturation of lymphocytes into T cells of the immune system. These mature cells are important in coordinating immune defenses.

Pathology and Treatment of the Thymus

- Thymitis (thigh-MY-tis) is an inflammation of the thymus gland (thym means thymus, and -itis means inflammation).
- A thymectomy (thigh-MECK-toh-mee) is the surgical removal of the thymus gland (thym means thymus, and -ectomy means surgical removal).

The Pancreatic Islets

The pancreas (PAN-kree-as) is a feather-shaped organ located posterior to the stomach that functions as part of both the digestive and the endocrine systems.
- The pancreatic islets (pan-kree-AT-ick EYE-lets) are those parts of the pancreas that have endocrine functions.

Functions of the Pancreatic Islets

The endocrine functions of these islets are to control blood sugar levels and glucose metabolism throughout the body.
- Glucose (GLOO-kohs), also known as blood sugar, is the basic form of energy used by the body.
- Glycogen (GLYE-koh-jen) is the form in which the liver stores the excess glucose.

Secretions of the Pancreatic Islets

- Glucagon (GLOO-kah-gon) is the hormone secreted by the alpha cells of the pancreatic islets in response to low blood sugar levels. Glucagon increases the glucose level by stimulating the liver to convert glycogen into glucose for release into the bloodstream.
- Insulin (IN-suh-lin) is the hormone secreted by the beta cells of the pancreatic islets in response to high blood sugar levels. It functions in two ways. First, insulin allows glucose to enter the cells for use as energy. When additional glucose is not needed, insulin stimulates the liver to convert glucose into glycogen for storage.

Pathology and Treatment of the Pancreas

- An insulinoma (in-suh-lin-OH-mah) is a benign tumor of the pancreas that causes hypoglycemia by secreting additional insulin (insulin means insulin, and -oma means tumor).
- Pancreatalgia (pan-kree-ah-TAL-jee-ah) is pain in the pancreas (pancreat means pancreas, and -algia means pain).
- Pancreatitis (pan-kree-ah-TYE-tis) is an inflammation of the pancreas (pancreat means pancreas, and -itis means inflammation). Long-term alcohol abuse is a leading cause of pancreatitis.
- A pancreatectomy (pan-kree-ah-TECK-toh-mee) is the surgical removal all or part of the pancreas (pancreat means pancreas, and -ectomy means surgical removal). A total pancreatectomy is performed to treat pancreatic cancer, and this procedure involves the spleen, gallbladder, common bile duct, and portions of the small intestine and stomach.

Abnormal Blood Sugar Levels

- Hyperglycemia (high-per-glye-SEE-mee-ah) is an abnormally high concentration of glucose in the blood (hyper- means excessive, glyc means sugar, and -emia means blood condition). Hyperglycemia is seen primarily in patients with diabetes mellitus. The symptoms include polydipsia, polyphagia, and polyuria. Hyperglycemia is the opposite of hypoglycemia.
- Polydipsia (pol-ee-DIP-see-ah) is excessive thirst (poly- means many, and -dipsia means thirst).
- Polyphagia (pol-ee-FAY-jee-ah) is excessive hunger (poly- means many, and -phagia means eating).
- Polyuria (pol-ee-YOU-ree-ah) is excessive urination (poly- means many, and -uria means urination).
- Hyperinsulinism (high-per-IN-suh-lin-izm) is the condition of excessive secretion of insulin in the bloodstream (hyper- means excessive, insulin means insulin, and -ism means condition). Hyperinsulinism can cause hypoglycemia.
- Hypoglycemia (high-poh-glye-SEE-mee-ah) is an abnormally low concentration of glucose in the blood (hypo- means deficient, glyc

means sugar, and -emia means blood condition). Symptoms include nervousness and shakiness, confusion, perspiration, or feeling anxious or weak. Hypoglycemia is the opposite of hyperglycemia.

Diabetes Mellitus

- Diabetes mellitus (dye-ah-BEE-teez MEL-ih-tus) is a group of metabolic disorders characterized by hyperglycemia resulting from defects in insulin secretion, insulin action, or both.
- This condition is described as type 1 and type 2.
- Many patients present with symptoms of both types of diabetes, and their treatment must be modified accordingly.
- In the past, when a child developed diabetes, this condition was referred to as juvenile diabetes; however, the condition in children in now described as being type 1 or type 2.
- The treatment goals for all types of diabetes are to most effectively control the blood sugar levels and prevent complications.

Type 1 Diabetes

- Type 1 diabetes is an autoimmune insulin deficiency disorder caused by the destruction of pancreatic islet beta cells. Insulin deficiency means that the pancreatic beta cells do not secrete enough insulin.
- Symptoms of type 1 diabetes include polydipsia, polyphagia, polyuria, weight loss, blurred vision, extreme fatigue, and slow healing.
- Type 1 diabetes is treated with diet and exercise as well as carefully regulated insulin replacement therapy administered by injection or pump.

Type 2 Diabetes

- Type 2 diabetes is an insulin resistance disorder. Insulin resistance means that insulin is being produced, but the body does not use it effectively. In an attempt to compensate for this lack of response, the body secretes more insulin.
- With the rise of childhood obesity, type 2 diabetes is increasingly common in children and young adults. Obese adults are also at high risk for this condition.
- Prediabetes is a condition in which the blood sugar level is higher than normal, but not high enough to be classified as type 2 diabetes. However, this condition indicates an increased risk of developing type 2 diabetes, heart disease, and stroke.
- Type 2 diabetes can have no symptoms for years. When symptoms do occur, they include those of type 1 diabetes plus recurring infections, irritability, and a tingling sensation in the hands or feet.
- Type 2 diabetes is usually treated with diet, exercise, and oral medications.

- Oral hypoglycemics lower blood sugar by causing the body to release more insulin.
- Glucophage (metformin hydrochloride) and similar medications work within the cells to combat insulin resistance and to help insulin let blood sugar into the cells.

Gestational Diabetes

- Gestational diabetes (jes-TAY-shun-al dye-ah-BEE-teez) is a form of diabetes mellitus that occurs during some pregnancies. This condition usually disappears after delivery; however, many of these women later develop type 2 diabetes. Diabetes Mellitus Diagnostic Procedures
- A fasting blood sugar test measures the glucose (blood sugar) levels after the patient has not eaten for 8–12 hours. This test is used to screen for diabetes. This test is also used to monitor treatment of this condition.
- An oral glucose tolerance test is performed to confirm a diagnosis of diabetes mellitus and to aid in diagnosing hypoglycemia.
- Home blood glucose monitoring measures the current blood sugar level. This test, which requires a drop of blood, is performed by the patient.
- The fructosamine test (fruck-TOHS-ah-meen) measures average glucose levels over the past 3 weeks. The fructosamine test is able to detect changes more rapidly than the HbA1c test.
- Hemoglobin A1c testing, also known as HbA1c and pronounced as "H-B A-one-C," is a blood test that measures the average blood glucose level over the previous 3–4 months.

Diabetic Emergencies

Diabetic emergencies are due to either too much or too little blood sugar. Treatment depends on accurately diagnosing the cause of the emergency.

- Insulin shock is caused by very low blood sugar (hypoglycemia). Oral glucose, which is a sugary substance that can quickly be absorbed into the bloodstream, is administered orally to rapidly raise the blood sugar level.
- A diabetic coma is caused by very high blood sugar (hyperglycemia). Also known as diabetic ketoacidosis, this condition is treated by the prompt administration of insulin.

Diabetic Complications

Most diabetic complications result from the damage to capillaries and other blood vessels due to long-term exposure to excessive blood sugar.

- Diabetic retinopathy (ret-ih-NOP-ah-thee) occurs when diabetes damages the tiny blood vessels in the retina, causing blood to leak into the posterior segment of the eyeball. This can cause the loss of vision.

- Heart disease occurs because excess blood sugar makes the walls of the blood vessels sticky and rigid. This encourages hypertension and atherosclerosis.
- Kidney disease can lead to renal failure because damage to the blood vessels reduces blood flow through the kidneys.
- Peripheral neuropathy is damage to the nerves affecting the hands and feet

The Adrenal Glands

The adrenal glands are also known as the suprarenals because they are located with one on top of each kidney. Each of these glands consists of an outer portion, known as the adrenal cortex, and the middle portion, which is the adrenal medulla. Each of these parts has a specialized role, and the entire gland is surrounded by an adrenal capsule.

Functions of the Adrenal Glands

One of the primary functions of the adrenal glands is to control electrolyte levels within the body.
- Electrolytes (ee-LECK-troh-lytes) are mineral substances, such as sodium and potassium, that are normally found in the blood.
-
- Other important functions of the adrenal glands include helping to regulate metabolism and interacting with the sympathetic nervous system in response to stress.

Secretions of the Adrenal Cortex

- Corticosteroids (kor-tih-koh-STEHR-oidz) are the steroid hormones produced by the adrenal cortex. The same term describes synthetically produced equivalents that are administered as medications.
- Aldosterone (al-DOSS-ter-ohn) regulates the salt and water levels in the body by increasing sodium reabsorption and potassium excretion by the kidneys. Reabsorption means returning a substance to the bloodstream.
- Androgens (AN-droh-jenz) are hormones that influence sex-related characteristics. Normally, in adults the production of androgens in the adrenal cortex is minimal; instead, these hormones are produced in the male and female gonads.
- Cortisol (KOR-tih-sol), also known as hydrocortisone, has an anti-inflammatory action, and it regulates the metabolism of carbohydrates, fats, and proteins in the body.

Secretions of the Adrenal Medulla

- Epinephrine (ep-ih-NEF-rin), also known as adrenaline, stimulates the sympathetic nervous system in response to stress or other stimuli. It makes the heart beat faster and can raise blood pressure. It also helps the liver release glucose (sugar) and limits the release of insulin.

- Norepinephrine (nor-ep-ih-NEF-rin) is both a hormone and a neurohormone. It is released as a neurohormone by the sympathetic nervous system and as a hormone by the adrenal medulla. It plays an important role in the "fight-or-flight response" by raising blood pressure, strengthening the heartbeat, and stimulating muscle contractions.

Pathology of the Adrenal Glands

- Addison's disease (AD-ih-sonz) occurs when the adrenal glands do not produce enough of the hormones cortisol or aldosterone. This condition is characterized by chronic, worsening fatigue and muscle weakness, loss of appetite, and weight loss.
- Adrenalitis (ah-dree-nal-EYE-tis) is inflammation of the adrenal glands (adrenal means adrenal glands, and -itis means inflammation).
- Aldosteronism (al-DOSS-teh-roh-niz-em) is an abnormality of electrolyte balance caused by the excessive secretion of aldosterone.
- Conn's syndrome is a disorder of the adrenal glands due to excessive production of aldosterone.
- A pheochromocytoma (fee-oh-kroh-moh-sigh-TOHmah) is a benign tumor of the adrenal medulla that causes the gland to produce excess epinephrine (phe/o means dusky, chrom/o means color, cyt means cell, and -oma means tumor).

Cushing's Syndrome

- Cushing's syndrome (KUSH-ingz SIN-drohm), also known as hypercortisolism, is caused by prolonged exposure to high levels of cortisol. The symptoms include a rounded or "moon face". This condition can be caused by overproduction of cortisol by the body or by taking glucocorticoid hormone medications to treat inflammatory diseases such as asthma and rheumatoid arthritis.

Treatment Procedures of the Adrenal Glands

- A laparoscopic adrenalectomy (ah-dree-nal- ECK-toh-mee) is a minimally invasive procedure to surgically remove one or both adrenal glands (adrenal means adrenal gland, and -ectomy means surgical removal).
- Cortisone (KOR-tih-sohn), also known as hydrocortisone, is the synthetic equivalent of corticosteroids produced by the body. Cortisone is administered to suppress inflammation and as an immunosuppressant.
- Epinephrine is a synthetic hormone used as a vasoconstrictor to treat conditions such as heart dysrhythmias and asthma attacks. A vasoconstrictor causes the blood vessels to contract.

The Gonads

- The gonads (GOH-nadz), which are ovaries in females and testicles in males, are gamete-producing glands.

- A gamete (GAM-eet) is a reproductive cell. These are sperm in the male and ova (eggs) in the female.
- Gonadotropin is any hormone that stimulates the gonads (gonad/o means gonad, and -tropin means to simulate).

Functions of the Gonads

- The gonads secrete the hormones that are responsible for the development and maintenance of the secondary sex characteristics that develop during puberty. The additional functions of these glands are discussed in Chapter 14.
- Puberty is the condition of first being capable of reproducing sexually. It is marked by maturing of the genital organs, development of secondary sex characteristics, and by the first occurrence of menstruation in the female. The average age at which puberty occurs is 12 years in females and 14 in males.
- Precocious puberty is the early onset of the changes of puberty. This is before age 9 years in females and before age 10 in males.

Secretions of the Testicles

- Testosterone (tes-TOS-teh-rohn), which is secreted by the testicles, stimulates the development of male secondary sex characteristics.
- The term virile (VIR-ill) means having the nature, properties, or qualities of an adult male.

Secretions of the Ovaries

- Estrogen (ES-troh-jen) is important in the development and maintenance of the female secondary sex characteristics and in regulation of the menstrual cycle.
- Progesterone (proh-JES-ter-ohn) is the hormone released during the second half of the menstrual cycle by the corpus luteum in the ovary. Its function is to complete the preparations for pregnancy.
- If pregnancy occurs, the placenta takes over the production of progesterone.
- If pregnancy does not occur, secretion of the hormone stops and is followed by the menstrual period.

The Placenta

- During pregnancy, the placenta secretes the hormone human chorionic gonadotropin (kor-ee-ON-ick gon-ahdoh- TROH-pin) to stimulate the corpus luteum to continue producing the hormones required to maintain the pregnancy. It also stimulates the hormones required to stimulate lactation after childbirth.

Pathology and Treatment of the Gonads
- Hypergonadism (high-per-GOH-nad-izm) is the condition of excessive secretion of hormones by the sex glands (hyper- means excessive, gonad means sex gland, and -ism means condition).
- Hypogonadism (high-poh-GOH-nad-izm) is the condition of deficient secretion of hormones by the sex glands (hypo- means deficient, gonad means sex gland, and -ism means condition).
- Gynecomastia (guy-neh-koh-MAS-tee-ah) is the condition of excessive mammary development in the male (gynec/o means female, mast means breast, and -ia means abnormal condition).

Abbreviations Related To The Endocrine System
- diabetes insipidus = DI
- diabetes mellitus = DM
- diabetic retinopathy = DR, DRP
- fasting blood sugar = FBS
- fructosamine test = FA
- Graves' disease = GD
- hypoglycemia = HG
- leptin = LEP, LPT
- pheochromocytoma = PC, PCC, Pheo

Critical Thinking Exercise

The following story and questions are designed to stimulate critical thinking through class discussion or as a brief essay response. There are no right or wrong answers to these questions.

By the time 14-year-old Jacob Tuls got home, he was sick enough for his mom to notice. He seemed shaky and confused, and was sweaty even though the fall weather was cool. "Jake, let's get you a glass of juice right away," his mother said as calmly as she could. She was all too familiar with the symptoms of hypoglycemia brought on by Jake's type 1 diabetes. Ever since he was diagnosed at age six, she had carefully monitored his insulin, eating, and exercise. But now that he was in middle school, the ball was in his court, and it really worried her that he often seemed to mess up.

"Yeah, I know I shouldn't have gone so long without eating," Jake muttered once he was feeling better. "But you don't understand. I don't want to be different from the other kids." Before he could finish, his mom was on the telephone to the school nurse's office.

Jacob needed to inject himself with insulin three times a day. He knew what happened when his blood sugar got too high or if he didn't eat on schedule and it got too low. But when he was on a field trip with his friends, he hated to go to the chaperone and say that he needed to eat something right away. And he hated it when some kid walked in while he was injecting. His mom had made arrangements with the school nurse for him to go to her office to get some privacy, but whenever he didn't show up between fourth and fifth period, she'd come into the classroom to get him as if he was some kind of sick "dweeb."

He was tired of having this disease, sick of shots, and angry that he couldn't sleep late and skip meals like other kids. He made a face at his mother as she talked on the telephone to the nurse, and slammed the back door on his way out to find his friend Joe.

Suggested Discussion Topics

1. Why is it more difficult for Jacob to maintain his injection routine in middle school than it was in elementary school?
2. Knowing that missing an insulin injection could cause a diabetic coma and possibly death. Why do you think Jacob isn't more conscientious in his self-care?
3. Do you think Jacob's schoolmates talk about him, or does he just think they do? Discuss both possibilities. What steps can Jacob take to help his classmates understand his condition?
4. Jacob is having problems coping with his diabetes in middle school. Do you think managing his diabetes will be easier, or more difficult, when he enters high school?

CHAPTER 14

THE REPRODUCTIVE SYSTEMS

This list contains essential word parts and medical terms for this chapter.

Word Parts
- cervic/o
- colp/o
- -gravida
- gynec/o
- hyster/o
- mast/o
- men/o
- nullihov/o
- ovari/o
- -para
- -pexy
- salping/o
- test/i, test/o
- vagin/o

Medical Terms
- amenorrhea (ah-men-oh-REE-ah)
- amniocentesis (am-nee-oh-sen-TEE-sis)
- andropause (AN-droh-pawz)
- Apgar score
- azoospermia (ay-zoh-oh-SPER-mee-ah)
- cervical dysplasia (SER-vih-kal dis-PLAY-see-ah)
- cervicitis (ser-vih-SIGH-tis)
- chlamydia (klah-MID-ee-ah)
- chorionic villus sampling (kor-ee-ON-ick VIL-us)
- colostrum (kuh-LOS-trum)
- colpopexy (KOL-poh-peck-see)
- colporrhaphy (kol-POR-ah-fee)
- colposcopy (kol-POS-koh-pee)

- dysmenorrhea (dis-men-oh-REE-ah)
- eclampsia (eh-KLAMP-see-ah)
- ectopic pregnancy (eck-TOP-ick)
- endocervicitis (en-doh-ser-vih-SIGH-tis)
- endometriosis (en-doh-mee-tree-OH-sis)
- epididymitis (ep-ih-did-ih-MY-tis)
- episiotomy (eh-piz-ee-OT-oh-mee)
- fibroadenoma (figh-broh-ad-eh-NOH-mah)
- fibrocystic breast disease (figh-broh-SIS-tick)
- galactorrhea (gah-lack-toh-REE-ah)
- gonorrhea (gon-oh-REE-ah)
- hemospermia (hee-moh-SPER-mee-ah)
- hydrocele (HIGH-droh-seel)
- hypomenorrhea (high-poh-men-oh-REE-ah)
- hysterectomy (hiss-teh-RECK-toh-mee)
- hysterosalpingography (hiss-ter-oh-sal-pin- GOG-rah-fee)
- hysteroscopy (hiss-ter-OSS-koh-pee)
- leukorrhea (loo-koh-REE-ah)
- mastalgia (mass-TAL-jee-ah)
- mastopexy (MAS-toh-peck-see)
- menarche (meh-NAR-kee)
- menometrorrhagia (men-oh-met-roh-RAY-jee-ah)
- metrorrhea (mee-troh-REE-ah)
- neonate (NEE-oh-nayt)
- nulligravida (null-ih-GRAV-ih-dah)
- nullipara (nuh-LIP-ah-rah)
- obstetrician (ob-steh-TRISH-un)
- oligomenorrhea (ol-ih-goh-men-oh-REE-ah)
- orchidectomy (or-kih-DECK-toh-mee)
- orchiopexy (or-keeoh-PECK-see)
- ovariectomy (oh-vay-ree-ECK-toh-mee)
- ovariorrhexis (oh-vay-ree-oh-RECK-sis)
- perimenopause (pehr-ih-MEN-oh-pawz)
- Peyronie's disease (pay-roh-NEEZ)
- placenta previa (plah-SEN-tah PREE-vee-ah)
- polycystic ovary syndrome (pol-ee-SIS-tick)
- preeclampsia (pree-ee-KLAMP-see-ah)
- priapism (PRYE-ah-piz-em)
- primigravida (prye-mih-GRAV-ih-dah)
- primipara (prye-MIP-ah-rah)
- pruritus vulvae (proo-RYE-tus VUL-vee)
- salpingo-oophorectomy (sal-ping-goh oh-ahf-oh- RECK-toh-mee)
- syphilis (SIF-ih-lis)
- trichomoniasis (trick-oh-moh-NYE-ah-sis)

- uterine prolapse (proh-LAPS)
- varicocele (VAR-ih-koh-seel)
- vasovasostomy (vay-soh-vah-ZOS-toh-mee)

Objectives

On completion of this chapter, you should be able to:
1. Identifyanddescribe the major functionsand structures of the male reproductive system.
2. Recognize, define, spell, and pronounce the terms related to the pathology and the diagnostic and treatment procedures of the male reproductive system.
3. Name at least six sexually transmitted diseases.
4. Identify and describe the major functions and structures of the female reproductive system.
5. Recognize, define, spell, and pronounce the terms related to the pathology and the diagnostic and treatment procedures of the female reproductive system.
1. Recognize, define, spell, and pronounce the terms related to the pathology and the diagnostic and treatment procedures of the female during pregnancy, childbirth, and the postpartum period.

Terms Related To The Reproductive Systems Of Both Sexes

- The genitalia (jen-ih-TAY-lee-ah) are the organs of reproduction and their associated structures. External genitalia are reproductive organs located outside of the body cavity. Internal genitalia are reproductive organs protected within the body.
- The perineum (pehr-ih-NEE-um) is the external surface region in both males and females between the pubic symphysis and the coccyx.
- The male perineum extends from the scrotum to the anus.
- The female perineum extends from the vaginal orifice to the anus.

Structures Of The Male Reproductive System

- The external male genitalia are the penis and the scrotum, which contains two testicles.
- The internal male genitalia includes the remaining structures of the male reproductive system.

The Scrotum and Testicles

- The scrotum (SKROH-tum) is the saclike structure that surrounds, protects, and supports the testicles. This scrotum is suspended from the pubic arch behind the penis and lies between the thighs. The testicles, also known as testes, are the two small, egg-shaped glands that produce the sperm (singular, testis). These glands develop within the abdomen of the male fetus and normally descend into the scrotum before, or soon after, birth.

- Sperm are formed within the seminiferous tubules (see-mih-NIF-er-us TOO-byouls) of each testicle.
- The epididymis (ep-ih-DID-ih-mis) is a coiled tube at the upper part of each testicle. This tube runs down the length of the testicle then turns upward toward the body. Here, it narrows to form the tube known as the vas deferens.
- The spermatic cord extends upward from the epididymis and is attached to each testicle. Each cord contains a vas deferens plus the arteries, veins, nerves, and lymphatic vessels required by each testicle.

The Penis

- The penis (PEE-nis) is the male sex organ that transports the sperm into the female vagina. The penis is composed of three columns of erectile tissue.
- During sexual stimulation, the erectile tissue fills with blood under high pressure. This causes the swelling, hardness, and stiffness known an erection.
- The adjectives penile and phallic both mean relating to the penis (both pen/i and phall/i mean penis).
- The glans penis (glanz PEE-nis), also known as the head of the penis, is the sensitive region located at the tip of the penis.
- The foreskin, also known as the prepuce, is a retractable double-layered fold of skin and mucous membrane that covers and protects the glans penis.

The Vas Deferens, Seminal Vesicles, and the Ejaculatory Duct

- The vas deferens (vas DEF-er-enz), also known as the ductus deferens, are the long, narrow continuations of each epididymis. These structures lead upward, eventually join the urethra.
- The seminal vesicles (SEM-ih-nal) are glands that secrete a thick, yellow substance to nourish the sperm cells. This secretion forms 60% of the volume of semen. These glands are located at the base of the urinary bladder and open into the vas deferens as it joins the urethra.
- The ejaculatory duct, which begins at the vas deferens, passes through the prostate gland, and empties into the urethra. During ejaculation, a reflex action caused by these ducts, semen passes into the urethra, which exits the body via the penis.
- Semen (SEE-men) is the whitish fluid containing sperm that is ejaculated through the urethra at the peak of male sexual excitement. The term ejaculate means to expel suddenly.

The Prostate Gland

- The prostate gland (PROS-tayt) lies under the bladder and surrounds the end of the urethra in the region where the vas deferens enters the urethra. During ejaculation, the prostate gland secretes a thick, alkaline fluid into the semen that aids themotility of the sperm. Motility means ability to move.

The Bulbourethral Glands

- The two bulbourethral glands (bul-boh-you-REE-thral), also known as Cowper's glands, are located just below the prostate gland. One of these glands is located on either side of the urethra, and they open into the urethra. During sexual arousal, these glands secrete a fluid known as pre-ejaculate. This fluid helps flush out any residual urine or foreign matter in the urethra. It also lubricates the urethra for sperm to pass through. This fluid can contain sperm and is able to cause pregnancy even if ejaculation does not occur.

The Urethra

- The urethra passes through the penis to the outside of the body. In the male, the urethra serves both the reproductive and the urinary systems.

Semen Formation

- Spermatogenesis (sper-mah-toh-JEN-eh-sis) is the process of sperm formation (spermat/o means sperm, and -genesis means creation).
- The ideal temperature for sperm formation is 93.2°F. The scrotum aids in maintaining this temperature by adjusting how closely it holds the testicles to the body.
- Sperm are the male gametes (reproductive cells). Also known as spermatozoa, these gametes are formed in the seminiferous tubules of the testicles.
- From here, the sperm move into the epididymis where they become motile and are temporarily stored. Motile means capable of spontaneous motion.
- From the epididymis, the sperm travel upward into the body and enter the vas deferens. Here, the seminal vesicles and the prostate gland add their secretions to form semen.

Medical Specialties Related To The Male Reproductive System

- A urologist (you-ROL-oh-jist) is a physician who specializes in diagnosing and treating diseases and disorders of the urinary system of females and the genitourinary system of males (ur means urine, and -ologist means specialist). The term genitourinary refers to both the genital and urinary organs.

Pathology Of The Male Reproductive System

The Penis

- Balanitis (bal-ah-NIGH-tis) is an inflammation of the glans penis that is usually caused by poor hygiene in men who have not had the foreskin

removed by circumcision (balan means glans penis, and -itis means inflammation).
- Phimosis (figh-MOH-sis) is a narrowing of the opening of the foreskin so it cannot be retracted (pulled back) to expose the glans penis. This condition can be present at birth or become apparent during childhood.
- Impotence (IM-poh-tens), also known as erectile dysfunction, is the inability of the male to achieve or maintain a penile erection. A penis that is not erect is referred to as being flaccid (limp).
- Peyronie's disease (pay-roh-NEEZ), also known as penile curvature, is a form of sexual dysfunction in which the penis is bent or curved during erection.
- Premature ejaculation is a condition in which the male reaches climax too soon, usually before, or shortly after, penetration of the female.

The Testicles and Related Structures

- Andropause (AN-droh-pawz), which is often referred to as male menopause, is marked by the decrease of the male hormone testosterone (andr/o means male or masculine, and -pause means stopping). This change is also referred to as ADAM (Androgen Decline in the Aging Male). It usually begins in the late 40s and progresses very gradually over several decades.
- Anorchism (an-OR-kizm) is the absence of one or both testicles (an- means without, orch means testicle, and -ism means abnormal condition). This condition can be congenital or caused by trauma or surgery.
- Cryptorchidism (krip-TOR-kih-dizm), also known as an undescended testicle, is a developmental defect in which one or both of the testicles fail to descend into their normal position in the scrotum (crypt/o means hidden, orchid means testicle, and -ism means abnormal condition).
- Epididymitis (ep-ih-did-ih-MY-tis) is inflammation of the epididymis that is frequently caused by the spread of infection from the urethra or the bladder (epididym means epididymis, and -itis means inflammation).
- A hydrocele (HIGH-droh-seel) is a fluid-filled sac in the scrotum along the spermatic cord leading from the testicles (hydr/o means relating to water, and -cele means a hernia or swelling). Note: The term hydrocele is also used to describe the accumulation of fluid in any body cavity.
- Priapism (PRYE-ah-piz-em) is a painful erection that lasts 4 hours or more but is not accompanied by sexual excitement. The condition can be caused by medications or by blood-related diseases such as sickle cell anemia or leukemia.
- A spermatocele (sper-MAH-toh-seel) is a cyst that develops in the epididymis and is filled with a milky fluid containing sperm (spermat/o means sperm, and -cele means hernia, tumor, or swelling).

- Testicular cancer is the most common cancer in American males between the ages of 15 and 34 years. This cancer is highly treatable when diagnosed early.
- Testicular pain, also known as orchalgia, is pain in one or both testicles. This pain can be due to an injury, testicular torsion, epididymitis, or a spermatocele.
- Testicular torsion is a sharp pain in the scrotum caused by twisting of the vas deferens and blood vessels leading into the testicle. Torsion means twisting.
- Testitis (test-TYE-tis), also known as orchitis, is inflammation of one or both testicles (test means testicle, and -itis means inflammation).
- A varicocele (VAR-ih-koh-seel) is a knot of varicose veins in one side of the scrotum (varic/o means varicose veins, and -cele means a hernia or swelling). Varicose veins are abnormally swollen veins.

Sperm Count

- A normal sperm count is 20–120 million or more sperm per milliliter (ml) of semen.
- Azoospermia (ay-zoh-oh-SPER-mee-ah) is the absence of sperm in the semen (a- means without, zoo means life, sperm means sperm, and -ia means abnormal condition).
- A low sperm count, also known as oligospermia (olih- goh-SPER-mee-ah), is a sperm count below 20 million/ml (olig/o means few, sperm means sperm, and -ia means abnormal condition).
- Hemospermia (hee-moh-SPER-mee-ah) is the presence of blood in the seminal fluid (hem/o means blood, sperm means sperm, and -ia means abnormal condition). This condition can be caused by infections of the seminal vesicles, prostatitis, urethritis, or urethral strictures.

Diagnostic Procedures Of The Male Reproductive System

- Sperm count, also known as a sperm analysis, is the testing of freshly ejaculated semen to determine the volume plus the number, shape, size, and motility of the sperm.
- Testicular self-examination is a self-help step in early detection of testicular cancer by detecting lumps, swelling, or changes in the skin of the scrotum.

Treatment Procedures Of The Male Reproductive System

General Treatment Procedures

- Circumcision (ser-kum-SIZH-un) is the surgical removal of the foreskin of the penis. This procedure is usually performed within a few days of birth.
- An orchidectomy (or-kih-DECK-toh-mee), also spelled as orchiectomy, is the surgical removal of one or both testicles (orchid means testicle, and -ectomy means surgical removal).

- Orchiopexy (or-kee-oh-PECK-see) is endoscopic surgery to move an undescended testicle into its normal position in the scrotum (orchi/o means testicle, and -pexy means surgical fixation). This procedure is usually performed on infants before the age of 1 year.
- A varicocelectomy (var-ih-koh-sih-LECK-toh-mee) is the removal of a portion of an enlarged vein to relieve a varicocele (varic/o means varicose vein, cel means swelling, and -ectomy means surgical removal).

Male Sterilization

- Sterilization is any procedure rendering an individual (male or female) incapable of reproduction.
- Castration (kas-TRAY-shun), also known as bilateral orchidectomy, is the surgical removal or destruction of both testicles.
- A vasectomy (vah-SECK-toh-mee) is the male sterilization procedure in which a small portion of the vas deferens is surgically removed (vas means vas deferens, and -ectomy means surgical removal). This prevents sperm from entering the ejaculate, but does not change the volume of semen.
- A vasovasostomy (vay-soh-vah-ZOS-toh-mee), also known as a vasectomy reversal, is a procedure performed as an attempt to restore fertility to a vasectomized male (vas/o means blood vessel, vas means the vas deferens, and -ostomy means surgically creating an opening).

Sexually Transmitted Diseases

Sexually transmitted diseases (STDs), alsoknownas venereal diseases (VD), are infections that affect both males and females. These conditions are commonly spread through sexual intercourse or other genital contact.

- A pregnant woman who is infected with one of these diseases can transmit it to her baby during birth. For this reason, all newborns receive one drop of silver nitrate or an antibiotic ointment in each eye immediately after birth to prevent ophthalmia neonatorum.
- This condition is a form of conjunctivitis that is caused by the bacteria responsible for chlamydia or gonorrhea.

Chlamydia

- Chlamydia (klah-MID-ee-ah), which is caused by the bacterium Chlamydia trachomatis, is the most commonly reported STD in the US. It is highly contagious and requires early treatment with antibiotics.
- In females, chlamydia can damage the reproductive organs. Even though symptoms are usually mild or absent, serious complications can cause irreversible damage, including infertility.
- In males, chlamydia is one of the causes of urethritis.

Other Sexually Transmitted Diseases

- Bacterial vaginosis (vaj-ih-NOH-sis) is a condition in women in which there is an abnormal overgrowth of certain bacteria in the vagina (vagin means vagina, and -osis means abnormal condition or disease). This condition can cause complications during pregnancy and an increased risk of HIV infection. Symptoms sometimes include a discharge, odor, pain, itching, or burning.
- Genital herpes (HER-peez) is caused by the herpes simplex virus type 2. Symptoms include itching or burning before the appearance of lesions (sores). This condition is highly contagious at all times, including when visible lesions are not present. Antiviral drugs ease symptoms and can suppress future outbreaks; however, currently there is no cure. Note: The herpes simplex virus type 1.
- Genital warts, which are caused by the human papilloma virus (HPV), are highly contagious. In the male, this virus infects the urethra. In the female, it infects the external genitalia, cervix, and vagina. It also increases the risk of cervical cancer.
- A human papilloma virus vaccine is available to prevent the spread of this disease. It is recommended that it be administered to girls between the ages 11 and 12 or before they become sexually active.
- Gonorrhea (gon-oh-REE-ah) is a highly contagious condition caused by the bacterium Neisseria gonorrhoeae. In women, this condition affects the cervix, uterus, and fallopian tubes. In men, it affects the urethra by causing painful urination and an abnormal discharge. It can also affect the mouth, throat, and anus of both men and women.
- The human immunodeficiency virus (HIV) is transmitted through exposure to infected body fluids, particularly through sexual intercourse with an infected partner. HIV and AIDS.
- Syphilis (SIF-ih-lis), which is caused by the bacterium Treponema pallidum, has many symptoms that are difficult to distinguish from other STDs. Syphilis is highly contagious and is passed from person to person through direct contact with a chancre, which is a sore caused by syphilis. This condition can be detected through the VDRL (Venereal Disease Research Laboratory) blood test before the lesions appear. The RPR test (Rapid plasma reagin) is another blood test for syphilis.
- Trichomoniasis (trick-oh-moh-NYE-ah-sis), also known as trich, is an infection caused by the protozoan parasite Trichomonas vaginalis. One of the most common symptoms in infected women is a thin, frothy, yellow-green, foul-smelling vaginal discharge. Infected men often do not have symptoms; however, when symptoms are present, they include painful urination or a clear discharge from the penis.

Structures Of The Female Reproductive System

The structures of the female reproductive system are described as being the external female genitalia and the internal female reproductive organs.

The External Female Genitalia
- The external female genitalia are located posterior to the mons pubis (monz PYOU-bis), which is a rounded, fleshy prominence located over the pubic symphysis. These structures are known collectively as the vulva (VULvah) or the pudendum. The vulva consists of the labia, clitoris, Bartholin's glands, and vaginal orifice.
- The labia majora and labia minora are the vaginal lips that protect the other external genitalia and the urethral meatus (singular, labium). The urethral meatus, which is the external opening of the urethra.
- The clitoris (KLIT-oh-ris) is an organ of sensitive, erectile tissue located anterior to the urethral meatus and the vaginal orifice.
- Bartholin's glands produce a mucus secretion to lubricate the vagina. These two small, round glands are located on either side of the vaginal orifice.
- The vaginal orifice is the exterior opening of the vagina. Orifice means opening. The hymen (HIGHmen) is a mucous membrane that partially covers this opening before a woman has had intercourse. However, this tissue can be absent in a woman who has not been sexually active.

The Mammary Glands
- Breasts are made up of fat, connective tissue, and the mammary glands (the word parts mamm/o and mast/o both mean breast). Each breast is fixed to the overlying skin and the underlying pectoral muscles by suspensory ligaments.
- Mammary glands, also known as the lactiferous glands, are the milk-producing glands that develop during puberty.
- The lactiferous ducts (lack-TIF-er-us), also known as milk ducts, carry milk from the mammary glands to the nipple (lact means milk, and -iferous means carrying or producing).
- Breast milk flows through the nipple, which is surrounded by the dark-pigmented area known as the areola (ah-REE-oh-lah).

The Internal Female Genitalia
The internal female genitalia are located within the pelvic cavity where they are protected by the bony pelvis. These structures include two ovaries, two fallopian tubes, one uterus, and the vagina.

The Ovaries
- The ovaries (OH-vah-rees) are a pair of small, almondshaped organs located in the lower abdomen, one on either side of the uterus.
- A follicle (FOL-lick-kul) is a fluid-filled sac containing a single ovum (egg). There are thousands of these sacs on the inside surface of the ovaries.
- The ova (OH-vah), also known as eggs, are the female gametes (singular, ovum). These immature ova are present at birth. Normally, after puberty, one ovum matures and is released each month.

- The ovaries also produce the sex hormones estrogen and progesterone.

The Fallopian Tubes
- There are two fallopian tubes (fal-LOH-pee-an), which are also known as uterine tubes. These tubes extend from the upper end of the uterus to a point near, but not attached to, an ovary.
- The infundibulum (in-fun-DIB-you-lum) is the funnelshaped opening into the fallopian tube near the ovary.
- The fimbriae (FIM-bree-ee) are the fringed, finger-like extensions of this opening. Their role is to catch themature ovum when it leaves the ovary (singular, fimbria).
- Each month, one of these tubes carries amatureovumfrom the ovary to the uterus. These tubes also carry sperm upward fromthe uterus toward the descending mature ovum so that fertilization can occur.

The Uterus
- The uterus (YOU-ter-us), formerly known as the womb, is a pear-shaped organ with muscular walls and a mucous membrane lining filled with a rich supply of blood vessels.
- The uterus is located between the urinary bladder and the rectum and midway between the sacrum and the pubic bone.
- In its normal position, which is known as anteflexion (an-tee-FLECK-shun), the body of the uterus is bent forward (ante- means forward, flex means bend, and -ion means condition).

The Parts of the Uterus
- The body of the uterus consists of three major anatomic areas.
- The fundus (FUN-dus) is the bulging, rounded part above the entrance of the fallopian tubes.
- The corpus (KOR-pus), also known as the body of the uterus, is the middle portion.
- The cervix (SER-vicks), also known as the cervix uteri, is the lower, narrow portion that extends into the vagina.

The Tissues of the Uterus
The uterus is composed of three major layers of tissue.
- The perimetrium (pehr-ih-MEE-tree-um) is the tough, membranous outer layer (peri- means surrounding, metri means uterus, and -um is a singular noun ending). Membranous means pertaining to a thin layer of tissue.
- The myometrium (my-oh-MEE-tree-um) is the muscular middle layer (my/o means muscle, metri means uterus, and -um is a singular noun ending).
- The endometrium (en-doh-MEE-tree-um), which is the inner layer of the uterus, consists of specialized epithelial mucosa that is rich in blood

vessels (endomeans within, metri means uterus, and -um is a singular noun ending). Mucosa means referring to mucous membrane.

Vagina

The vagina (vah-JIGH-nah) is the muscular tube lined with mucosa that extends from the cervix to the outside of the body. The word parts colp/o and vagin/o both mean vagina.

Menstruation

- Menstruation (men-stroo-AY-shun), also known as menses, is the normal periodic discharge of the endometrial lining and unfertilized egg from uterus.
- Menarche (meh-NAR-kee) is the beginning of the menstrual function (men means menstruation, and -arche means beginning). This function begins after the maturation that occurs during puberty.
- The average menstrual cycle consists of 28 days. These days are grouped into four phases.
- Menopause (MEN-oh-pawz) is the normal termination of the menstrual function (men/o means menstruation and -pause means stopping). Menopause is considered to be confirmed when a woman has gone 1 year without having a period.
- Perimenopause (pehr-ih-MEN-oh-pawz) is the term used to designate the transition phase between regular menstrual periods and no periods at all (peri- means surrounding, men/o means menstruation, and -pause means stopping). During this phase, which can last as long as 10 years, changes in hormone production can cause symptoms including irregular menstrual cycles, hot flashes, mood swings, and disturbed sleep.

Medical Specialties Related To The Female Reproductive System And Childbirth

- A gynecologist (guy-neh-KOL-oh-jist) is a physician who specializes in diagnosing and treating diseases and disorders of the female reproductive system (gynec means female, and -ologist means specialist).
- An obstetrician (ob-steh-TRISH-un) is a physician who specializes in providing medical care to women during pregnancy, childbirth, and immediately thereafter. This specialty is referred to as obstetrics.
- A neonatologist (nee-oh-nay-TOL-oh-jist) is a physician who in diagnosing and treating disorders of the newborn (neo- means new, nat means born, and -ologist means specialist).
- A pediatrician (pee-dee-ah-TRISH-un) is a physician who specializes in diagnosing, treating, and preventing disorders and diseases of children. This specialty is known as pediatrics.

Pathology Of The Female Reproductive System

The Ovaries, Fallopian Tubes, and Ovulation

- Anovulation (an-ov-you-LAY-shun) is the absence of ovulation when it would be normally expected (an- means without, and ovulation means the release of a mature egg). This condition can be caused by stress, inadequate nutrition, or hormonal imbalances. Menstruation can continue, although ovulation does not occur.
- Oophoritis (oh-ahf-oh-RYE-tis) is inflammation of an ovary (oophor means ovary, and -itis means inflammation). This condition frequently occurs when salpingitis or pelvic inflammatory disease are present.
- Ovarian cancer originates within the cells of the ovaries. These cancer cells can break away from the ovary and spread (metastasize) to other tissues and organs within the abdomen or travel through the blood stream to other parts of the body.
- Ovariorrhexis (oh-vay-ree-oh-RECK-sis) is the rupture of an ovary (ovari/o means ovary, and -rrhexis means to rupture).
- Pelvic inflammatory disease (PID) is any inflammation of the female reproductive organs that is not associated with surgery or pregnancy. This condition occurs most frequently as a complication of a sexually transmitted disease and can lead to infertility, ectopic pregnancy, and other serious disorders.
- Polycystic ovary syndrome (pol-ee-SIS-tick), also known as Stein-Leventhal syndrome, is a condition caused by a hormonal imbalance in which the ovaries are enlarged by the presence of many cysts formed by incompletely developed follicles.
- Pyosalpinx (pye-oh-SAL-pinks) is an accumulation of pus in the fallopian tube (py/o means pus, and -salpinx means fallopian tube).
- Salpingitis (sal-pin-JIGH-tis) is an inflammation of a fallopian tube (salping means fallopian or eustachian tube, and -itis means inflammation).

The Uterus

- Endometriosis (en-doh-mee-tree-OH-sis) is a condition in which patches of endometrial tissue escape the uterus and become attached to other structures in the pelvic cavity (endo- means within, metri means uterus, and -osis means abnormal condition). It is a leading cause of infertility.
- Metrorrhea (mee-troh-REE-ah) is an abnormal discharge, such as mucus or pus, from the uterus (metr/o means uterus, and -rrhea means flow or discharge).
- Uterine cancer involves cancerous growth on the lining of the uterus. One of the earliest symptoms of this cancer that frequently occurs after menopause is abnormal bleeding from the uterus.
- A uterine fibroid, also known as a myoma, is a benign tumor composed of muscle and fibrous tissue that occurs in the wall of the uterus.

- A uterine prolapse (proh-LAPS), also known as a pelvic floor hernia, is the condition in which the uterus slides from its normal position in the pelvic cavity and sags into the vagina. Prolapse means the falling or dropping down of an organ or internal part.

The Cervix

- Cervical cancer is the second-most common cancer in women and usually affects women between the ages of 45 and 65 years. It can be detected early through routine Pap tests.
- Cervical dysplasia (SER-vih-kal dis-PLAY-see-ah), also known as precancerous lesions, is the growth of abnormal cells in the cervix, which can be detected by a Pap smear. Without early detection and treatment, these cells can become malignant.
- Cervicitis (ser-vih-SIGH-tis) is an inflammation of the cervix that is usually caused by an infection (cervic means cervix, and -itis means inflammation).
- Endocervicitis (en-doh-ser-vih-SIGH-tis) is an inflammation of the mucous membrane lining of the cervix (endo- means within, cervic means cervix, and -itis means inflammation).

The Vagina

- Colporrhexis (kol-poh-RECK-sis) means tearing or laceration of the vaginal wall (colp/o means vagina, and -rrhexis means to rupture). A laceration is a torn, ragged wound or an accidental cut.
- Leukorrhea (loo-koh-REE-ah) is a profuse, whitish mucus discharge from the uterus and vagina (leuk/o means white, and -rrhea means flow or discharge). Women normally have a vaginal discharge; however, leukorrhea describes a change and increase in this discharge that can be due to an infection, malignancy, or hormonal changes.
- Vaginal candidiasis (kan-dih-DYE-ah-sis), also known as vaginal thrush or a yeast infection, is a vaginal infection caused by the yeast-like fungus Candida albicans. The growth of this fungus in the vagina is usually controlled by the bacteria normally present there. When these bacteria are not able to control the fungal growth, symptoms occur that include burning, itching, and a "cottage cheese-like" vaginal discharge.
- Vaginitis (vaj-ih-NIGH-tis), also known as colpitis, is an inflammation of the lining of the vagina (vagin and colp both mean vagina, and -itis means inflammation). The most common causes of a vaginal inflammation are bacterial vaginosis, trichomoniasis, and vaginal candidiasis.

The External Genitalia

- Pruritus vulvae (proo-RYE-tus VUL-vee) is a condition of severe itching of the external female genitalia. Pruritus means itching.

- Vulvodynia (vul-voh-DIN-ee-ah) is a syndrome of unknown cause that is characterized by chronic burning, pain during sexual intercourse, itching, or stinging irritation of the vulva (vulv/o means vulva, and -dynia means pain).
- Vulvitis (vul-VYE-tis) is an inflammation of the vulva (vulv means vulva, and -itis means inflammation). Possible causes include fungal or bacterial infections, chafing, skin conditions, or allergies to products such as soaps and bubble bath.

Breast Diseases

- Breast cancer, its diagnosis and treatment.
- A fibroadenoma (figh-broh-ad-eh-NOH-mah) is a round, firm, rubbery mass that arises from excess growth of glandular and connective tissue in the breast. These masses, which can grow to the size of a small plum, are benign and usually painless. Fibroadenomas often enlarge during pregnancy and shrink during menopause.
- Fibrocystic breast disease (figh-broh-SIS-tick) is the presence of single or multiple benign cysts in the breasts. This condition occurs more frequently in older women. A cyst is a closed sac containing fluid or semisolid material.
- Galactorrhea (gah-lack-toh-REE-ah) is the production of breast milk in a woman who is not breastfeeding (galact/o means milk, and -rrhea means flow or discharge). This condition is caused by a malfunction of the thyroid or pituitary gland.
- Mastalgia (mass-TAL-jee-ah), also known as mastodynia, is pain in the breast (mast means breast, and -algia means pain).
- Mastitis (mas-TYE-tis) is a breast infection that is most frequently caused by bacteria that enter the breast tissue during breastfeeding (mast means breast, and -itis means inflammation).

Menstrual Disorders

- Amenorrhea (ah-men-oh-REE-ah) is an abnormal absence of menstrual periods for 3 or more months (a- means without, men/o means menstruation, and -rrhea means flow or discharge). This condition is normal only before puberty, during pregnancy, while breastfeeding, and after menopause.
- Dysmenorrhea (dis-men-oh-REE-ah) is pain caused by uterine cramps during a menstrual period (dys- means bad, men/o means menstruation, and -rrhea means flow or discharge). This pain, which occurs in the lower abdomen, can be sharp, intermittent, dull, or aching.
- Hypermenorrhea (high-poh-men-oh-REE-ah), also known as menorrhagia, is an excessive amount of menstrual flow over a period of more than 7 days (hyer- means excessive, men/o means menstruation, and -rrhea means flow or discharge). Hypermenorrhea is the opposite of hypomenorrhea.

- Hypomenorrhea (high-poh-men-oh-REE-ah) is an unsually small amount of menstrual flow during a shortened regular menstrual period (hypo- means deficient, men/o means menstruation, and -rrhea means flow or discharge). Hypomenorrhea is the opposite of hypermenorrhea.
- Menometrorrhagia (men-oh-met-roh-RAY-jee-ah), also known as intermenstrual bleeding, is excessive uterine bleeding at both the usual time of menstrual periods and at other irregular intervals (men/o means menstruation, metr/o means uterus, and -rrhagia means abnormal bleeding).
- Oligomenorrhea (ol-ih-goh-men-oh-REE-ah) is the term used to describe infrequent or very light menstruation in a woman with previously normal periods (olig/o means scanty, men/o means menstruation, and -rrhea means flow or discharge). Oligomenorrhea is the opposite of polymenorrhea.
- Polymenorrhea (pol-ee-men-oh-REE-ah) is the occurrence of menstrual cycles more frequently than is normal (poly- means many, men/o means menstruation, and -rrhea means flow or discharge). Polymenorrhea is the opposite of oligomenorrhea.
- Premature menopause is a condition in which the ovaries cease functioning before age 40 years due to disease, a hormonal disorder, or surgical removal. This causes infertility and often bringing on menopausal symptoms.
- Premenstrual syndrome (PMS) is a group of symptoms experienced by some women within the 2-week period before menstruation. These symptoms can include bloating, swelling, headaches, mood swings, and breast discomfort.
- Premenstrual dysphoric disorder (PMDD) is a condition associated with severe emotional and physical problems that are closely linked to the menstrual cycle. Symptoms occur regularly in the second half of the cycle and end when menstruation begins or shortly thereafter.

Diagnostic Procedures Of The Female Reproductive System

- Colposcopy (kol-POS-koh-pee) is the direct visual examination of the tissues of the cervix and vagina (colp/o means vagina, and -scopy means direct visual examination). This examination is performed using a binocular magnifier known as a colposcope.
- In an endometrial biopsy, a small amount of the tissue from the lining the uterus is removed for microscopic examination. This test is most often used to determine the cause of abnormal vaginal bleeding.
- Endovaginal ultrasound (en-doh-VAJ-ih-nal) is performed to determine the cause of abnormal vaginal bleeding. This test is performed by placing an ultrasound transducer in the vagina so that the sound waves can create images of the uterus and ovaries.
- Hysterosalpingography (hiss-ter-oh-sal-pin-GOG-rahfee) is a radiographic examination of the uterus and fallopian tubes (hyster/o

means uterus, salping/o means tube, and -graphy means the process of producing a picture or record). This test requires the instillation of radiopaque contrast material into the uterine cavity and fallopian tubes to make them visible. Instillation means slowly pouring a liquid onto a body part or into a body cavity.
- Hysteroscopy (hiss-ter-OSS-koh-pee) is the direct visual examination of the interior of the uterus and fallopian tubes (hyster/o means uterus, and -scopy means direct visual examination). This examination is performed by using the magnification of a hysteroscope.
- A Papanicolaou test (pap-ah-nick-oh-LAY-ooh), also known as a Pap smear, is an exfoliative biopsy for the detection of conditions that can be early indicators of cervical cancer. As used here, exfoliative means that cells are scraped from the tissue and examined under a microscope.
- Ultrasound and laparoscopy, which are also used to diagnose disorders of the reproductive system.

Treatment Procedures Of The Female Reproductive System

Medications

- A contraceptive is a measure taken, or a device used, to lessen the likelihood of conception and pregnancy. Birth control pills are a form of hormones that are administered as a contraceptive.
- An intrauterine device is a molded plastic contraceptive inserted through the cervix into the uterus (intrameans within, and uterine means uterus).
- Hormone replacement therapy is the use of the female hormones estrogen and progestin to replace those the body no longer produces during and after perimenopause. Progestin is a synthetic form of the female hormone progesterone.

The Ovaries and Fallopian Tubes

- An ovariectomy (oh-vay-ree-ECK-toh-mee), also known as an oophorectomy, is the surgical removal of one or both ovaries (ovari mean ovary, and -ectomy means surgical removal). If both ovaries are removed in a premenopausal woman, the patient experiences surgical menopause.
- A salpingectomy (sal-pin-JECK-toh-mee) is the surgical removal of one or both fallopian tubes (salping means tube, and -ectomy means surgical removal).
- A salpingo-oophorectomy (sal-ping-goh oh-ahf-oh- RECK-toh-mee) (SO) is the surgical removal of a fallopian tube and ovary (salping/o means tube, oophor means ovary, and -ectomy means surgical removal). A bilateral salpingo-oophorectomy is the removal of both of the fallopian tubes and ovaries.
- Tubal ligation is a surgical sterilization procedure in which the fallopian tubes are sealed or cut to prevent sperm from reaching a mature ovum.

The Uterus, Cervix, and Vagina

- A colpopexy (KOL-poh-peck-see), also known as vaginofixation, is the surgical fixation of a prolapsed vagina to a surrounding structure such as the abdominal wall (colp/o means vagina, and -pexy means surgical fixation in place).
- Conization (kon-ih-ZAY-shun), also known as a cone biopsy, is the surgical removal of a cone-shaped specimen of tissue from the cervix. This is performed as a diagnostic procedure or to remove abnormal tissue.
- Colporrhaphy (kol-POR-ah-fee) is the surgical suturing of a tear in the vagina (colp/o means vagina, and -rrhaphy means surgical suturing).
- Dilation and curettage (dye-LAY-shun and kyou-reh- TAHZH), commonly known as a D & C, is a surgical procedure in which the cervix is dilated and the endometrium of the uterus is scraped away. This can be performed as a diagnostic or a treatment procedure. Dilation means the expansion of an opening. Curettage is the removal of material from the surface by scraping with an instrument known as a curette.
- A myomectomy (my-oh-MECK-toh-mee) is the surgical removal of uterine fibroids (myom means muscle tumor, and -ectomy means surgical removal).

Hysterectomies

- A hysterectomy (hiss-teh-RECK-toh-mee) is the surgical removal of the uterus (hyster means uterus, and -ectomy means surgical removal). The procedure is further described depending upon the structures that are removed.
- In a total hysterectomy, also known as a complete hysterectomy, the uterus and cervix are removed. This procedure can be performed through the vagina or laparoscopically through the abdomen.
- In a partial or subtotal hysterectomy, the uterus is removed and the cervix is left in place.
- A radical hysterectomy, also known as a bilateral hysterosalpingo-oophorectomy, is most commonly performed to treat uterine cancer. This procedure includes the surgical removal of the ovaries and fallopian tubes, the uterus and cervix, plus nearby lymph nodes. If this surgery is performed before natural menopause, the patient immediately experiences surgical menopause.

Mammoplasty

- Mammoplasty (MAM-oh-plas-tee), also spelled mammaplasty, is a general term for a cosmetic operation on the breasts (mamm/o means breast, and -plasty means surgical repair).
- Breast augmentation is mammoplasty performed to increase breast size. Augmentation means the process of adding to make larger. Breast augmentation is the opposite of breast reduction.

- Breast reduction is mammoplasty performed to decrease and reshape excessively large, heavy breasts. Breast reduction is the opposite of breast augmentation.
- Mastopexy (MAS-toh-peck-see) is mammoplasty to affix sagging breasts in a more elevated position (mast/o means breast, and -pexy means surgical fixation).

PREGNANCY AND CHILDBIRTH

Ovulation

- Ovulation (ov-you-LAY-shun) is the release of a mature egg from a follicle on the surface of the ovary.
- After the ovum is released, it is caught up by the fimbriae of the fallopian tube. Wave-like peristaltic actions move the ovum down the fallopian tube toward the uterus.
- It usually takes an ovum about 5 days to pass through the fallopian tube. If sperm are present, fertilization occurs within the fallopian tube.
- After the ovum has been released, the ruptured follicle enlarges, takes on a yellow fatty substance, and becomes the corpus luteum.
- The corpus luteum (KOR-pus LOO-tee-um) secretes the hormone progesterone during the second half of the menstrual cycle. This maintains the growth of the uterine lining in preparation for the fertilized egg.
- If the ovum is not fertilized, the corpus luteum dies, and the endometrium lining of the uterus sloughs off as the menstrual flow occurs.
- If the ovum is fertilized, the corpus luteum continues to secrete the hormones required to maintain the pregnancy.

Fertilization

- During coitus (KOH-ih-tus), also known as copulation or sexual intercourse, the male ejaculates approximately 100 million sperm into the female's vagina. The sperm travel upward through the vagina, into the uterus, and on into the fallopian tubes.
- Conception occurs when a sperm penetrates and fertilizes the descending ovum. This union, which is the beginning of a new life, forms a single cell known as a zygote (ZYE-goht).
- After fertilization occurs in the fallopian tube, the zygote travels to the uterus where it is implanted. Implantation is the embedding of the zygote into the lining of the uterus.
- From implantation through the 8th week of pregnancy, the developing child is known as an embryo (EM-breeoh).
- From the 9th week of pregnancy, to the time of birth, the developing child in utero is known as a fetus (fet means unborn child, and -us is a singular noun ending). In utero means within the uterus.

Multiple Births
- If more than one egg is passing down the fallopian tube when sperm are present, the fertilization of more than one egg is possible.
- Fraternal twins result from the fertilization of separate ova by separate sperm cells. These develop into two separate embryos.
- Identical twins are formed by the fertilization of a single egg cell by a single sperm that divides to from two embryos. Each of these twins receives exactly the same genetic information from the parents.
- The term multiples is used to describe a birth involving more than two infants.

The Chorion and Placenta
- The chorion (KOR-ee-on) is the thin outer membrane that encloses the embryo. It contributes to the formation of the placenta.
- The placenta (plah-SEN-tah) is a temporary organ that forms within the uterus to allow the exchange of nutrients, oxygen, and waste products between the mother and fetus without allowing maternal blood and fetal blood to mix. The placenta also produces hormones necessary to maintain the pregnancy.
- After delivery of the newborn, the placenta is expelled as the afterbirth.

The Amniotic Sac
- The amniotic sac (am-nee-OT-ick), which is alsoknownas the amnion, is the innermost membrane that surrounds the embryo inthe uterus. The commonname for this structure is the bag of waters.
- The developing embryo is surrounded by the amniotic cavity. This is the fluid-filled space between the embryo and the amniotic sac.
- Amnionic fluid (am-nee-ON-ick), also known as amniotic fluid, is the liquid that protects the fetus and makes possible its floating movements.

The Umbilical Cord
- The umbilical cord (um-BILL-ih-kal) is the tube that carries blood, oxygen, and nutrients from the placenta to the developing child. It also transports waste from the fetus to be disposed of through the mother's excretory system. This cord is cut soon after the birth of the infant and before the delivery of the placenta.
- After birth, the navel, also known as the belly button, is formed where the umbilical cord was attached to the fetus.

Gestation
- Gestation (jes-TAY-shun), which lasts approximately 280 days, is the period of development of the child in the mother's uterus. Upon completion of this developmental time, the fetus is described as being at term and should be ready for birth.

- The term pregnancy, which is often used interchangeably with gestation, means the condition of having a developing child in the uterus.
- The length of pregnancy is described according to the number of weeks of gestation (usually 40 weeks total). For descriptive purposes, pregnancy can also be divided into three trimesters of about 13 weeks each.
- The due date, or estimated date of confinement, is calculated from the first day of the last menstrual period (LMP). Confinement is an old-fashioned term describing the period of rest for the mother that followed childbirth.
- quickening is the first movement of the fetus in the uterus that can be felt by the mother. This usually occurs during the 16th to 20th week of pregnancy.
- Braxton Hicks contractions are intermittent painless uterine contractions that occur with increasing frequently as the pregnancy progresses. These contractions are not true labor pains and are usually infrequent, irregular, and essentially painless.
- The fetus is described as being viable when it is capable of living outside the uterus. Viability depends on the developmental age, birth weight, and developmental stage of the lungs of the fetus.
- The term antepartum (an-tee-PAHR-tum) refers to the final stage of pregnancy just before the onset of labor.

The Mother

- A nulligravida (null-ih-GRAV-ih-dah) is a woman who has never been pregnant (nulli- means none, and -gravida means pregnant). Compare with nullipara.
- A nullipara (nuh-LIP-ah-rah) is a woman who has never borne a viable child (nulli- means none, and -para means to bring forth). Compare with nulligravida.
- A primigravida (prye-mih-GRAV-ih-dah) is a woman during her first pregnancy (primi- means first, and -gravida means pregnant). Compare with primipara.
- A primipara (prye-MIP-ah-rah) is a woman who has borne one viable child (primi- means first, and -para means to bring forth). Compare with primigravida.
- Multiparous (mul-TIP-ah-rus) means a woman who has given birth two or more times (multi- means many, and -parous means having borne one or more children).

Childbirth

Labor and delivery, also known as childbirth or parturition, occurs in three stages. These are dilation, delivery of the baby, and expulsion of the afterbirth.

The First Stage
- During the first, and longest, stage of labor, the changes that occur include the gradual dilatation and effacement of the cervix and the rupture of the amniotic sac. Effacement is the process by which the cervix prepares for delivery as it gradually softens, shortens, and becomes thinner.
- Fetal monitoring is the use of an electronic device to record the fetal heart rate and the maternal uterine contractions during labor.

The Second Stage
The second stage is the delivery of the infant. As the uterine contractions become stronger and more frequent, the mother pushes to help expel the child through the birth canal (vagina). Normally, the baby's head presents first. Crowning describes when the head can be seen at the vaginal opening.

The Third Stage
The third stage is the expulsion of the placenta as the Afterbirth.

Postpartum
The term postpartum (pohst-PAR-tum) means after childbirth.

The Mother
- Puerperium (pyou-er-PEE-ree-um) is the time from the delivery of the placenta through approximately the first 6 weeks after the delivery. By the end of this period, most of the changes in the mother's body due to pregnancy have resolved, and the body has reverted to the nonpregnant state.
- Lochia (LOH-kee-ah) is the postpartum vaginal discharge that typically continues for 4–6 weeks after childbirth (loch means childbirth, and -ia means pertaining to). It consists of blood, mucus, and placental tissue.
- Uterine involution is the return of the uterus to its normal size and former condition after delivery. Involution means the return of an enlarged organ to its normal size.
- Colostrum (kuh-LOS-trum) is a specialized form of milk that delivers essential nutrients and antibodies in a form that the newborn can digest. Colostrum is produced by the mammary glands in late pregnancy and during the first few days after giving birth.
- Lactation (lack-TAY-shun) is the process of forming and secreting milk from the breasts as nourishment for the infant. The breast milk develops a few days after giving birth to replace the colostrum.
- Postpartum depression is a mood disorder characterized by feelings of sadness and the loss of pleasure in normal activities that can occur shortly after giving birth. One cause of this depression is the rapid change in the hormone levels that occurs after giving birth. When the depression is severe, treatment is required.

The Baby
- The newborn infant is known as a neonate (NEE-oh-nayt) during the first 4 weeks after birth.
- Vernix(VER-nicks) is a greasy substance that protects the fetus in utero and can still be present at birth.
- Meconium (meh-KOH-nee-um) is the greenish material that collects in the intestine of a fetus and forms the first stools of a newborn.

Apgar Scores
An Apgar score is a scale of 1–10 to evaluate a newborn infant's physical status at 1 and 5 minutes after birth. The newborn is evaluated by assigning numerical values (0–2) to each of five criteria: (1) heart rate, (2) respiratory effort, (3) muscle tone, (4) response stimulation, and (5) skin color. A total score of 8–10 indicates the best possible condition.

PATHOLOGY OF PREGNANCY AND CHILDBIRTH

Pregnancy
- An abortion (ah-BOR-shun) is the interruption or termination of pregnancy before the fetus is viable. A spontaneous abortion, also known as a miscarriage, usually occurs early in the pregnancy and is due to an abnormality or genetic disorder.
- An induced abortion, caused by human intervention, is achieved through the use of drugs or suctioning. When done for medical purposes, it is known as known as a therapeutic abortion.
- An ectopic pregnancy (eck-TOP-ick), also known as an extrauterine pregnancy, is a potentially dangerous condition in which a fertilized egg is implanted and begins to develop outside of the uterus. Ectopic means out of place.
- Preeclampsia (pree-ee-KLAMP-see-ah), also known as pregnancy-induced hypertension or toxemia, is a complication of pregnancy characterized by hypertension (high blood pressure), edema (swelling), and proteinuria (an abnormally high level of protein in the urine).
- Eclampsia (eh-KLAMP-see-ah), which is a more serious form of preeclampsia, is characterized by convulsions and sometimes coma. Treatment for this condition is delivery of the fetus.

Childbirth
- Abruptio placentae (ab-RUP-shee-oh plah-SEN-tee) is an abnormal disorder in which the placenta separates from the uterine wall before the birth of the fetus.
- Breech presentation is one in which the buttocks or feet of the fetus are positioned to enter the birth canal first instead of the head.
- Placenta previa (plah-SEN-tah PREE-vee-ah) is the abnormal implantation of the placenta in the lower portion of the uterus. Previa

means appearing before or in front of. Symptoms include painless, suddenonset bleeding during the third trimester.
- A premature infant, also known as a preemie, is a fetus born before the 37th week of gestation.
- A stillbirth is the birth of a fetus that died before, or during, the delivery.

Diagnostic Procedures Related to Pregnancy and Childbirth

- A pregnancy test is performed to detect an unusually high level of the human chorionic gonadotropin hormone in either a blood or urine specimen, which is usually an indication of pregnancy. A "home pregnancy test" uses a urine specimen. A pregnancy test based on a blood specimen usually provides more reliable results.
- First trimester screening, also known as combined screening, is performed between 11 and 13 weeks of pregnancy and involves an ultrasound and a fingerstick blood test. The combined results of these two measurements, plus the mother's age, detect most of the fetuses at risk for Down syndrome. Diagnostic tests, such as amniocentesis or chorionic villus sampling, are recommended for those at increased risk for this condition.
- Chorionic villus sampling (kor-ee-ON-ick VIL-us) is the examination of cells retrieved from the chorionic villi, which are minute, vascular projections on the chorion. This test is performed between the 8th and 10th weeks of pregnancy to search for genetic abnormalities in the developing fetus.
- Amniocentesis (am-nee-oh-sen-TEE-sis) is a surgical puncture with a needle to obtain a specimen of amniotic fluid (amnio means amnion and fetal membrane, and -centesis means a surgical puncture to remove fluid). This specimen, which is obtained after the 14th week of pregnancy, is used to evaluate fetal health and to diagnose certain congenital disorders.
- Pelvimetry (pel-VIM-eh-tree) is a radiographic study to measure the dimensions of the pelvis to evaluate its capacity to allow passage of the fetus through the birth canal (pelvi means pelvis, and -metrymeans tomeasure).

Treatment Procedures Related to Pregnancy and Childbirth

- A cesarean section (seh-ZEHR-ee-un SECK-shun), also known as a C-section, is the delivery of the child through an incision in the maternal abdominal and uterine walls. This is usually performed when a vaginal birth would be unsafe for either the mother or baby.
- VBAC is the acronym used to describe Vaginal Birth After a Cesarean.
- An episiotomy (eh-piz-ee-OT-oh-mee) is a surgical incision made through the perineum to enlarge the vaginal orifice to prevent tearing of the tissues as the infant moves out of the birth canal (episi means vulva, and -otomy means a surgical incision).

- An episiorrhaphy (eh-piz-ee-OR-ah-fee) is the surgical suturing to repair an episiotomy (episi/o means vulva, and -rrhaphy means surgical suturing).

ASSISTED REPRODUCTION
- Infertility is the inability of a couple to achieve pregnancy after 1 year of regular, unprotected intercourse, or the inability of a woman to carry a pregnancy to a live birth.
- An infertile couple may seek the help of an infertility specialist, also known as a fertility specialist, who diagnoses and treats problems associated with conception and maintaining pregnancy.

Abbreviations Related To The Reproductive Systems
- amniocentesis = AMN
- bacterial vaginosis = BV
- chorionic villus sampling = CVS
- circumcision = CIRC, circum
- digital rectal examination = DRE
- erectile dysfunction = ED
- hormone replacement therapy = HRT
- human papilloma virus = HPV
- hysterosalpingography = HSG
- hysteroscopy = HYS
- intrauterine device = IUD
- labor and delivery = L & D
- pelvic inflammatory disease = PID
- trichomoniasis = Trich

Critical Thinking Exercise

The following story and questions are designed to stimulate critical thinking through class discussion or as a brief essay response. There are no right or wrong answers to these questions.

"But Sam, you promised!" Jamie Chu began.

"Please do not get so upset," her husband interrupted. "I know I agreed to a vasectomy, but Grandmother may have a point. I do not have a son. Our family name has to be considered. I just feel that we should think about this."

"But Sam, we already discussed it. You're scheduled for the procedure." It seemed to Jamie that they had already spent plenty of time considering the number of children they wanted and talking about various contraceptive methods. Jamie had problems taking the pill, and Sam didn't like using a condom. A tubal ligation could have been the answer, but Jamie had a fear of not waking up from the anesthesia. Besides, she had been the one to go through two pregnancies and childbirths. Sam had reluctantly agreed that it was his turn to take responsibility for family planning.

Their two daughters, 2-year-old Nanyn and her big sister Nadya, made the perfect size family, Jamie thought. She had grown up in a large family. A lot of her childhood was spent taking care of her brothers and sisters, and she rarely had her mother's undivided attention. She didn't want that for her children.

Sam's story was different. Before his parents immigrated to America, they had had four daughters. His father was so proud when Sam was born, a son to carry on the family tradition. It had taken quite a long time to convince Sam that a family of only daughters could be considered complete. And now Grandmother was questioning that decision.

Suggested Discussion Topics

1. In a sexual relationship, which partner is responsible for birth control and why?
2. If a couple cannot agree about family size or birth control methods, what options are available to them?
3. Discuss how cultural differences and religious beliefs influence choices like family size and birth control.
4. Some cultures value male children over female children. Discuss why you think this is so and how the changing cultural role of women may affect these values.

CHAPTER 15

DIAGNOSTIC PROCEDURES AND PHARMACOLOGY

This list contains essential word parts and medical terms for this chapter.

Word Parts
- albumin/o
- calc/i
- -centesis
- creatin/o
- glycos/o
- -graphy
- hemat/o
- lapar/o
- -otomy
- phleb/o
- radi/o
- -scope
- -scopy
- son/o
- –uria

Medical Terms
- acetaminophen (ah-seet-ah-MIN-oh-fen)
- albuminuria (al-byou-mih-NEW-ree-ah)
- analgesic (an-al-JEE-zick)
- antipyretic (an-tih-pye-RET-ick)
- arthrocentesis (ar-throh-sen-TEE-sis)
- auscultation (aws-kul-TAY-shun)
- bacteriuria (back-tee-ree-YOU-ree-ah)
- bruit (BREW-ee)
- calciuria (kal-sih-YOU-ree-ah)
- computed tomography (toh-MOG-rah-fee)

- contraindication
- creatinuria (kree-at-ih-NEW-ree-ah)
- echocardiography (eck-oh-kar-dee-OG-rah-fee)
- endoscope (EN-doh-skope)
- fluoroscopy (floo-or-OS-koh-pee)
- glycosuria (glye-koh-SOO-ree-ah)
- hematocrit (hee-MAT-oh-krit)
- hematuria (hee-mah-TOO-ree-ah)
- hyperthermia (high-per-THER-mee-ah)
- hypothermia (high-poh-THER-mee-ah)
- idiosyncratic reaction (id-ee-oh-sin-KRAT-ick)
- intradermal injection
- intramuscular injection
- intravenous injection
- ketonuria (kee-toh-NEW-ree-ah)
- laparoscopy (lap-ah-ROS-koh-pee)
- lithotomy position (lih-THOT-oh-mee)
- magnetic resonance imaging
- ophthalmoscope (ahf-THAL-moh-skope)
- otoscope (OH-toh-skope)
- palliative (PAL-ee-ay-tiv)
- parenteral (pah-REN-ter-al)
- percussion (per-KUSH-un)
- perfusion (per-FYOU-zuhn)
- pericardiocentesis (pehr-ih-kar-dee-oh-sen-TEE-sis)
- phlebotomist (fleh-BOT-oh-mist)
- phlebotomy (fleh-BOT-oh-mee)
- placebo (plah-SEE-boh)
- positron emission tomography
- potentiation (poh-ten-shee-AY-shun)
- prone position
- proteinuria (proh-tee-in-YOU-ree-ah)
- pyuria (pye-YOU-ree-ah)
- radiolucent (ray-dee-oh-LOO-sent)
- radiopaque (ray-dee-oh-PAYK)
- rale (RAHL)
- recumbent (ree-KUM-bent)
- rhonchus (RONG-kus)
- Sims' position
- single photon emission computed tomography
- speculum (SPECK-you-lum)
- sphygmomanometer (sfig-moh-mah-NOM-eh-ter)
- stethoscope (STETH-oh-skope)
- stridor (STRYE-dor)

- subcutaneous injection
- transdermal
- transesophageal echocardiography (trans-eh-sofah- JEE-al eck-oh-kar-dee-OG-rah-fee)
- ultrasonography (ul-trah-son-OG-rah-fee)
- urinalysis (you-rih-NAL-ih-sis)

Objectives

On completion of this chapter, you should be able to:

1. Describe the vital signs recorded for most patients.
2. Recognize, define, spell, and pronounce the terms associated with basic examination procedures.
3. Identify and describe the basic examination positions.
4. Recognize, define, spell, and pronounce terms associatedwith frequently performed blood and urinalysis laboratory tests.
5. Recognize, define, spell, and pronounce terms associated with radiography and other imaging techniques.
6. Differentiate between projection and position, and describe basic radiographic projections.
7. Recognize, define, spell, and pronounce the pharmacology terms introduced in this chapter.

Vital Signs

Vital signs are the four key indications that the body systems are functioning. These signs, which are recorded for most patient visits, include temperature, pulse, respiration, and blood pressure.

Temperature

An average normal temperature is 98.6°F (Fahrenheit) or 37.0°C (Celsius).

- Temperature readings are named for the location in which they are taken: oral (in the mouth), aural (in the ear), axillary (under the arm), and rectal (in the rectum). Caution: oral and aural sound alike; however, they require different equipment and are taken in different locations.
- Temperature readings vary slightly depending upon the location where they are taken.
- Hypothermia (high-poh-THER-mee-ah) is an abnormally low body temperature (hypo- means deficient, therm means heat, and -ia means pertaining to).
- Hyperthermia (high-per-THER-mee-ah) is an extremely high fever (hyper- means excessive, therm means heat, and -ia means pertaining to).

Pulse

The pulse is the rhythmic pressure against the walls of an artery caused by the contraction of the heart. The pulse rate reflects the number of times the heart beats each minute and is recorded as bpm (beats per minute.
- Normal resting pulse rates differ by age group. In adults, a normal resting pulse is from 50 to 80 bpm. Generally pulse rates are higher in younger people and for a newborn the pulse rate ranges from 100 to 160 bpm.

Respiration

Respiration, also known as the respiratory rate (RR), is the number of complete respirations per minute. One inhalation and one exhalation are counted as a single respiration. The normal respiratory rate for adults ranges from 12 to 20 respirations per minute.

Blood Pressure

Blood pressure is the force of the blood against the walls of the arteries.
- This force is measured using a sphygmomanometer (sfig-moh-mah-NOM-eh-ter). When using manual style, a stethoscope is required to listen to the blood sounds. A digital sphygmomanometer is automated and does not require the use of a stethoscope.
- Blood pressure is recorded as a ratio with the systolic over the diastolic reading. For example, 120/80. Memory aid: SSSS-systolic is like steam going up. DDDD-diastolic as in going down.

Pain

In certain settings, such as a hospital, pain is considered to be the fifth vital sign. Since this is a subjective symptom that cannot be measured objectively, it must be determined as reported by the patient.
- Using a pain rating scale, the patient is asked to describe his or her level of pain.
- Acute pain, which comes on quickly, can be severe and lasts only a relatively short time.
- Chronic pain, which can be mild or severe, persists over a long period of time.

Auscultation

- The term auscultation (aws-kul-TAY-shun) means listening for sounds within the body and is usually performed n Rhonchus (RONG-kus), also known as wheezing, is an abnormal sound heard while listening to the chest during inspiration, expiration or both (plural, rhonchi). These sounds, which are low-pitched, whistle-like, or similar to snoring, are caused are partial obstruction of the airway. Memory aid: Rhonchus occurs in a partially blocked bronchus. Compare rhonchus with stridor.

- Stridor (STRYE-dor) is an abnormal high-pitched harsh sound heard during inhalation. Stridor is the result of a partial blockage of the pharynx, larynx, and trachea. Memory aid: Stridor is a harsh sound. Compare stridor with rhonchus.

Heart Sounds

- The heartbeat heard through a stethoscope has two distinct sounds. These are known as the "lubb dupp" or "lub dub" sounds. The lubb sound is heard first. This is caused by the tricuspid and mitral valves closing between the atria and the ventricles. The dupp sound, which is shorter and higher pitched, is heard next. It is caused by the closing of the semilunar valves in the aorta and pulmonary arteries as blood is pumped out of the heart.
- A bruit (BREW-ee) is an abnormal sound heard during auscultation of an artery. These sounds are usually due to a partially blocked, narrowed, or diseased artery. These sounds are also produced by the blood flowing though a graft, fistula, or shunt.
- A heart murmur is an abnormal heart sound that is most commonly a sign of abnormal function of the heart valves.

Abdominal Sounds

Abdominal sounds, also known as bowel sounds, are normal noises made by the intestines. Auscultation of the abdomen is performed to evaluate these sounds and to detect abnormalities. For example, increased bowel sounds can indicate a bowel obstruction. The absence of these sounds can indicate ileus, which is the stopping of intestinal peristalsis.

Palpation and Percussion

- Palpation (pal-PAY-shun) is an examination technique in which the examiner's hands are used to feel the texture, size, consistency, and location of certain body parts.
- Percussion (per-KUSH-un) is a diagnostic procedure designed to determine the density of a body part by the sound produced by tapping the surface with the fingers.

Basic Examination Instruments

- An ophthalmoscope (ahf-THAL-moh-skope) is an instrument used to examine the interior of the eye (ophthalm/o means eye, and -scope means instrument for visual examination).
- An otoscope (OH-toh-skope) is an instrument used to visually examine the external ear canal and tympanic membrane (ot/o means ear, and -scope means instrument for visual examination).
- A speculum (SPECK-you-lum) is an instrument used to enlarge the opening of any canal or cavity to facilitate inspection of its interior.

- A stethoscope (STETH-oh-skope) is an instrument used to listen to sounds within the body.

Basic Examination Positions

Specific positions are used to examine different areas of the body.

Recumbent Positions

The term recumbent (ree-KUM-bent) describes any position in which the patient is lying down. This can be on the back, front, or side. In radiography the term decubitus is used to describe the patient lying in a recumbent position.

Prone Position

In a prone position, the patient is lying on the belly with the face down. The arms may be placed under the head for comfort. This position is used for the examination and treatment of the back and buttocks.

Horizontal Recumbent Position

In the horizontal recumbent position, also known as the supine position, the patient is lying on the back with the face up. This position is used for examination and treatment of the anterior surface of the body and for x-rays.

Dorsal Recumbent Position

In the dorsal recumbent position, the patient is lying on the back with the knees bent. This position is used for the examination and treatment of the abdominal area and for vaginal or rectal examinations.

Sims' Position

In the Sims' position, the patient is lying on the left side with the right knee and thigh drawn up with the left arm placed along the back. This position is used in the examination and treatment of the rectal area. The name of this position is also spelled as Sims position.

Knee-Chest Position

In the knee-chest position, the patient is lying face down with the hips bent so that the knees and chest rest on the table. This position is used for rectal examinations.

Lithotomy Position

In the lithotomy position (lih-THOT-oh-mee) the patient is lying on the back with the feet and legs raised and supported in stirrups. This position is used for vaginal and rectal examinations and during childbirth.

The term lithotomy is also used to describe the removal of a stone from the urinary bladder.

Laboratory Tests

When a laboratory test is ordered stat, the results are needed immediately, and the tests have top priority in the laboratory. Stat comes from the Latin word meaning immediately.

Blood Tests

When used in regard to laboratory tests, the term profile means tests that are frequently performed as a group on automated multichannel laboratory testing equipment. Specimens are :

- A phlebotomist (fleh-BOT-oh-mist) is an individual trained and skilled in phlebotomy.
- Phlebotomy (fleh-BOT-oh-mee), which is also known as venipuncture, is the puncture of a vein for the purpose of drawing blood (phleb means vein, and -otomy means a surgical incision).
- A capillary puncture is the technique used when only a smallamount of blood is needed as a specimen for a blood test.Named forwhere it is performed, a capillary puncture is usually known as a finger, heel, or an earlobe stick.

Complete Blood Cell Counts

A complete blood cell count is a series of tests performed as a group to evaluate several blood conditions.

- Erythrocyte sedimentation rate (eh-RITH-roh-site), also known as a sed rate, is a test based on the speed at which the red blood cells separate from the plasma and settle to the bottom of the container. An elevated sed rate indicates the presence of inflammation in the body.
- The term hematocrit (hee-MAT-oh-krit) describes the percentage, by volume, of a blood sample occupied by red cells (hemat/o means blood, and -crit means to separate). This test is used to diagnose abnormal states of hydration (fluid levels in the body), polycythemia (excess red blood cells), and anemia (deficient red blood cells).
- A platelet count measures the number of platelets in a specified amount of blood and is a screening test to evaluate platelet function. It is also used to monitor changes in the blood associated with chemotherapy and radiation therapy. These changes include thrombocytosis (an abnormal increase in the number of platelets) and thrombocytopenia (an abnormal decrease in the number of platelets).
- A red blood cell count is a determination of the number of erythrocytes in the blood. A depressed count can indicate anemia or a hemorrhage lasting more than 24 hours.
- A total hemoglobin test (Hg) is usually part of a complete blood count (hem/o means blood, and -globin means protein). Elevated Hg levels indicate a higher than normal hemoglobin concentration in the plasma due to polycythemia or dehydration. Low Hg indicates lower then

normal hemoglobin concentration due to anemia, recent hemorrhage, or fluid retention.
- A white blood cell count is a determination of the number of leukocytes in the blood. An elevated count can be an indication of infection or inflammation.
- A white blood cell differential test determines what percentage of the total count is composed of each of the five types of leukocyte. This test provides information about the patient's immune system, detects certain types of leukemia, and determines the severity of infection.

Additional Blood Tests

- A basicmetabolic panel is a group of eight specific blood tests that provide important information about the current status of the patient's kidneys, electrolyte balance, blood sugar, and calcium levels. Significant changes in these test results can indicate acute problems such as kidney failure, insulin shock or diabetic coma, respiratory distress, or heart rhythm changes.
- A blood urea nitrogen test measures the amount of nitrogen in the blood due to the waste product urea. This test is performed to obtain an indication of kidney function. Urea (you-REE-ah) is the major end product of protein metabolism found in urine and blood.
- Crossmatch tests are performed to determine the compatibility of donor and recipient blood before a transfusion. Agglutination is a positive reaction that indicates the donor unit is not a suitable match. Agglutination is the clumping together of the red blood cells.
- A C-reactive protein test (CRP) is performed to identify high levels of inflammation within the body. The information is obtained by the presence of the C-reactive protein, which is produced by the liver only during episodes of acute inflammation. Although this test does not identify the specific cause of the inflammation, an elevated level can be indicative of a heart attack or coronary artery disease.
- A lipid panel measures the amounts of total cholesterol, high-density lipoprotein (HDL), low-density lipoprotein (LDL), and triglycerides in a blood sample.
- Prothrombin time (proh-THROM-bin), also known as pro time, is a test used to diagnose conditions associated with abnormalities of clotting time and to monitor anticoagulant therapy. A longer prothrombin time can be caused by serious liver disease, bleeding disorders, blood-thinning medicines or a lack of vitamin K.
- A serum bilirubin test measures the ability of the liver ability to take up, process, and secrete bilirubin into the bile. This test is useful in determining whether a patient has liver disease or a blocked bile duct.
- A thyroid-stimulating hormone assay measures circulating blood levels of thyroid-stimulating hormone that can indicate abnormal thyroid activity.

Urinalysis

- Urinalysis (you-rih-NAL-ih-sis) is the examination of the physical and chemical properties of urine to determine the presence of abnormal elements.
- Routine urinalysis is performed to screen for urinary and systemic disorders. This test utilizes a dipstick. This is a plastic strip impregnated with chemicals that react with substances in the urine and change color when abnormalities are present.
- Microscopic examination of the specimen is performed when more-detailed testing of the specimen is necessary, for example to identify casts. Casts are fibrous or protein materials, such as pus and fats, that are thrown off into the urine in kidney disease.

pH Values of Urine

The average normal pH range of urine is from 4.5 to 8.0. The abbreviation pH describes the degree of acidity or alkalinity of a substance.

- A pH value below 7 indicates acid urine and is an indication of acidosis. Acidosis is excessive acid in the body fluids.
- A pH value above 7 indicates alkaline urine and can indicate conditions such as a urinary tract infection.

Specific Gravity

The specific gravity of urine reflects the amount of wastes, minerals, and solids that are present.

- Low specific gravity (dilute urine) is characteristic of diabetes insipidus.
- High specific gravity (concentrated urine) occurs in conditions such as dehydration, liver failure, or shock. Conditions Identified through Urinalysis
- Acetone (ASS-eh-tohn), which has a sweet, fruity odor, is found in small quantities in normal urine and in larger amounts in the urine of a diabetic.
- Albuminuria (al-byou-mih-NEW-ree-ah) is the presence of the protein albumin in the urine and is a sign of impaired kidney function (albumin means albumin or protein, and -uria means urine). Albumin is a form of protein found in most body tissues.
- Bacteriuria (back-tee-ree-YOU-ree-ah) is the presence of bacteria in the urine (bacteri means bacteria, and -uria means urine).
- Calciuria (kal-sih-YOU-ree-ah) is the presence of calcium in the urine (calci means calcium, and -uria means urine). Abnormally high levels can be diagnostic for hyperparathyroidism.
- Creatinuria (kree-at-ih-NEW-ree-ah) is an increased concentration of creatine in the urine (creatin means creatinine, and -uria means urine). Creatinine is a waste product of muscle metabolism that is normally removed by the kidneys. The presence of excess creatinine is an

indication of increased muscle breakdown or a disruption of kidney function.
- A drug-screening urine test is a rapid method of identifying the presence in the body of one or more drugs of abuse such as cocaine, heroin, and marijuana. These tests are also used to detect the use of performance-enhancing drugs by athletes.
- Glycosuria (glye-koh-SOO-ree-ah), which is the presence of glucose in the urine, is most commonly caused by diabetes (glycos means glucose, and -uria means urine).
- Hematuria (hee-mah-TOO-ree-ah) is the presence of blood in the urine (hemat means blood, and -uria means urine). This condition can be caused by kidney stones, infection, damage to the kidney, or bladder cancer.
- In gross hematuria, the presence of blood can be detected without magnification because the urine is pink, brown, or bright red in color. In microscopic hematuria, the urine is clear; however, the blood cells can be seen under a microscope.
- Ketonuria (kee-toh-NEW-ree-ah) is the presence of ketones in the urine (keton means ketones, and –uria means urine). Ketones are formed when the body breaks down fat. Their presence in urine can indicate starvation or uncontrolled diabetes.
- Proteinuria (proh-tee-in-YOU-ree-ah) is the presence of an abnormal amount of protein in the urine (protein means protein, and -uria means urine). This condition is usually a sign of kidney disease.
- Pyuria (pye-YOU-ree-ah) is the presence of pus in the urine (py means pus, and -uria means urine). When pus is present, the urine has a turbid appearance. Turbid means a cloudy or smoky appearance.
- Urine culture and sensitivity tests are laboratory tests that are used to identify the cause of a urinary tract infection and to determine which antibiotic would be the most effective treatment.

Endoscopy

Endoscopy (en-DOS-koh-pee) is the visual examination of the interior of a body cavity (endo- means within, and -scopy means visual examination). These procedures are usually named for the organs involved.
The termendoscopic surgery describes a surgical procedure performed through very small incisions with the use of an endoscope and specialized instruments. These procedures are named for the body parts involved, for example, arthroscopic surgery.

Endoscopes

An endoscope (EN-doh-skope) is a small flexible tube with a light and a lens on the end. These fiber optic instruments are named for the body parts they are designed to examine. For example, a hysteroscope is used to examine the interior of the uterus while a laparoscope is used to examine the interior of the abdomen.

Laparoscopic Procedures

Laparoscopy (lap-ah-ROS-koh-pee) is the visual examination of the interior of the abdomen with the use of a laparoscope that is passed through a small incision in the abdominal wall (lapar/o means abdomen, and -scopy means visual examination).

Laparoscopic surgery involves the use of a laparoscope plus specialized instruments inserted into the abdomen through small incisions. A laparoscope is used to:

- Explore and examine the interior of the abdomen.
- Take specimens to be biopsied.
- Perform surgical procedures.

Centesis

- Centesis (sen-TEE-sis) is a surgical puncture to remove fluid for diagnostic purposes or to remove excess fluid.
- Note: Centesis is used alone as a noun or as a suffix in conjunction with the combining form describing the body part being treated.
- Abdominocentesis (ab-dom-ih-noh-sen-TEE-sis) is the surgical puncture of the abdominal cavity to remove fluid (abdomin/o means abdomen, and -centesis means a surgical puncture to remove fluid).
- Amniocentesis, which is a diagnostic test performed during pregnancy.
- Arthrocentesis (ar-throh-sen-TEE-sis) is a surgical puncture of the joint space to remove synovial fluid for analysis to determine the cause of pain or swelling in a joint (arthr/o means joint, and -centesis means a surgical puncture to remove fluid).
- Cardiocentesis (kar-dee-oh-sen-TEE-sis), also known as cardiopuncture, is the puncture of a chamber of the heart for diagnosis or therapy (cardi/o means heart, and -centesis means a surgical puncture to remove fluid).
- Pericardiocentesis (pehr-ih-kar-dee-oh-sen-TEE-sis) is the puncture of the pericardial sac for the purpose of removing fluid (peri- means surrounding, cardi/o means heart, and -centesis means a surgical puncture to remove fluid). This procedure is performed to treat pericarditis.
- Tympanocentesis (tim-pah-noh-sen-TEE-sis) is the surgical puncture of the tympanic membrane with a needle to remove fluid or pus from an infected the middle ear (tympan/o means eardrum, and -centesis means a surgical puncture to remove fluid).

Contrast Medium

A contrast medium is administered by swallowing, via an enema, or intravenously to make specific body structures visible. Specialized substances are

used depending upon the imaging systems and the body parts to be enhanced. These media are either radiopaque or radiolucent.
- Radiopaque (ray-dee-oh-PAYK) means that the substance does not allow x-rays to pass through and appears white or light gray on the resulting film. Radiopaque is the opposite of radiolucent.
- Radiolucent (ray-dee-oh-LOO-sent) means that the substance, such as air or nitrogen gas, does allow x-rays to pass through and appears black or dark gray on the resulting film. Radiolucent is the opposite of radiopaque.
- An intravenous contrast medium is injected into a vein to make the flow of blood through blood vessels and organs visible.

Radiology

In conventional radiology, also known as x-rays, an image of hard-tissue internal structures is created by the exposure of sensitized film to x-radiation (radi/o means radiation, and -graphy means the process of producing a picture or record). The resulting film is known as a radiograph or radiogram; however, it is commonly referred to as an x-ray.
- X-radiation, which is also referred to as ionizing radiation, is beneficial in producing diagnostic images and in treating cancer; however, excess exposure to this radiation is dangerous, and the effects are cumulative. Because x-radiation is invisible, has no odor, and cannot be felt, appropriate precautions must always be taken to protect the technician and the patient.
- Radiographs are made up of shades of gray. Radiopaque hard tissues, such as bone and tooth enamel, appear white or light gray on the radiograph. Radiolucent soft tissues appear as shades of gray to black on the radiograph.
- A radiologist (ray-dee-OL-oh-jist) is a physician who specializes in diagnosing and treating diseases and disorders with x-rays and other forms of radiant energy (radi means radiation, and -ologist means specialist).

Radiographic Positioning

The term radiographic positioning describes the body placement and the part of the body closest to the x-ray film. For example, in a left lateral position, the left side of the body is placed nearest the film.

Radiographic Projections

The term radiographic projection describes the path that the x-ray beam follows through the body from entrance to exit.
- When the name of the projection combines two terms into a single word, the term listed first is the one that the x-ray penetrates first.

- The basic projections described in the next section can be used for most body parts. These projections can be exposed with the patient in a standing or recumbent position.

Basic Radiographic Projections

- An anteroposterior projection (AP) has the patient positioned with the back parallel to the film (anter/o means front, poster means back, and -ior means pertaining to). The x-ray beam travels from anterior (front) to posterior (back).
- A posteroanterior projection (PA) has the patient positioned facing the film and parallel to it (poster/o means back, anter means front, and -ior means pertaining to). The x-ray beam travels through the body from posterior to anterior.
- A lateral projection (LAT) has the patient positioned at right angles to the film. This view is named for the side of the body nearest the film.
- An oblique projection (OBL) has the patient positioned so the body is slanted sideways to the film. This is halfway between a parallel and a right angle position. This view is named for the side of the body nearest the film. Oblique means slanted sideways.

Dental Radiography

Specialized techniques and equipment are used in obtaining dental radiographs.

- The term extraoral radiography means that the film is placed and exposed outside of the mouth.
- Intraoral radiography means that the film is placed within the mouth and exposed by a camera positioned next to the exterior of the cheek.
- Periapical radiographs show the entire tooth and some surrounding tissue (peri- means surrounding, apic means apex, and -al means pertaining to). These films are used to detect abnormalities, such as an abscess at the tip of the root.
- Bite-wing radiographs show the crowns of teeth in both arches on one side of the mouth. These films are used primarily to detect dental decay (cavities) between the teeth.

Computed Tomography

- Computed tomography (toh-MOG-rah-fee) uses a thin, fan-shaped x-ray beam that rotates around the patient to produce multiple cross-sectional views of the body (tom/o means to cut, section, or slice, and -graphy means the process of recording a picture or record).
- Information gathered by radiation detectors is downloaded to a computer, analyzed, and converted into gray-scale images corresponding to anatomic slices of the body. These images are viewed on a monitor, stored as digital files, or printed as films.

- Computed tomography is more effective than MRI at imaging compact bone and is frequently preferred for patients with head injuries or strokes.
- Tomotherapy is the combination of tomography with radiation therapy to precisely target the tumor being treated, avoiding healthy tissue.

Magnetic Resonance Imaging

Magnetic resonance imaging, also known as MRI, uses a combination of radio waves and a strong magnetic field to create signals that are sent to a computer and converted into images of any plane through the body.
- These images can be produced in coronal, sagittal, or oblique planes and are created without the use of ionizing radiation (x-rays).
- These images have excellent low-contrast resolution, which is useful for differentiating soft tissue densities such as the tissues of the heart, blood vessels, brain, spinal cord, joints, muscles, and internal organs.
- Because of the use of powerful magnets, the presence of metal implants such as a knee replacement, an artificial pacemaker, or metal stents can be contraindications for using an MRI on a patient.
- Closed architecture MRI, which is the most commonly used type of equipment, produces the most accurate images; however, patients can be uncomfortable because of the noise generated by the machine and the feeling of being closed in. As an alternative open architecture MRI is designed to be less confining and is more comfortable for some patients.
- Magnetic resonance angiography (MRA), also known as magnetic resonance angio, combines MRI with the use of a contrast medium to locate problems within blood vessels throughout the body. This diagnostic imaging is frequently used as an alternative to conventional angiography.

Fluoroscopy

- Fluoroscopy (floo-or-OS-koh-pee) is the visualization of body parts in motion by projecting x-ray images on a luminous fluorescent screen (fluor/o means glowing, and -scopy means visual examination). Luminous means glowing.
- Cineradiography (sin-eh-ray-dee-OG-rah-fee) is the recording of images as they appear in motion on a fluorescent screen (cine- means relationship to movement, radi/o means radiation, and -graphy means process of recording a picture or record).
- Fluoroscopy can also be used in conjunction with conventional x-ray techniques to capture a record of parts of the examination.

Ultrasonography

Ultrasonography (ul-trah-son-OG-rah-fee), commonly referred to as ultrasound or diagnostic ultrasound, is imaging of deep body structures by recording the echoes of pulses of sound waves that are above the range of human hearing (ultra- means beyond, son/o means sound, and -graphy means the process of recording a picture or record).

- A sonogram (SOH-noh-gram) is the image created by ultrasonography (son/o means sound, and -gram means a picture or record). These images are created by a sonographer who is a technician specifically trained in this technique.
- This technique is most effective for viewing solid organs of the abdomen and soft tissues where the signal is not stopped by intervening bone or air. Common uses of ultrasound include evaluating fetal development, detecting the presence of gallstones, or confirming the presence of a mass found on a mammogram.
- Carotid ultrasonography is the use of sound waves to image the carotid artery to detect an obstruction that could cause an ischemic stroke.
- Echocardiography (eck-oh-kar-dee-OG-rah-fee) is an ultrasonic diagnostic procedure used to evaluate the structures and motion of the heart (ech/o means sound, cardi/o means heart, and -graphy means the process of recording a picture or record). The resulting record is an echocardiogram.
- A Doppler echocardiogram is performed in the same way as an echocardiogram; however, this procedure measures the speed and direction of the blood flow within the heart.
- Fetal ultrasound is a noninvasive procedure used to image and evaluate fetal development during pregnancy that uses specialized equipment to create photograph- like images of the developing child.
- Transesophageal echocardiography (trans-eh-sof-ah- JEE-al eck-oh-kar-dee-OG-rah-fee), also known as TEE, is an ultrasonic imaging technique used to evaluate heart structures. This diagnostic test is performed from inside the esophagus, and because the esophagus is so close to the heart, this technique produces clearer images than those obtained with echocardiography.

Nuclear Medicine

- In nuclear medicine radioactive substances known as radiopharmaceuticals are administered for either diagnostic or treatment purposes. When used for diagnostic purposes, this is referred to as nuclear imaging, and these images document the structure and function of the organ or organs being examined.
- Each radiopharmaceutical contains a radionuclide tracer, also known as a radioactive tracer, which is specific to the body system being examined.
- Radiopharmaceuticals emit gamma rays that are detected by a gamma-ray camera attached to a computer. These data are used to generate an image showing the pattern of absorption that can be indicative of pathology.

Nuclear Scans

A nuclear scan, also known as a scintigram, is a diagnostic procedure that uses nuclear medicine technology to gather information about the structure and function of organs or body systems that cannot be seen on conventional x-rays.

Bone Scans

A bone scan is a nuclear scanning test that identifies new areas of bone growth or breakdown. The results are obtained after a radionuclide tracer is injected into the bloodstream, and the patient then waits while the material travels through the body tissues. This testing can be done to evaluate damage to the bones, detect cancer that has metastasized (spread) to the bones, and monitor conditions that can affect the bones. A bone scan can often detect a problem days to months earlier than a regular x-ray.

Thyroid Scans

For a thyroid scan, a radiopharmaceutical containing radioactive iodine is administered. This scan makes use of the thyroid gland's ability to concentrate certain radioactive isotopes to generate images of it. A thyroid scan provides information about the size, shape, location, and relative activity of different parts of the thyroid gland.

Single Photon Emission Computed Tomography

Single photon emission computed tomography, also known as SPECT, is a type of nuclear imaging test that produces 3D computer-reconstructed images showing perfusion through tissues and organs. Perfusion (per- FYOU-zuhn) means the flow of blood through an organ.
SPECT scanning is used primarily to view the flow of blood through arteries and veins in the brain.
It is also useful in diagnosing blood-deprived areas of brain following a stroke, and tumors.

Positron Emission Tomography

Positron emission tomography, also known as PET imaging, combines tomography with radionuclide tracers to produce enhanced images of selected body organs or areas. PET scans of the whole body are often used to detect cancer and to examine the effects of cancer therapy.
PET scans of the heart are used to determine blood flow to the heart muscle. This procedure helps to evaluate signs of coronary artery disease or to differentiate nonfunctional heart muscle from tissue that would benefit from a procedure such as angioplasty or coronary artery bypass surgery.
PET scans of the brain are used to evaluate patients who have memory disorders of an undetermined cause, suspected or proven brain tumors, or seizure disorders that are not responsive to medical therapy and are therefore candidates for surgery.

Pharmacology

Pharmacology is the study of the nature, uses, and effects of drugs for medical purposes (pharmac means drug, and -ology means study of). A pharmacist is a licensed specialist who formulates and dispenses prescribed medications.

Prescription and Over-the-Counter Drugs

- A prescription drug is a medication that can legally be dispensed only by a pharmacist with an order from a licensed professional such as a physician or dentist.
- An over-the-counter drug, also known as an OTC, is a medication that can be purchased without a prescription.

Generic and Brand-Name Drugs

- A generic drug is usually named for its chemical structure and is not protected by a brand name or trademark. For example, diazepam is the generic name of a drug frequently used as skeletal muscle relaxant, sedative, and antianxiety agent.
- A brand-name drug is sold under the name given the drug by the manufacturer. A brand name is always spelled with a capital letter. For example, Valium is a brand name for diazepam.

Terminology Related to Pharmacology

- An addiction is compulsive, uncontrollable dependence on a drug, alcohol, or other substance. It can also be a habit, or practice, which cannot be stopped without causing severe emotional, mental, or physiologic reactions.
- An adverse drug reaction (ADR), also known as a side effect, is an undesirable reaction that accompanies the principal response for which the drug was taken.
- Compliance is the patient's consistency and accuracy in following the regimen prescribed by a physician or other health care professional. As used here, regimen means directions or rules.
- A contraindication is a factor in the patient's condition that makes the use of a medication or specific treatment dangerous or ill advised.
- A drug interaction is the result of drugs reacting with each other, often in ways that are unexpected or potentially harmful. Such interactions can also occur when medications are taken along with herbal remedies.
- An idiosyncratic reaction (id-ee-oh-sin-KRAT-ick) is an unexpected reaction to a drug that is peculiar to the individual.
- A palliative (PAL-ee-ay-tiv) is a substance that eases the pain or severity of the symptoms of a disease, but does not cure it.
- A paradoxical reaction is the result of medical treatment that yields the exact opposite of normally expected results. Paradoxical means not being normal or the usual kind.

- A placebo (plah-SEE-boh) is an inactive substance, such as a sugar pill or liquid, that is administered only for its suggestive effects. In medical research, a placebo is administered to one group and the drug being studied is administered to another group.
- In medicine, potentiation (poh-ten-shee-AY-shun) is a drug interaction that occurs when the effect of one drug is increased by another drug, herbal remedy, or other treatment. Potentiate means to enhance the effects of a drug.
- An antipyretic (an-tih-pye-RET-ick) is medication administered to prevent or reduce fever (anti- means against, pryet means fever, and -ic means pertaining to). These medications, such as aspirin and acetaminophen, act by lowering a raised body temperature; however, they do not affect a normal body temperature when a fever is not present.
- An anti-inflammatory relieves inflammation and pain without affecting consciousness.

Medications for Pain Management

Acute pain generally comes on suddenly as the result of disease, inflammation, or injury to tissues. When the cause of the pain is diagnosed and treated, the pain goes away. Chronic pain persists over a longer period of time than acute pain and is resistant to most medical treatments. It often causes severe problems for the patient.

Analgesics

- The term analgesic (an-al-JEE-zick) refers to the class of drugs that relieves pain without affecting consciousness. These include such drugs as aspirin, acetaminophen, and ibuprofen.
- Nonnarcotic analgesics, such as aspirin, are sold over the counter for mild to moderate pain. Prescription pain relievers, sold through a pharmacy under the direction of a physician, are used for more moderate to severe pain.
- Narcotic analgesics, such as morphine, Demerol, and codeine are available by prescription only to relieve severe pain. These medications also have a sedative (calming) effect, and can cause physical dependence or addiction.
- Acetaminophen (ah-seet-ah-MIN-oh-fen) is an analgesic that reduces pain and fever, but does not relieve inflammation; however, it does not have the negative side effects of NSAIDS. This substance is basic ingredient found in Tylenol® and its generic equivalents.
- Nonsteroidal anti-inflammatory drugs, commonly known as NSAIDs, are nonnarcotic analgesics administered to control pain by reducing inflammation and swelling. NSAIDS, such as aspirin and ibuprofen, are available over the counter. Stronger NSAIDs are available by

prescription. Medications in this group can cause side effects, including attacking the stomach lining and thinning the blood.
- Ibuprofen (eye-byoo-pro-fen) is a nonsteroidal antiinflammatory medicine that is sold over the counter under the brand names of Advil and Motrin. This medication acts an analgesic to relieve the pain of arthritis. It also acts as an antipyretic.
- Although pain management is not their primary roles, anticonvulsants and antidepressants have been found to be effective as part of some chronic pain management programs. Anticonvulsants are traditionally administered to prevent seizures such as those associated with epilepsy. Antidepressants are primarily administered to prevent or relieve depression.

Addition Pain Control Methods

Pain-relieving creams are applied topically to relieve pain due to conditions such as osteoarthritis and rheumatoid arthritis. The primary active ingredient in these ointments is capsaicin, a chemical found in chili peppers. Transcutaneous electronic nerve stimulation, also known as TENS, is a method of pain control by wearing a device that delivers small electrical impulses, as needed, to the nerve endings through the skin (trans- means across, cutane means skin, and -ous means pertaining to). These electrical impulses cause changes in muscles, such as numbness or contractions, which produce temporary pain relief. The term transcutaneous means performed through the unbroken skin.

Methods of Drug Administration

- Inhalation administration describes vapors and gases taken in through the nose or mouth and absorbed into the bloodstream through the lungs. One example is the use of a metered-dose inhaler to treat asthma or the gases used for general anesthesia.
- Oral administration refers to medications taken by mouth to be absorbed through the walls of the stomach or small intestine. These drugs can be in the form of liquids, tablets (pills), or capsules. Medications to be released in the small intestine are covered with an enteric coating to prevent them from being absorbed in the stomach.
- Rectal administration is the insertion of medication in the rectum either in the form of a suppository or a liquid. A suppository is medication in a semisolid form that is introduced into the rectum. The suppository melts at body temperature, and the medication is absorbed through the surrounding tissues.
- Sublingual administration is the placement of medication under the tongue where it is allowed to dissolve slowly (sub- means under, lingu means tongue, and -al means pertaining to). Because the sublingual tissues are highly vascular, the medication is quickly absorbed directly into the bloodstream. Highly vascular means containing many blood vessels.

- A topical application is a liquid or ointment that is rubbed into the skin on the area to be treated. Examples: cortisone ointment is applied topically to relieve itching and to speed healing; antibiotic ointments are applied over minor wounds to prevent infection.
- A transdermal medication is administered from a patch that is applied to unbroken skin (trans- means through or across, derm means skin, and -al means pertaining to). The medication, which is continuously released by the patch, is absorbed through the skin and transmitted to the bloodstream so that it can produce a systemic effect. These multilayered patches are used to convey medications, such as nitroglycerin for angina, hormones for hormone replacement therapy, or nicotine patches for smoking cessation.

Parenteral Administration

- The term parenteral (pah-REN-ter-al) means taken into the body, or administered, in a manner other than through the digestive tract. The most common use of parenteral administration is by injection through a hypodermic syringe.
- A subcutaneous injection (SC) is made into the fatty layer just below the skin.
- An intradermal injection is made into the middle layers of the skin.
- An intramuscular injection (IM) is made directly into muscle tissue.
- An intravenous injection (IV) is made directly into a vein. A peripherally inserted central catheter, commonly known as a PICC line, may be used for a patient who will need IV therapy for more than 7 days.
- A bolus (BOH-lus), also known as a bolus infusion, is a single, concentrated dose of drug usually injected into a blood vessel over a short period of time.

Abbreviations Related To The Diagnostic Procedures And Pharmacology

- beats per minute = bpm
- blood pressure = BP
- blood urea nitrogen = BUN
- complete blood count = CBC
- endoscopy = endo
- erythrocyte sedimentation rate = ESR
- hematocrit = Hct, hct
- red blood count = RBC
- respiratory rate = RR
- temperature, pulse, respiration = TPR
- white blood count = WBC

Critical Thinking Exercise

The following story and questions are designed to stimulate critical thinking through class discussion or as a brief essay response. There are no right or wrong answers to these questions.

Terrance Ortega had finally made it. Standing behind the counter of the pharmacy at SuperDrug, he thought back on his years at pharmacology school. He had studied hard, and it paid off when he landed this job.

A young man approached the counter and said, "I'm James Tirendale, and I'm here to pick up my mom Ginny's prescription for MS Contin." He flashed a handwritten scrawled note from his mother. "Sure thing James, let me just find that for you."

Terrance headed to the counter where filled prescriptions were kept and grabbed the one marked "Ginny Tirendale." Sure enough, there was a prescription for MS Contin; a palliative usually prescribed for pain.

He explained to James the adverse affects that this drug could have, that it was to be administered orally, and that it was not to be crushed or cut. James paid cash and headed out of the store in a hurry.

Later that day, a woman on crutches came up to the pharmacy counter. She explained that her name was Ginny Tirendale and that she needed to pick up some pain medication because she'd just had knee surgery. A confused look came over Terrance's face. "Your son already picked that up, Ms. Tirendale," he explained. "Oh no!" Ginny replied, "I knew I shouldn't have told him I was coming here this afternoon. He must have realized which drug I was prescribed and got here before me." Suddenly Terrance realized that he should have looked at the note more closely or called Ms. Tirendale before giving out a prescription for a drug with such a high "street value." It occurred to him that potentiation would occur if MS Contin was taken with alcohol, and it could easily lead to psychological and physical dependence if abused. What if her son didn't know that and died, or sold it to someone else who abused it?

Suggested Discussion Topics

1. What precaution had James taken in case the pharmacist asked questions?
2. Suppose Terrance was suspicious about allowing James to pick up the prescription. Discuss the steps Terrance might have taken, including involving his supervisor.
3. Terrance appears to blame himself for what happened with the MS Contin prescription. Discuss what might have happened if another pharmacist was on duty when Ms. Tirendale came to pick up her prescription?
4. Ms. Tirendale is obviously suspicious of her son's actions regarding the prescription. Discuss the steps she might take to help him if she thinks he is abusing drugs.

***

Scott J. Barnard

CONCLUSION

Before a person attempts to memorize any medical term, it is essential that he/she learns the fundamental arrangement and base of medical words. It would be difficult for people without the knowledge of Latin and Greek to learn these expressions, since most of them are based on these languages.

When students who wish to enter the field of medicine learn some fundamental terminologies, they will be in a position to take apart a word to identify its meaning.

In addition to being a good learner, it is essential that people should be good spellers since there are some words with the same spelling in the field of medicine, but with different pronunciation and vice versa.

To begin with the learning process, he/she can enroll in an introductory medical terminology class, since these courses enable them to learn how some of the medical terminologies are created and what are the words used for denoting different parts of the human body, etc...

These courses are being offered by some technical schools, vocational and community colleges and even some training institutions offer them; not only under classroom training method, but also under online training method.

It would be better for the learners to check the class description before taking up the course with an institution, since some institutions might incorporate fundamental terminology into introductory and other courses.

For people who are already taking up some form of courses or for working professionals, it would be better to take medical terminology classes online and some institutions are offering this facility.

These people can also enhance their skills by studying on their own with the help of many tools and books sold online by some of the institutions. The books offered by these institutions don't just provide a list of terminologies to memorize, but they also they lay attention on the foundation of learning different expressions.

To make the process of learning medical terms easier, it would be better for learners to take up some fundamental language training course on Greek and Latin languages since most of the words used in the field of medicine are combinations of adjectives and verbs in these languages.

This will enable them to understand the structure and foundation of medical terms.

During the process of learning, they can get hold of some dictionaries pertaining to these languages to make the process easier.

For a person who wishes to shine in the field of health care, it is better to learn medical terminology. Health care is a field where unfamiliar words are used frequently, and to get out of the confusing medical language a medical terminology course can be taken up.

With some hard work any person can expose this niche and excel in medical field.

The best thing about this course is that it is not just for nurses and physicians, but it is meant for any person working in the health care industry.

This course will be of great use to people who wish to enter medical transcription field since they will have to transcribe different medical terms. Not only medical transcriptionists, but also radiological technicians can benefit from this course. Even though any person who can easily memorize words can memorize medical terms, only when a person takes up a medical terminology course he will be in a position to understand the meaning of the terms.

Once the meaning of a word is understood, it can be easily remembered and there will not be any requirement for memorizing the term. A person interested in medical terminologies can learn them easily if he/she can understand the meaning of the words on the basis of word roots, suffixes and prefixes.

The meaning of longer terms can be sensed out, if the person can understand the meaning of commonly used parts of words. This logic is well understood by institutes offering these courses and therefore they teach the trainees accordingly.

Nowadays, a person can learn medical terminology by taking up the course online and some institutes are offering online courses in addition to classroom training in such a way that a person can learn medical terms regardless of wherever he lives.

With these courses, students will be able to learn terms pertaining to therapeutics, pharmacology, diagnoses, diseases, physiology and anatomy. Generally, it is hard to learn medical terminologies and any person taking up this course should be committed to study every day.

Just like learning a foreign language, learning medical terms is also difficult unless regular revision takes place. To become proficient in medical language several hours of review is highly essential.

Ask anyone that has taken medical terminology and they'll tell you it is like learning a second language.

The method for constructing words is similar and some of the terminology can be confusing. The good news is that there is some logic to how medical terms are constructed and many of the terms will be familiar.

If you know the meaning of arthritis or pneumonia, then you already know two medical terms.

The use of everyday terms makes medical terminology much easier to learn than a second language.

Apart from the wide application of medical terminology in the medical field there is a lot of demand for the people that are working depending on this field to get to know the medical terms themselves.

Medical transcription is one department where it is very important for the transcriptionist to be aware of the medical terminology. The work of the medical transcriptionist is to type out medical reports as dictated by the doctor, which will contain anything from a surgical procedure through prescription medication. If a transcriptionist is going to make a minor error it can lead to a lot of complications.

The work strategy of a medical transcriptionist is never complete without the use of medical terminology.

Truly, medical terminology is the foundation stone for the medical transcriptionist.

Even the most trained medical transcriptionist would need to refer the medical terminology when they are unsure about a particular work.

Referring medical terminology books is an important attribute that adds to the skill level of any medical transcriptionist.

Since the transcriptionist does the typing based on contextual thinking they need to correlate the terms and dictations based on the meaning of the medical terminology dictated by the doctor.

Learning medical terminology can be an extremely valuable experience. Mastering word building principles will make the process easier and help you to retain the knowledge for a long time to come.

Keep in mind to use a reputable accredited company and pick a course delivery option that's right for you.

Scott J. Barnard

Medical Terminology for Health Professions 4.0

AUTHOR BIO

Scott J. Barnard

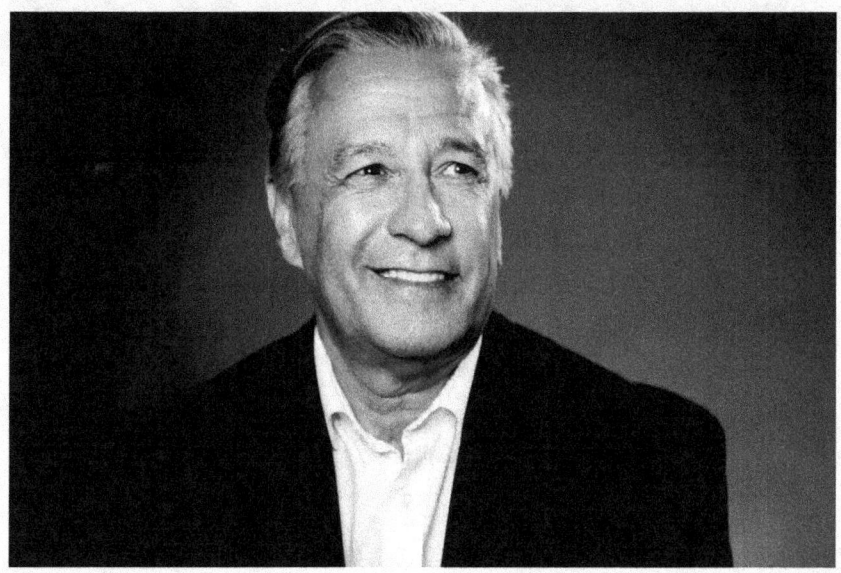

SCOTT J. BARNARD

Scott J. Barnard is an author and medical expert with years of experience as a GP and health consultant. He has worked for countless years in the medical field, dealing with patients and working with the cardiovascular system, immune system, respiratory system, and more.

Scott has personally trained hundreds of students through courses and face-to-face, and he's coached countless more to help them pass their medical exams and break into the field. Armed with a wide range of knowledge, he has helped his students become doctors, nurses, paramedics, physicians, and more.

With his book, *Medical Terminology for Health Professions 4.0*, he hopes to inspire and empower a new wave of medical students to reach the next level by passing their exams and succeeding in their careers.

Scott has condensed his knowledge and research into a comprehensive list of terminology which will help students understand, pronounce, and memorize thousands of medical terms.

Scott J. Barnard is the author of several books, including:
- MEDICAL TERMINOLOGY FOR HEALTH PROFESSIONS 4.0
- THE METABOLIC APPROACH TO OBESITY 4.0
- THYROID SYMPTOMS 4.0
- ANTI-INFLAMMATORY HERBAL HEALING 4.0
- REVERSING YOUR CHILD'S EATING DISORDER 4.0

LinkedIn: www.linkedin.com/in/scottjbarnard/
email: scottbarnard1959@gmail.com

Thank you for reading this book.

If you enjoyed it please visit the site where you purchased it and write a brief review. Your feedback is important to me and will help other readers decide whether to read the book too.

Thank you!
Scott J. Barnard

Do you want more?
Grab "Reversing Your Child's Eating Disorder 4.0" for free

Instructions

Scan the Qr code or click on the link and click BUY NOW, click on Add a Coupon and enter this coupon that gives you the **100% discount code**

BY2HZUA5ZD

Now Download the book for Free

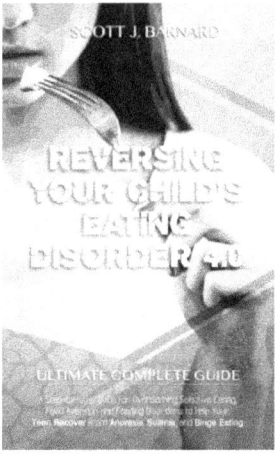

So don't wait! This is the book for you!

https://mgdluxurybooks.com/b/8x0rK

Scott J. Barnard

BONUS

Download **FREE** and listen to the audiobook "Medical Terminology for Health Professions 4.0" wherever you are.

You will download the audiobook in MP3 format and divided by chapters.

Instructions

Scan the Qr code or click on the link and click BUY NOW, click on Add a Coupon and enter this coupon that gives you the **100% discount code**

NA6KTSB2JY

Now Download the audiobook for Free

https://mgdluxurybooks.com/b/JbTRK

www.ingramcontent.com/pod-product-compliance
Lightning Source LLC
Chambersburg PA
CBHW052341220526
45465CB00003BA/895